1994

WHAT DOCTORS CAN'T
HEAL

WHAT DOCTORS CAN'T HEAL

The Unflattering Truth about Sexual Diseases and Individual Responsibility

BERNARD JACKSON

Strictly Honest
815 N. La Brea Avenue
Suite 187
Inglewood, CA 90302

LCCN 92-62048

ISBN 0-9634505-4-9

ATTENTION: CORPORATIONS, GOVERNMENT AGENCIES, PROFESSIONAL ORGANIZATIONS, AND EDUCATIONAL INSTITUTIONS: Quantity discounts are available on bulk purchases of this book for educational purposes, gifts, or fund raising. Special books or book excerpts can also be created to fit specific needs. For information, please contact Strictly Honest, 815 N. La Brea Avenue, Suite 187, Inglewood, CA 90302, or call 800-578-2284.

ACKNOWLEDGMENTS

I would like to thank my wife D Renee Brooks for her support and encouragement during the many years of struggling and doubt that I endured while writing this book. Furthermore, I wish to publicly acknowledge her for being willing to serve as that independent analyst/reviewer/critic, without whom I would have lost my way many more times than I did. What I discovered was that losing my way was not the end of the world with her in my corner.

I would also like to thank my parents for guiding me through the first 17 years of my life and providing me with the basic values of decency, goodness and respect for my elders.

I would like to thank my spiritual teachers, particularly Dr. Homer Johnson, Rev. Juanita Dunn and Bessie Pickett for exemplifying patience that goes far beyond reasonable understanding.

Finally, I wish to give thanks to that nameless Source that spawned all life, created all potentialities and colored my world with an endless variety of love and joy and wonderment.

TABLE OF CONTENTS

PREFACE

Any discussion of modern day STD's (Sexually Transmissible Diseases) begins with AIDS. We all hear and read so much about AIDS, but there are other STD's — syphilis, gonorrhea, herpes, human papilloma virus (sexual warts) and chlamydia being the most prevalent. I know, because at one time or another I have had about half of them. Though AIDS has dominated the limelight in the last decade, the pain borne by those suffering from these less publicized, more survivable STD's is just as serious.

In the wake of the AIDS crisis, some long-term and chronic sufferers of diseases such as herpes simplex type 2 (HS2) may feel forgotten. It is for these forgotten people that I have written this book. I also wrote this book because, as an avid fan of talk shows, I grew tired of watching a steady stream of "experts" parade across the stage to give people like me advice. It always struck me as less than convincing when unblemished experts could stand over there and disseminate what is considered to be objective advice about the life of someone (me) standing over here. The so-called experts have no idea what it's like to live through the prime of one's life with HS2. Hiding behinds masks of professional detachment, their lives never seem to have been touched by the disorders that they so dispassionately advise. I thought, "Wouldn't it be nice if someone who is credible, balanced, reasonably objective *and* happy would write a book and tell people how it really is to live with HS2?"

In spite of the new openness with which AIDS is being addressed, the most prevalent STD, HS2, remains society's Great Unmentionable. Said to be incurable, HS2 afflicts an estimated 30 million people, and yet barely a whisper is spoken about it. In the course of a month, you'd be hard-pressed to find a single talk show, newspaper or major magazine broaching the subject.

Clearly when 30 million people, or one out of eight Americans, suffer from a common affliction, a great toll is being paid in terms of unresolved suffering, hurt and pain, an emotional burden which undergirds the psychological health of this country. There is a need for purging, redemption and healing by bringing this problem out into the open and releasing the personal shame associated with the bearing of this disease. To put it bluntly, there are literally millions of people whose lives are stuck because they have HS2, and they need to be liberated. They need to talk openly about this thing so that they can be purged, but they sense that for some inexplicable reason HS2 is still a taboo subject in polite society. Unfortunately, they are right. HS2 remains taboo for five main reasons:

* It is considered to be incurable.
* There exists the unchallenged — and false — presumption that only people of low breeding, who aren't too smart and have questionable morals could be stupid enough to catch something like HS2.
* Among the huge number of people who have it, many are highly-educated, high-achiever types who are used to taking charge of their lives and solving problems of every sort.
* Unlike AIDS, dealing with HS2 in one's private life can be deferred indefinitely without ever having to be found out.
* No matter how enlightened one is, having to deal honestly with HS2 in one's private, intimate relationship is very embarrassing, so many people never do. The result of this behavior is that it perpetuates the taboo.

Of course, none of these are sufficient reasons to harbor shame for having HS2. An outsider might think: "Hey, what's the big deal? AIDS is so much more deadly and threatening than HS2. You people should be glad that you *only* have HS2 and that you don't have AIDS."

WHAT DOCTORS CAN'T HEAL

The argument can further be made: When people are dying from AIDS, what right do those with something as trivial as HS2 have to complain and draw attention to themselves? But the argument is flawed and has nothing to do with the truth. It is true that many who have HS2 feel that, out of respect for AIDS sufferers, it is not politically- or socially-correct to complain about their plight, but that doesn't mean that the pain has gone away. Conversely, the pain has grown larger as they have suppressed their need to be heard, attended to, loved, accepted and forgiven.

Case in point: In October of 1991, two women in Michigan made national news for committing suicide after conferring on videotape with Dr. Jack Kevorkian, the physician who invented the suicide machine. Reportedly, one of the women, Margorie Wantz, tired of suffering from the STD known as human papilloma virus. Her suicide simply highlights the depth of the depression and psychological burden borne by some whose sexual identity has been compromised. I suspect that Margorie Wantz's case is just the tip of the iceberg. Over the past 19 years, I have read cases of many people with HS2 who were depressed and suicidal because they believed their lives to be over.

It is for all of these people that I am writing this book. I have absolutely no shame about my horrendously unflattering sexual past or about my present HS2 condition, and I defy anyone to try to levy guilt upon me. Now that I've admitted my past ignorance and learned my lessons, I feel WONDERFUL about myself and I intend to liberate other HS2 (and other STD) sufferers so that they may feel the same.

Though HS2, like any other disease, should not be trivialized, a good portion of the amazing tales and anecdotes recounted from my life is humorous and should make you laugh. Indeed it is time to lighten up and laugh a little. But I trust that you'll be laughing *with* me, and not *at* me. It is time to clear up some misconceptions, admit some truths about our mistakes and limited human power, and get on with our lives. Then being so liberated, our new motto may become: Stuck no more!

INTRODUCTION

I have herpes simplex, type 2 (HS2), a sexually-related disease for which there is reportedly no known cure. Despite it all, I am a well-adjusted, happy person who is living not just a normal life, but a marvelous, exciting and meaningful life. This is the story that I have come forth to share. It is clear to me that there are many who need to hear this story told in the first person singular. To tell it in any other voice would not do it justice. Though HS2 is a bummer — and granted, it is — it is strictly a physical thing. Among the articles and paltry offering of books that have been written on the medical aspects of HS2, no comprehensive work has been published about the practical aspects of day-to-day living with HS2 — the emotional, mental and spiritual factors. How does one cope with this disease? Can you be happy with HS2? If so, how? Can you live a normal life, date and eventually get married, or are such expectations unrealistic?

OF COURSE YOU CAN LIVE A NORMAL LIFE WITH HS2! Of course you can be happy, date and get married! And yes, you should by all means have such expectations, assuming these are your desires. I'm not coming to you as an aloof professional or book-of-the-month "expert" from talk show heaven. Not at all. I'm a real person just like you who happened to acquire HS2 at the age of 25, which is some 19 years ago for me. Afterwards, I believed that my life was over. There was no way that anybody could have convinced me that I would ever have a normal social life after that. But after years of indulging in self pity, I got tired of being an outsider looking in on life, and I began to construct a consistent philosophy for being victorious in every aspect of life. After treading a long, rocky, desolate road for many years, at 38 I married the woman of my dreams. And no, she does not have HS2. Once I got my head straight, I realized that (1) there is a Power in this universe that will fulfill our wildest expectations...within reason, of course, and (2) we don't have to compromise our standards as a consequence of having HS2, or any other condition.

I wrote this book to help put the widespread problem of HS2 in perspective. In stark contrast to the 30 million people in the United States who are estimated to have HS2, there is a strange dearth of writing and open discourse on this subject. In this book I have written about major portions of my life before and after acquiring HS2. The objective is to assist those whose lives have been stymied, put on hold or dead-ended by HS2 to gain some measure of needed relief by connecting with a fellow HS2 subject (as opposed to *victim* or *sufferer*) who has mastered the challenge of living a normal, happy, loving and optimistic life *with* HS2.

In the absence of a solid medical cure, the vast millions with HS2 have been left to conjure up their own medical, psychological and emotional salves. This has given rise to over 90 herpes support groups (known as "HELP" groups) across the nation. I've never attended one, but I'm glad they exist. To compound the matter and add to their collective despair, AIDS has taken center stage and garnered the bulk of attention and research dollars in the area of sexually transmissible diseases (STD's). When all else failed, people, in learning to cope with HS2, have done as people have always done. They have turned to God in one way or another.

But wait! The spread and distribution of HS2 has revealed an unexpected, but interesting, feature: Many of its hosts are well-educated, college bred, I-can-control-my-own-destiny type of intellectuals, like myself. OUCH! It wouldn't be too far-fetched to think of HS2 as a YUPPIE disease. These tormented intellectuals have been turning in droves to various spiritually-tinged New Age/metaphysical philosophies in last ditch, desperate attempts to revalidate their senses of self worth. As free-thinking intellectuals, they aren't necessarily seeking the punitive, illogical God of most orthodox religions. Instead they are attracted to movements that emphasize their inherent perfection and innate goodness, that they are spiritual beings first and foremost, as opposed to physical beings. Thus we have the basis for the popularity of Shirley MacLaine's books and others of that genre (Dr. Bernie Segal's book on cancer, Dr. M. Scott Peck's book *The Road Less Travelled*, Louise Hay's self-published book *You Can Heal Your Life*, etc.).

But there is a hook. As one who earned a license as a practitioner of spiritual healing in one of the popular New Thought/metaphysical religions during the '80s (Religious Science), I've been there. Millions of HS2 subjects see these enlightenment teachings as their last shred of hope. Countless numbers have been lured in by false promises, thinking that there is a guru, avatar, healer or super-evolved mystic somewhere who can speak special words or lay hands on them and render them instantly healed. This is their secret longing, though they enter under the guise of "searching for God," asseverating that "I just want to know God," while denying the obvious. As they sally forth, uttering affirmations such as: "I am spiritual; I am perfect; I am not a body," they are, in effect, denying their bodies altogether because they see their bodies as having deceived them. After a few years in their respective organizations, many of these seekers have become totally detached from reality. The pain of being "stigmatized" by HS2 is too great for them to bear, so they totally escape into a new, enlightened persona under lofty pretenses. Others have become even more deeply embittered after spending thousands of dollars and finding that their specially-anointed teachers cannot heal them.

This inner conflict is the core of what this book is about. It shines the light on the many foggy aspects of the enlightened spiritual ruse from an insider's point of view. Regardless of my personal disillusionment with religious and New Age organizations, I remain an unwavering believer in the Divine Presence. Nonetheless, I, too, thought that I would be able to earn or purchase my way to a healing by enmeshing myself in the New Age/metaphysical subculture. So, yes...I, too, became bitterly disappointed.

Few would want to read a story solely about HS2, for it would be too depressing and one-dimensional. Thus I have written what I hope is an amusing story of my many private, prodigal experiences as they relate to HS2. To arrive at a complete understanding of how one individual could overcome one of the most psychologically-devastating challenges of our time, you have to wade through the myriad experiences that shaped his life. I feel the story of HS2 needs to be told in this broader perspective, because then it can help others who have HS2 see that it is possible to live a normal, happy, fulfilled, social and positive life with HS2 — without shame! — even if one is NOT healed in the conventional medical sense.

It is important that the person who has HS2 understand that she (or he) is not just a walking herpesvirus. It is important that she begins to see herself as the marvelous and wonderfully-made human being that she is. She has a whole life, a large percentage of which has absolutely nothing to do with HS2. This is what I am trying to convey. It is all too easy for an HS2 subject, burdened by the self-imposed, and, for the most part, assumed stigma of his or her condition, to see every aspect of life tainted by HS2. What I want to tell people is that life can be wonderful — yes, even *with* HS2. Many wonderful people will still gravitate to you — yes, even though you have HS2. And you can still develop idyllic relationships — yes, even with HS2.

Far too many people with HS2 are withdrawing from society with deep wounds, and divorcing their partners and becoming bitter and angry, refusing to forgive those who infected them. Far too many people are living shadowy lives, going to great extremes to protect this great, dark secret — which, justifiable or not, only reflects how they feel about themselves. The very word *herpes* has been imputed with such an immensely overwhelming and deleterious power that people are afraid to even utter the word in polite company. Just the sound of the word makes them shudder. In Truth, this word has no power at all, but we've been conditioned to respond to the public's perception of sexual herpes as some kind of horrible curse. Well it isn't.

Thus I have gone into great detail to describe my earliest socio-sexual development, as well as many errors in judgment and choice that I made during adolescence, college and young adulthood. I began life with an unhealthy, negative image of myself, as well as of sexuality, society and women. I didn't just wake up one day at age 25 with HS2. Not at all. That's why you will seldom find me using the word *victim* in this book. Make no mistake about this one point: I AM NOT A VICTIM! I may be the first person to admit this, but I deserved HS2. Anyone who lives the way I lived and believes the way I believed will eventually attract HS2 or something of a commensurate nature. It is pure law. Oh, I had warnings. It took many erroneous thoughts, bad choices, an assortment of other diseases and embarrassing situations to run as precursors to HS2. It was pretty hard to catch HS2, but I did it anyway. The Universe, God, or what have you, kept trying to warn me, but I wouldn't listen. Life is always that way. We always get many subtle forewarnings. This is the greater, untold part of the story about the experience called HS2.

There is so much meaning in the experience of HS2. Life hasn't made any mistakes. It's not about just getting cured from some horrible condition. We have to review our whole lives, but from a healthy perspective, to learn all of the lessons that HS2 has brought to our attention. Then we can move on healthily and happily, and be the better for it. Then we can be truly healed.

When the day arrives that you can sit down with a friend or acquaintance and discuss HS2 just as normally as you would the weather, you will know then that you are healed, for then HS2 will have no power over you.

It would be so easy for me to feed you a line about how virtuous I am, what a model citizen I have striven to be, my generosity and sensitivity. I could show you pictures of me holding cute little babies and working with kids, and I would not be lying. I could evoke your sympathy and cast myself among the world's endless chain of innocent, undeserving victims. The world would look at me through filtered lenses and see the archetype of a good human being. Nevertheless, the world would be judging from appearances.

There is one particular flaw possessed by all humans which primarily concerns me: our propensity for judging by appearances. We can't help it. We can work to become more aware of this problem and improve meritoriously in this regard, but we cannot completely eradicate this most compelling of all human flaws. I do it; I have little doubt but that you do it; everyone that I have ever met does it — and I have met some of the more enlightened people on Earth.

One of my objectives in writing this book is to pick at the sore of humankind's most fundamental, and thus most ignored, flaw. A consistent interlacing thesis throughout these pages is this: We are NOT what we appear to be. Though I have carved out an exemplary public image in the community, business environment and church, I am also aware that I am not the person that most people believe me to be. Besides the admirable attributes, I am also a person with a deeply troubled history, involving all kinds of deprivations, imbalances and diseases. I'm talking HS2, sickle cell tendency (allegedly, if I believe the doctor), heart murmur (again, if I believe the doctor), osteomyelitis, atrophied testicle (which can lead to cancer, if I believe the doctor), gonorrhea, syphilis, nonspecific urethritis, alcoholism, marijuana usage and deep-rooted, congenital anger, yet I am what a consensus of my acquaintances today would call a "nice" guy.

This has led me to ponder, "Just what in the world is a nice guy, anyway, and how much is such a moniker worth?" If I can be a nice guy, anybody can, including murderers, child molesters, rapists, religious charlatans, extortionists, scheming politicians, demented policemen, sadistic school teachers, racist bosses, chauvinistic husbands and wife-beaters, self-absorbed mothers and deserting fathers, my best friend and your worst enemy — I mean anyone! It's a nebulous label used by lazy people to cover virtually everyone, while describing no one.

It means nothing to label someone as "nice," for we can never see into the core of another's heart or read the imprint of his brain, which is where truth is centered. Such erroneous presumptions only add to the plethora of sexual confusion and fear that is associated with avoiding AIDS, HS2, and other unwelcome concomitants of sex. I have met modern women who believe that they can interview a guy, observe him, or have a private investigator check him out and confirm that he is indeed professional, employed and straight, the presumption being that they would then know for sure that the prospective suitor is "safe." Such people are still laboring under the illusion that nice guys don't have AIDS or HS2. Well, I am a nice guy and I have HS2. This is just the point that this book purports to make: You can never gather enough information based upon your own devices to know anything for certain. For this reason we must reach higher and bank upon principles that are more exact than our thinking, which is limited.

Today, I do not smoke, drink, use drugs, stay out late, sleep around or inflict guilt on people. I believe in God as Universal, All-Creative Spirit, but I do not belong to any particular religion. Thus I don't have "the answer" that would "save" everyone or bring the whole world into harmony.

I love America, respect the police and believe that we should seek out the wisdom of our elders. If a friend has a need, he or she knows that he or she can always call upon me day or night and I will respond with a cheerful countenance. When friends are down, they often call upon me, for they know that I can always help them believe in a brighter day with new possibilities.

All of this has been transpiring for the last 10 years for this archetypal "nice" guy, with rarely a whimper or a complaint registered in protest. With few exceptions, these friends haven't had a clue that I have been dealing with the likes of HS2. This is why I eschew the "nice" guy connotation. As you can see, it means absolutely nothing! We don't tend to look upon white collar professionals who smile and hug children as the type of people who have HS2. Though they may seem to manage life effortlessly with nary a complaint, and though they may always be there to encourage others, they may still be the sort who have engaged in every kind of deviancy know to humankind. They may still be grappling with deep-seated mental and physical challenges. "Nice" has nothing to do with it.

So "nice" isn't all it's cracked up to be. I am content to be classified as a human being just like everyone else, sometimes riddled with conflicts and continuously burdened by choices. This puts the lie to the well-manicured, monolithic image. If there is anything about me that is worth modeling, it is that I absolutely refuse to use my humanness as an excuse for any of my shortcoming whatsoever, past or present. Though I face the same challenges as everyone else, I don't have to act according to common standards and expectations. I can *do* better, *act* better and *be* better than I was yesterday.

This is the message that I am trumpeting. Ostensibly, this is a book about HS2 — not so much about the medical aspects, for there is no known medical cure. Instead, it is about the emotional, mental and spiritual aspects of living a perfectly harmonious and victorious life *in spite of* HS2. Remember: It's all right to be human, but never, never use that as an excuse. Rather, let your humanness be your launching pad for aspiring heavenward. This you can do, but not if you insist on seeing things only for what they appear to be and finding contentment in present images that limit you to labels like "nice," "good," "generous," "victim".... No, no, no! — never settle for that. Break out of the mold at whatever cost, and venture to be all that you can be — sometimes good, sometimes bad, and, when it is warranted, sometimes as ugly as hell.

This is my story. I have nothing to hide. I choose to stand up and be accountable. The world has enough teachers and preachers lecturing from on high. If my story is to be of any utility at all, let it be by example.

I have a message which is not a simple tale of good versus evil, or right versus wrong. Nor is it a veiled religious preachment. My message is that each of our lives is a complex accumulation of all past experiences, and not just the simple, too-easy-to-sum-up picture that casts its image before us at the present moment. As a result I hope that my presentation will not distance you from me, but lead you to see a little bit of yourself in me. That way, we will both be dealing on equal ground and we can both grow — you by having read this book, and I by having written it.

WHAT DOCTORS CAN'T HEAL

The Unflattering Truth about Sexual Diseases and Individual Responsibility

CHAPTER 1: MY PREDICAMENT

For about 19 years now, I have been among the millions of Americans with herpes. That's herpes simplex type 2 (HS2), the sexual kind. Oh, I'm not ashamed to admit it. We're not inhabitants of a fantasy land. This is the real world in which we live, and this is my predicament.

HS2 is the acronym that I've chosen to use for herpes simplex type 2, and shall use throughout this book. Chances are you can relate to what I'm talking about, and if not you, someone you know. After all, health authorities estimate that approximately 30 million Americans currently have HS2. That's 12 percent of the entire population! Among sexually-active teen-agers and adults the percentage is even higher.

What I'm here to tell you is that even if you do have HS2, big deal! Your life isn't over. Oh, I'm not trivializing this condition.

9

During the past 19 years, I have been forced to accept a few inevitables, but none have stopped me from living a wonderful and fulfilling life. It wouldn't be fair for me to expect everyone else with HS2 to be where I am in consciousness concerning this condition. This is my attempt to give a balanced and honest account about a prevalent, vexatious condition.

I have suffered the devastating agony and pain that HS2 can put a person through. Like so many others, I went desperately in search of medical, herbal, vitamin and mineral cures. When none of these worked, I reached rock bottom in faith and hope and seriously asked myself: Is life under these conditions worth living? Once I decided that suicide was not a viable option, I got on with my life, which included dating and socializing in an attempt to live as normally as possible. But my life was not normal. I was continuously haunted by the ravages of this great dark secret. After so many years of living on the fringe of sanity, I picked myself up, remembering my early spiritual upbringing, and made a conscious decision to try to get back to Truth. But that was just the beginning of a long and arduous journey that left me confused, disappointed and very much unhealed. It seemed that everyone else in the churches, New Age and metaphysical organizations and therapy sessions were bubbling over with happiness, while there was obviously something askew in me. I could only assume that I was hopelessly deficient and cursed with the most pernicious kind of karma, and that it must have been my fate to live out this life under the unhappiest of circumstances.

This is not a book about healing as the world at large is accustomed to defining it. Let me be crystal clear and honest about this. I am not healed in any medical sense of the word. Regardless, I am content, I am at peace and I am joyful. I have found that peace which passes all understanding, but it is not the kind of answer that can be readily packaged and sold. This is a book about victory over HS2, for I can say to you without equivocation that through my long and grueling search I have achieved knowledge, wisdom and understanding. Not only that, but I have found my true purpose in life. Today, I am balanced and grounded. In fact, I am happier and more balanced now than I was even *before* I contracted HS2. Even if I have to live out my life as it presently is, I will consider it to have been a whopping success. This is my story. What I want others who have HS2 to know is that they, too, can achieve the same level of comfort and peace, and that they, too, can achieve this victory.

HOW IT HAPPENED

Among the various case histories that I have read about people with HS2, there have been many who weren't sure how they acquired it. It seems that no one has ever given it to anyone else. The storyteller is always the innocent victim. Some of them say they got it from kissing, communal towels or toilet seats. Well, the best I can figure is that I got it from sex. My problem was forcing my way into situations when I shouldn't have, being with people that I shouldn't have been with and doing things that I shouldn't have done.

Today, I have absolutely no concern about the woman from whom I acquired HS2. This is not repression or denial in my case. You have to bear in mind that I have been processing my feelings and attitudes on this issue for some 19 years at this juncture. If the truth be told, I'm not 100 sure how I contracted HS2. I *think* I know. There was a woman. The woman whom I believe passed it on to me had just moved back to the States from Ghana, where she had just been divorced from a full-bloodied African. I had known her back in my hometown of Augusta, Georgia, before she married and moved to Ghana.

The year was 1974 and at 25, I was in my sexual prime. Being fresh out of college and living in the Boston area, I was attempting to make up for everything that I thought I'd missed during college. My only goal in life was to get out there and sow wild oats, and I mean with abandon — a not uncommon, yet still peculiar male affliction.

Anyhow, I received this call from New York and this old heartthrob of mine was back on the scene and available. It's strange looking back. When a young man is 25 and full of fire, a weekend drive from Boston to New York for a carefree romp in the hay is about as close to heaven as he ever hopes to get. There are no obstacles that he won't work around to keep such an appointment. He'll call in sick or lie to his mama, if necessary. Today, if I were single, I wouldn't drive 10 blocks in Los Angeles to spend a night with Miss Universe! What a difference a few years of wisdom make.

But that's the way it was in those days. I was carefree, hot to trot, and constantly on the move. I broke lots of hearts and lots of hearts broke me. But finally — and Hollywood couldn't have written it any better — I met my match. It seems that, in the end, we always do.

When one is young, hot-blooded, and continuously horny, things that should be obvious aren't. I hope I remember this when I'm counseling my children — not that they will listen.

During another trip to New York to visit my brother, after partying and drinking heavily, I called up my New York connection and literally begged her to let me come over. She was alone and she was lonely, so how could she resist the opportunity for some company? I understand this very well now after having been confused so many times by the insidious nature of desire. Many times I have said yes when I felt deeply within my soul that I should have said no.

Anyway, when I got over there and began to put the move on my lady-friend (or was she putting the move on me?), I distinctly remember her trying to tell me no. It's strange how I can remember that now. She was protesting, but none too vehemently. Her lips were repeating the words no, no, no, but her body language was most definitely saying yes. I'm not saying that it is right, but when a young man is horny and gaming, it is very difficult to listen to the spoken word. It's the body's own special language that he heeds.

All the while she was saying no, she was clutching desperately and pulling me closer. She wanted me and she wanted me bad, but I couldn't figure out why she kept saying no. So I queried her. When I asked if she was on her period, she said no. It would be my luck that I would be dealing with somebody who was too honest to lie. All she had to do was say yes, and that would have stopped me cold, body language or no body language. Though I was a rascal, I was not uncivilized. God has equipped women with an eternal alibi when they don't want to be bothered. All they have to do is say, "I'm on my period." Oh I've heard of the existence of beasts among men who aren't even fazed by that, but I am not among them.

As I said, she wasn't any clearer about her desires than I have been at times about mine. As it was, I kept pressuring her with flattery, skewed arguments and kisses until I wore her down, but I could tell during the inevitable, subsequent physical encounter that she wasn't comfortable. I don't think she wanted to go all the way, at least not in her mind, but she had the same problem as so many men: she couldn't help herself. In retrospect, I believe her objectivity was distorted by her desire. Consequently, she probably rationalized that God would be on her side and make everything all right. Oh, how I understand such irrational behavior, for how many times have I played the odds the very same way!

How can otherwise intelligent human beings think that God will intervene to protect them when they aren't even using common sense? What a ludicrous way of reasoning.

How could I blame my New York friend, assuming she was the source from whom I acquired HS2? She was no different than I during those years of darkness when I was motivated solely by pleasure. We all want to do good, while simultaneously wanting to have what we want to have when we want to have it. Thus is the making of a dilemma. Until we really learn about life and our true relationship to it, issues such as this will continually arise in our consciousness to challenge our judgment and sense of moral right versus carnal desire.

Anyhow, within a few weeks I did break out with HS2. Of course, I had no idea what it was. There weren't that many doctors in 1974 who could have immediately identified HS2. When I called my friend long distance a few weeks later to find out about the condition that I presumably had acquired from her, she flatly denied that she could have been the donor of anything of the sort. I guess I shouldn't have been surprised, but I was. Now I knew that I had not slept with anyone else during a period of some months before that particular rendezvous — which, I admit, doesn't conclusively prove anything — but I thought I was right. Maybe I picked it up from a towel or a casual kiss...tsk, tsk!

Regardless, my friend denied it, and eventually, I forgave her, forgave myself, and went on to forget about it. Sort of. After that experience, I never heard from her again. That's the way it is. Beyond that singular incident, I've also had to forgive myself for the crazy, irresponsible lifestyle that I lived during those prodigal years. I wasn't wise, but what's done is done. You get no credit for lamenting the past.

Today, I don't blame a soul or hold a grudge against anyone. There are some 30 million people out there dealing with HS2 today, and I hope to God they aren't all holding grudges. However, my research has revealed that many are still unreasonably angry with previous lovers many years after the fact. They are not yet able to appreciate their lovers, boyfriends, girlfriends, husbands or wives for passing on this gift of great value to them. That's right, HS2 is a gift! More on that later, but those who haven't been able to forgive have become severely hardened and crippled by the effects of harboring long-term anger. They are angry with people, they are angry with life, and in some cases they are angry with God. Let's face it. If we aren't mature enough to take the responsibility ourselves, many times it comes down to being angry with God for letting this horrible thing happen to us.

As far as I am concerned, it is totally unreasonable to prolong anger against anyone in a situation such as this. Of course, you will be angry at first. Nevertheless, if you sincerely want to grow spiritually and accomplish your mission in this life, the day will arrive when you will come to a higher understanding about what your experience really represents and realize that, in reality, there are no victims. Let me repeat this important corollary to spiritual principle:

THERE ARE NO VICTIMS!

I realize that some of the recipients of HS2 *appear* to be "innocent victims." I cannot debate appearances. They were not callously pursuing pleasure, they will tell you. Though I sincerely empathize with those who see themselves as "victims," still, I know for myself that life is fair and everything that happens is totally justified. To continuously think of yourself as a victim is to ingest a poison that will serve to prevent your own eventual healing. It will become clearer later why I feel this way. For now, it must suffice for me to say that I care about these people and I wish to see them get on with their lives. Unfortunately – or fortunately – life moves in only one direction and that's forward. No one can turn back the clock to reverse the afflictions of yesterday.

INITIAL QUESTIONS

Following is a questionnaire that can help you decide if this book will be able to assist you, and if so, exactly how. They represent some of the most difficult and emotionally-tinged issues which arise in the lives of HS2 subjects. These are the questions that are not always pleasant to broach, for their substance is rooted in that part of the subconscious mind that we'd just as soon suppress. These are the questions that I've had to ask myself over the past 19 years. They are the ones that I will answer in this book by sharing and story-telling from my near endless stream of experiences. Though much of this may seem funny now (I certainly hope so), you can bet I wasn't laughing at the time that it was happening.

1. Are you ashamed because you allowed yourself to catch HS2?

2. Are you embarrassed about it to the degree that it would just kill you if anybody found out? Would you be able to handle it if it became public knowledge?

3. Do you feel that your prospects for dating, meeting a mate or living a happy life are nonexistent now?

4. Do you become deeply depressed every time you have an outbreak?

5. When HS2 causes you to reach your lowest ebbs, do you sometimes feel that your life, for all practical purposes, is over?

6. Do you sometimes feel sorry for yourself, envying friends who seem to be happy and jovial while having "normal" sex lives, wishing that you could have the same options and freedom that they have?

7. Have you ever confided in a new or potential mate about your condition only to be rejected?

8. Have you ever been intimate with someone without telling him or her that you have HS2? Did you feel guilty afterwards?

9. Have you ever transmitted HS2 to an unknowing partner and then lied about it when queried? Did you feel guilty?

10. Have you ever broken off a developing relationship with someone because you were afraid to tell him or her, or because you feared that he or she would reject you after finding out?

11. Have you ever evaded truth by using any of the following coverups with your mate? "I'm a very private person." "I'm different." "I'm not what you think I am." "You wouldn't want to get too attached to me." "You have to understand that I'm just not that interested in sex." "I can see you, but only if you allow me lots of space when I need it without questioning me."

12. Have you ever separated from or divorced a spouse because one of you brought home HS2?

13. Does your level of stress and anxiety increase when you feel that you are going to be put into a situation where you could be seduced — e.g., a planned weekend trip with a mate, or a planned Friday night date where you know you will be expected to perform sexually? In these circumstances, is it difficult for you to be

straightforward with your mate about what is really going on with you?

14. During outbreaks, are you moody and asocial?

15. Does it irritate you if an uninformed mate tries to caress you during an HS2 outbreak? Do you try to avoid even nonsexual physical contact during those times?

16. Have you become more interested in religious, spiritual, New Age or metaphysical pursuits since acquiring HS2?

17. Have you experimented with metaphysical healing techniques such as transcendental meditation, chanting, affirmations, visualization, channeling, rebirthing, energy balancing, forgiveness exercises, hands-on healing, crystal healing, fasting, vegetarianism, herb treatment or vitamin therapy as possible means for healing HS2?

18. Have you ever changed your diet to try to control HS2?

19. If you were previously religious or a believer in God, have you ever questioned your faith in God as a result of having HS2?

20. Have you ever considered trying to find a mate who also has HS2, and if so, was it because you thought it would be a convenient answer to your problem?

21. Are you ashamed to admit to doctors that you have HS2, especially when visiting them for other ailments?

22. Have you ever lied on a medical questionnaire when asked if you have or have ever had a sexually-transmissible disease (STD) in general, or HS2, in particular?

23. Did you or do you have trouble overcoming your anger towards the person who gave you HS2? Do you believe that he or

she is responsible for your having HS2?

24. Does it make you uncomfortable when comedians or water fountain humorists crack jokes about people with HS2?

25. Do you try to avoid stress in hopes that it will prevent or reduce HS2 outbreaks?

26. Do you believe HS2 to be the greatest problem in your life?

27. Do you long, hope or pray for a miracle drug that will cure HS2 and restore you to normalcy once and for all?

28. Do you believe that if you could be cured of HS2, you would be happy?

29. Has HS2 led you to be more honest, faithful and committed towards your spouse, mate or dates?

30. Have you ever seriously considered suicide as the easiest way out of your predicament?

If you have entertained any of the above questions or acts, I just want you to know that you are not alone. Except for questions 9, 12 and 20, at one time or another I have been guilty of each of these issues. I considered number 20 at one time, but quickly overruled it. Fortunately, during my dating years, I never tried to evade responsibility by lying to a date. But I was deceptive and less than straightforward at times, and I admit to having backed out of relationships because I was afraid of confessing the truth about my condition. Furthermore, I have lied in impersonal ways, such as when filling out medical questionnaires. During those early years, I was no saint. I engaged in all kinds of devious behavior and tactics, but in the end I learned that honesty is indeed the best policy.

What I have set out to do in this book is answer these essential 30 questions — not by rote or boring numerical order, but by extruding the answers out of the intricate matter that comprises my life story. My thesis is that it is the story more than the answers that matters, so I will dwell on the story, the context and the philosophy behind the thoughts. If you have HS2, I believe that to come to grips with these 30 questions can represent the starting point in your healing. It has for me.

CHAPTER 2: WAS IT DESTINY?

As a kid, there were lots of ideas implanted in my subconscious, mental picture of how life was supposed to be when I grew up. HS2 was not one of them. It wasn't even a runner up. In 1955 when I began grade school, HS2 just wasn't one of the things that people worried about. Judging by the medical literature, it didn't even exist. I remember worrying about the mumps, or perhaps measles or chicken pox. I remember feeling blessed that I didn't have polio. It was around 1975 when people *en masse* began to worry about the sexual manifestation of HS2. But then, in 1975 people were not worrying about AIDS either. Wasn't it just yesterday (around 1981) when Americans *en masse* began worrying about AIDS? Either way, the point is that every few years some new medical threat with epidemic potential sweeps across the horizon. Though the type 2 herpesvirus was widely unknown in 1955, one thing is certain: Herpesviruses were widespread among us. I know, because I had it. That's right, in 1955 at age six! So did just about everyone else!

How many times I recall having acutely painful, highly uncomfortable lesions in my gums and being told, "Don't worry, it's only a fever blister. It'll go away." I am thankful that nobody corrected my parents by saying, "Are you crazy, lady? That kid's got HERPES!!!" — which would have been true, mind you. It is well known, medically, that cold sores are caused by herpes simplex type 1. Similarly, shingles, chicken pox and a number of other common diseases are caused by this broad family of herpesviruses. While these

20

facts do not render HS2 trivial, they should certainly help to put it in its rightful perspective among life's list of things which cause us grief.

CHILDHOOD REVISITED

We all grow up with our own dreams of how life is going to be. Our physical evolution is filled with such excitement and expectancy concerning the world of adulthood. Gradually, those dreams become our mental tapes, and like audio cassettes they play over and over in our minds as we grow into maturity. Every time something in the world "out there" does not align with our little picture of how it *should* be, those old cassettes start turning on our little mental capstans.

From the time I was in elementary school back in my hometown of Augusta, Georgia, I can remember my first teacher, Miss Tindell, prompting each of us kiddies to "Stand up and tell the class what you wanna be when you grow up." Whether I was aware of it or not back then, I was formulating my own mental picture of what I expected life to look like when I grew up.

Like all upwardly mobile little six-year-old ghetto boys — i.e., those who were not retarded — I wanted to be a fireman, or policeman, or teacher — and this was well before Yuppies, Puppies and Bumps (Young Urban Professionals, the kids of Yuppies, and Black Upwardly Mobile Professionals, respectively). Actually, we didn't refer to poor Black neighborhoods as ghettos in the South when I was growing up. Neither is that nomenclature used there today. Government-subsidized housing developments, such as where I lived, were simply referred to as "the projects."

Well, here I am some 30-plus years later, and though the path has been circuitous, I came pretty close to fulfilling my promise to Miss Tindell. No, I didn't become a fireman, policeman or teacher. I became an engineer, and later, a writer. The object of those early exercises was not so much to become a particular, predetermined type as it was to become SOME-THING — ANY-THING — as opposed to NO-THING! It was to become SOME-BODY as opposed to NO-BODY. Miss Tindell was simply planting seeds.

For kids brought up in dire poverty in the South in the mid-'50s, planting any kind of higher aspiration in their minds could be considered an accomplishment of the highest magnitude. So, in essence, I achieved that which I had envisioned. There were, however, a few things that came with the picture that I had not counted on.

Being dirt poor as child, I cannot say with great conviction that I expected to live in a column-decked mansion, replete with servants, regularly-served meals and limo service. I paid my annual homage to the "Wizard of Oz" as much as any other kid, but the dreams of Dorothy and the Tin Man were not the kind that were encouraged in my neighborhood. Wishful thinking, we had never heard of. Grandiose dreams were ridiculed, not encouraged. Maybe our teachers and elders had a point. They taught us that before you run, you've got to walk, but everybody I knew was still crawling.

I still have trouble believing that there are kids in this world who actually expect their parents to reach into their pockets and give them an allowance every week. I can envision myself being a millionaire one day, yet eccentric enough to deny my kids an allowance — for their own good, of course. Out of the nearly 2200 weeks that I have been alive on this planet, I think I can remember one in which my father gave me a dollar one week as an allowance. I'll never forget that week back in nineteen fifty...er, something. It was special.

Unlike the kids of today, back in the projects in Georgia we didn't have many well-to-do role models. In large city ghettos such as I encounter daily in my current town, Los Angeles, the big challenge in the school system is to give kids some positive role models to counteract the ubiquitous negative ones, such as the flashy, Rolls Royce-driving dope pushers.

Back where I grew up, even the hustlers and con artists were poor. Based on income, most of them could have qualified for welfare. They were basically twopenny hustlers and pimps, not the slick, cash-pregnant, big city dealers of modern lore. During the era in which I was a child, dope pushers were virtually unheard of in the projects. We would hear tell in hushed adult terms of guys going up to big cities like New York or somewhere in "Jersey" and getting involved with stuff like that. Back then, New York was "The Naked City," and tales were passed on without question about all kinds of deliciously shady characters who were known to proliferate nowhere else but there. Unfortunately, all of this has changed today, even in small town Augusta, Georgia. The age of innocence has passed, even amongst hustlers and thieves. The streets are too tough today for two-penny hustlers, and the price of everything is at least a dime.

To be sure, there were tough guys aplenty in my day, but they didn't walk around with wads of hundred dollar bills stuffed in their pockets, like the most insignificant adolescent hustler of today. The point is that at the top of life's hierarchy — looking at the legal, respectable route to success, as opposed to other options — there was nothing up there that I could relate to as a child that might have painted a picture of white mansions, meals on call and chauffeured limos. There was no way, based on the narrow perspective of life that I was exposed to during my first 15 years, that I could envision a Bernard Jackson in my future enjoying those kinds of trappings of success.

Neither did I have a picture of myself betrothed to some long-haired beauty who was there to respond to my every desire, or who would provide for me the missing element of love and demonstrable affection that had been so mysteriously absent from my prepubescent years. As far as I was concerned at that time, I would have gladly passed on the long-haired beauty in favor of demonstrable affection. A lot of my life, including the deeply-ingrained programming that put me on a collision course with HS2, was characterized by an obsessive search for love and affection. This is what everyone is searching for. Of course, I didn't know that until recently, and if someone had pointed it out to me back then I would have loudly denied it. It took me a long, long time to stumble upon a means by which I could receive my proper share of demonstrable affection from one of the world's two-and-a-half billion members of the fairer sex, but that did not deter my search. What I did not receive as a child, I tried to negotiate from every woman whose fate it was for me to meet.

According to some of today's New Age theories, I figure I must have had one hell of a past life to have created a present characterized by such grueling struggle and perpetual despair.

Not only was I was brought up dirt poor, but mine was a home where there were parents constantly struggling to survive, and where there was paternal alcoholism, a fair share of cursing, screaming, fighting, pain and perpetual suffering. Other than that, it was a normal household. Now I'm not blaming my parents. Considering that there were 10 kids and opportunities were limited for Blacks in the Old South, they did a wonderful job raising us as well as they did. Looking back, I feel blessed. As an adult, I realize that my parents are not responsible for how my life turned out, at least not totally or ultimately. What I have done with my life since I left their household is my responsibility, and that's the proverbial bottom line. Both my parents are outstanding individuals in their own right and I thank them profusely for providing me with the essential stuff necessary for success, something that was not available to them in their time.

Even so, it was embarrassing and degrading to be brought up seldom having clothes that fit, or shoes without holes in them, or items to wear that were either handed down or across. "Down" meant that my older brother or one of my cousins probably wore them. "Across" meant that my Mama received them from one of the White ladies for whom she did day work. Clothes handed across were very nice in terms of quality, but style-wise, they left a lot to be desired. They were both aesthetically incongruous and publicly embarrassing. They were just too much out of my league. Woolen plaid pants and tan and white saddle shoes with tassels are still out of my league. I'm talking about clothes that told on themselves. They screamed out, "Hey ya'll. I used to be worn by Southern White boys!"

Please understand that I don't have anything against Southern White boys or White people from whatever region of the United States. I'm simply describing my upbringing.

The period that I'm talking about spans from 1955 to about 1965 in a medium-sized Southern town. Strangely enough, I didn't hate White people back then, mainly because I never knew any. The only time I ever saw any was when the insurance man came to the house once a week to collect his premium. Other than that, the society that I knew was totally separate and unequal.

As far as my upbringing was concerned, I'm sure it's sort of redundant to say that I never saw my parents in a loving embrace. As a matter of fact, I never saw *anybody's* parents in my neighborhood in a loving embrace, yet hordes of kids were being hatched all the time. How could this be? As a child, I used to try to imagine my parents making love — No!...having sex. I could not. Psychology must have a name for this: the "Not Being Able to Imagine your Parents Having Sex" syndrome. I'm sure others have pondered the same enigma. It's the weirdest thing. Not being able to understand something is one thing, but not being able to imagine it, especially if you have the kind of fertile imagination that I had as a child, is indicative of a serious problem.

As a result of my early upbringing, I'm sure that I made the connection somewhere in my subconscious mind, perhaps deeply embedded, that large families, fighting, poverty, anger and hostility went together as a package deal. Love, I didn't know a thing about. The subject never came up in my neighborhood. Therefore, since I didn't want to witness any more fighting, and didn't want a large family, I concluded at an early age that I would never need to marry. And since I didn't know a thing about love, I didn't need a wife. For a long time I intellectualized that I didn't even need female companionship, but that was before I discovered the sweet nectar of amour.

I remember quite clearly when the age of innocence ended for me — in 1958 after my family moved to the projects. I was nine. It was then that the boys in the street began to instruct me in the ways of the world. That is, they hounded me and hounded me about sex. You see, I was an obedient and studious kid. Thus I was different, and if there's one thing that is not tolerated in the lower economic echelons of life, it's being different. Your very survival depends on blending in.

I was a virgin. That was my crime. So the guys hounded me

ceaselessly about this. Actually, they badgered me. It was something that they became obsessed with putting an end to. I mean I couldn't quite comprehend what the big deal was all about. They all thought that it was such an urgent crisis that I was still a virgin. For crying out loud, I was only nine years old! The day that we moved to the projects was the day when I was abruptly thrust out of my Garden of Eden fairyland: November 22, 1958. It's a day that I'll always remember. For me, the age of innocence had just ended.

Before the move, we were poor for sure. We didn't even have hot water, gas for cooking or heating, a bathtub or an indoor bathroom — but we were not *ghettoized*. In Delta Manor, which was the name of the housing project where I grew up, I was exposed to hard core kids. These were kids who swore and cursed and engaged in sex freely and indiscriminately, kids who had never known any semblance of parental control, at least compared with what was normal in my previous neighborhood. These were kids who couldn't comprehend why I, at the advanced age of nine, was still a virgin.

At nine, I didn't even know how the birds and the bees did whatever the birds and the bees were supposed to be doing. The fact that certain parts of my body could be used for more than one purpose was still a mystery to me, and an abstract one at that. Who could have ever imagined all of these new, adult possibilities? Those hardened little street people that I ran with in the projects were telling me that I had to hurry up and become initiated or else certain weird things were going to happen to my body.

Oh, by the way, in the '50s and '60s down South, sex education was neither taught in the schools nor in the home, so far as I knew. Although I was an "A" student in school, nothing that I learned was of much use down in the bowels of the projects. Those kids were my only source of early sex education. Of course I was skeptical at many of the things that they told me. I mean, I probably only believed about one-half of the crap that they fed me, but that was enough to serve me like a bad sentence for the next 20 years. Thank God I didn't swallow the whole pill.

BULLIES

I was fairly strong in those days, which came in handy since the local bullies thought it their duty to beat the hell out of studious little nerds like me. If anything was worse for a young boy living in the projects than being a virgin, it had to be being an "A" student. You could make book on such a one having to fight daily to prove his masculinity. Only sissies were supposed to be good at books and school-type of things. And since I wasn't a sissy, I had to fight.

Every time I looked around, some thug was trying to kick my butt. You can imagine how astonished they were to find out that, despite the stuffy-looking glasses, I was far from being a pushover. In fact, for the sake of survival I evolved into one mean kid. I certainly didn't run away from any fights. They thought I was crazy. What I lacked in brute strength, I more than made us for in sheer meanness and vindictiveness. If you crossed me, you'd better wear a lamp in the back of your head and walk backwards, because I was about as likely to forget as an elephant. During my Delta Manor years, forgiveness was a word that was not yet in my vocabulary. Along with that other foreign word, love, it just wasn't a concept that people talked about in my neck of the woods.

I am not proud of it, but honest to goodness I tried to kill a few people during my formative years. Fortunately, unsuccessfully. I didn't think about tomorrow, even though homework was due. There must be a God because something of a higher nature obviously wanted me to grow up into adulthood. I'm amazed that I did. If someone made me angry, I'd simply try to hurt him right then and there while I still had a full head of steam. I used to deliberately try to prolong my anger after getting all pumped up. I wanted to do my dirty work before having a chance to cool off.

Even back then, I realized how difficult it was to maintain anger. In fact, that was one of the things that I thought was wrong with life: Time tended to dissipate one's hostility. Life seems to have inherent in it a leveling tendency that makes you want to forgive people, which I thought was grossly unfair of life. I mean, what kind of world is this if you can't even enjoy a full head of steam? If someone turned you a grievous injustice, I thought it was a shame to cool down before you got even. As I said, forgiveness was simply not in my vocabulary at that time.

So yes, I was deliberately vindictive. I won't go into detail about it, but I remember cutting one guy with a meat cleaver, stabbing a second one, and lying in wait for yet another one with a big "Merry Brothers" in my hand. Merry Brothers is a well-known manufacturer of masonry bricks in Augusta, Georgia, the kind that are so popular for building brick houses. When this guy passed through the valley of ambush, I threw a large Merry Brothers at his head, and it was only through the grace of God that I missed his big head by a few inches. He probably became a born again at that very moment. Two inches to the right and instead of going to MIT, I probably would have graduated from Tobacco Road (the location of the local prison).

Life couldn't have been any worse for me growing up. As I think about this, I realize that I was extremely lucky that I never got beat up too badly despite almost daily fights. Some of the guys that I had to defend myself against were significantly larger than I and had a whole lot less to lose. The only reason I attribute for my success was that I was always so angry that I always had more than a fair share of adrenalin coursing through my blood. Plus there was Mama, who continuously tried to steer me in the right direction.

Anyhow, these were the experiences that shaped my view of life. The boys in the streets likened me to some kind of a Samson. They told me that it was totally unnatural for me to be as strong as I was, suggesting that the source of my strength was my virginity. I remember feeling like I must have been some kind of an ox. You can well believe that I was confused. For a long time, I didn't know whether they were complimenting me or putting me down. As I grew older, I was caught between wanting to maintain the purity of my strength and wanting to get laid. I didn't want to become weak, but I wanted to be accepted.

There was another experience that comes to mind when I think about those days. Some of the guys whom I was able to defeat during fisticuffs were bent on seeing me whipped into a public state of ridicule. One of the things that they used to do is go down to the jailhouse to visit some of their hardcore, older friends and feed them all kinds of vicious lies about me. The favorite one would be for one of my so-called enemies to tell whoever was in jail from our end of town that Bernard said such and such about his mama.

I know it sounds trite, so much so that you probably doubt that anybody would ever fall for it. If you think that, then you don't know life in the projects. These were hardcore recidivists that I'm talking about. Back then we used to call them plain ol' thugs, but actually, they were just street-hardened dudes with a strong criminal bent. They tended to vacillate back and forth between terrorizing their own communities and serving time in jail. While in jail, they would plan and scheme new mischief that they could get into as soon as they got out. It sort of gave 'em something to look forward to.

For those hard core recidivists, the worse thing that could happen to them would be to get out of jail and not be able to think of any new crimes to immediately get into. They knew that such a fate could only happen due to lack of planning. So it was wildly exciting for some of these near Neanderthals to hear that Bernard said something about their mamas. It gave them a new incentive to try to make parole. That's what is referred to in the trade as a good day in jail.

Now I clearly remember the case of one particular bully who was set up like that against me. He put out the word that he was going to rip me a new rear orifice when he got out. This was the same guy whose mother turned him in to the police. She turned him in for beating her up and tearing up his own house, and yet this guy wanted to kick my butt for allegedly saying something about his mama. Show me the logic.

My criterion for selecting a college was to go somewhere far enough away that no one from my neighborhood could drive to where I was in one weekend, especially bullies fresh out of jail. I was tired of fighting.

You're probably wondering what ever happened when my Neanderthal friend got out of jail. So am I. All I know is that he never bothered me. Maybe he found some other crimes to commit.

I heard recently that he got in the way of a bullet a few years ago and is now confined to a wheelchair. I can name a number of guys from my past who are either dead or shot or paralyzed or any two of the above, but that would only account for about half of them. Half of the other 50 percent went to Vietnam and got shot there. That leaves 25 percent unaccounted for. Those are the ones that wound up either in jail or college. Very few men died from natural causes in my neighborhood. It still shocks me in a stranglely pleasant way whenever I hear that someone back home has died from a natural cause.

To be fair, I will admit that there were a few who didn't suffer any of the above fates, but turned out all right anyhow. A few.

Actually, I'm fairly sure I know what happened to ward off the bully who was supposed to tear me apart when he got out of jail. There was this guy in the neighborhood who, though not of impressive physical stature, was regarded as the de facto kingpin of the projects. He was charismatic, charming and even good-looking, but he gained a reputation for being one of the meanest and toughest of them all, especially if he didn't like you. His scouting report would have read, "If he comes after you, don't try to reason with this one; you'll simply have to kill him."

Paradoxically, he had another side to him. He was extremely intelligent and fun-loving. He'd been brought up in a loving, supportive household. As it was, his parents and mine were good friends, and so were he and I. That is, he liked me. He was sort of like my private mentor in the streets. He thought that I might amount to something some day, so he tried to keep me on the right track. Believe it or not, he taught me the first algebra that I learned, by scribbling right out there in the dirt on the playground. He liked me, and I think the word was out that if you messed with me, you had to go up against "The Law." In our neighborhood he was The Law.

Now this held true when it came to protecting me against the hard core recidivists, i.e., the heavyweight criminals, but none of this was ever discussed. The Law never used his influence between me and the little lightweight, everyday bullies that I faced. He must have figured that I could handle them myself. Plus he didn't want me to be a sissy.

It occurs to me that I never even told him thanks. To do that would have been to acknowledge that I knew that he was protecting me, and The Law wouldn't have liked that. It's a strange code of ethics that governs life in the projects.

BED-WETTING

Sometimes it seems as if I have been sentenced to a life of physical challenges from prepuberty. Some of the earliest memories that I have of myself is that of a bed-wetter. Whereas it isn't unusual for little boys of five or six — or maybe even eight or nine — to wet the bed, this embarrassing habit plagued me until I was 15! I am not proud of this. My greatest childhood fear was that I'd never outgrow it.

Its effects were amplified by the fact that I had to share a bed with at least one of my other brothers. Prior to age nine when the then 11 members of my household lived in two rooms, not counting the kitchen, it was common for three of us children to share a bed. Afterwards, when we moved to the relatively spacious accommodations of the projects, I only had to share a bed with one other brother.

It's difficult for me to revivify the experience or recall the extent of the embarrassment I felt during those awful, malodorous, soggy years. What I do recall are the morning bed checks that drove my poor mother to near hysteria as she alone dealt with the sodden aftermath each day. It was she who had to figure out a way to dry the mattress and bed linen each day, which was virtually impossible during the all too frequent rainy spells. It would have been burdensome enough if she had only one child to worry about, but by the time the bio-clock stopped ticking, there were 10 of us. I felt bad about causing all of these problems but there was nothing under my power that I could do. I used to dream of being like normal children — i.e., *dry* in the morning.

It's difficult enough for parents being poor without having to endure the extra hardship of having children with chronic illnesses and other dysfunctions that drain their already scanty resources. This is the great dilemma of being poor. More often than could ever be explained by the law of averages, subsistence-level parents seem to be beset with these extra burdens. It does something to a parent, I'm sure, to see a child of theirs suffer while knowing that they don't have the resources to do anything for him or her. This is the source of much anger, frustration, and even child abuse among the under-privileged class. If a parent either doesn't know how to or isn't accustomed to giving love at such times of material dearth — which is true of many — my experience has indicated that there is a high probability that they will act hostilely or abusively towards their children. As the child grows up and becomes independent, he has two choices: either he can take it personally and hold a grudge against his parents forever, or he can understand the dynamics of their dilemma and forgive them. As we all are aware, it is quite fashionable today for many privileged young adults to persistently blame their parents for everything that has gone awry in their lives. And, no matter our problems, we are all so privileged.

Since I lived in a house without indoor plumbing when I was in grammar school, there was no way to wash myself effectively each morning. As a consequence, I distinctly remember the experience of going to school with the strong smell of urine literally standing me off from the crowd like a pariah. There was this offensive aura like intense, invisible rays of heat radiating from white hot charcoals. Every time I heard someone blurt out, "Whew! You smell like pee!" not only would I blanch from the embarrassment, but the message would become reinforced in my psyche that I wasn't normal like other kids. There was no question in my mind but that they were right. Not only that, but as far as I could tell, I was never going to be normal, and that's the part that was so depressing.

How many times I remember recoiling from embarrassment at the sight of bed sheets hanging from the clothesline in our back yard with huge yellow-brown stains permanently etched in them like some form of abstract, yet highly perverse, art. Those sheets were like giant billboards advertising our internal business to the entire neighborhood. It's only now as I strive to recall the particulars that I realize how much of my early bed-wetting experience had been blocked out for two decades. It must have been more painful than I realized heretofore.

Again, physical dysfunctions are not new to me. Besides HS2 and bed-wetting, my life has been a continuous string of physical challenges of the embarrassing kind. I have also experienced gonorrhea, syphilis and osteomyelitis. Furthermore, I was born with an undescended testicle. This may not immediately seem significant, but let me tell you, every little boy wants to be symmetrical in that department! Adolescent boys do a whole lot of comparing as they spring into the awareness of their newfound sexuality, forming stigmas that may carry over well into adulthood.

Long before I knew what sexuality was all about, I remember the embarrassment of my testicular situation. I was taken to the welfare clinic, where an endless parade of White doctors and interns would come around and pull my shorts down to examine my little budding private parts. Of course, I was only 4 or 5 years old and poor and it was around 1954 in the evolution of America's social conscience, so who in the world would have thought that it bothered me? Even at that young, nonverbal age, I can tell you that it hurt like the dickens that nobody bothered to talk to me or consider my feelings. The medical practitioners would converse with my parents (at best), or to each other (more often), while I stood there exposed for all the world to see. I don't even know why I was so humiliated. I certainly didn't know anything about sex at that age. It doesn't quite make sense. Maybe it's an inbred thing, or perhaps it was a reaction based on learned behavior. Whatever the cause, I certainly remember the humiliation. In the poor folks' clinic down in Georgia during the early '50s, there was no privacy. I was examined right out in the open floor of a huge ward lined with small beds. Of course, I'm grateful but geez...

Finally, at the age of five the doctors performed surgery on me to correct my congenital testicular deformity and provide me with some semblance of symmetry. Given that I've never attempted to have children, I can only assume that I'm at least half fertile.

How I stopped bed-wetting is a remarkable story that I've never shared with my parents. A very special man, who was also my mentor, played an important role. One of my best friends is life is Dr. Leonard E. Dawson, now president of Voorhees College in Denmark, South Carolina. I am so proud of him. My God, I had some great Black educators to take interest in me down in small town Georgia during my early childhood, and I want the whole world to know it. I don't brag about many things, but when I talk about Dr. Dawson I feel no shame. During his entire life, this man has demonstrated nothing but pure, unadulterated love when it comes to helping under-privileged Black children rise up from literally nowhere. I, for one, was not an easy kid to love. I was angry, sullen and profane just about all the time.

Anyhow, I met Dr. Dawson in junior high school, where he served as my counselor and went on to take great interest in me and what he alone saw as my potential. From that day forward, he brought me under his wing as his protege. Having left Georgia briefly to take a master's at Columbia University in New York City, he knew the value of broadening one's educational experience in a way that few of my peers could appreciate in the early, pre-civil rights '60s. Thus as I was completing tenth grade, he greased the skids for me to go to an advanced summer math program at what used to be Norfolk State College in Norfolk, Virginia — which could just as well have been a foreign country to me at the time.

Though I projected the image of one possessing street wisdom and intrepidity, the truth was that I was afraid. I had never slept under any roof beside my parents' and I wasn't about to let anybody else in on my ignominious secret — that I was a bed-wetter. I absolutely refused to go to Norfolk. Mr. Dawson (he had not yet earned his Ph.D.) was dumbfounded, but there was no way he could have known my real reason for turning down that golden window of opportunity.

If I had been a prisoner of war, I could not have been subjected to a more intense interrogation than that which took place in Mr. Dawson's office over the next week. I can vividly picture myself sitting there being assaulted by my mentor's 1,001 reasons why I should go to Norfolk for the summer, and they were all valid. All that was missing were intense, hot klieg lights focused on my pupils and the threat of the rack to make it legitimate torture. Regardless, I held my ground for at least three days before he finally pummeled me into surrendering. Every excuse that I hurled at him, he countered. My need to work and earn money during the summer was the most legitimate. To answer that need — now get this — he actually purchased a small neighborhood grocery store and offered me the job of running the store upon my return. He had been looking for something to occupy the time of his retired, aged father, as well, so it was perfect. The old man could run the store during the day while I was in school. Finally, he had me in checkmate. My bluff had been called. Scared out of my wits, I found myself on a Greyhound bus to Norfolk, cursing to the high heavens all the way that I had let this guy finagle me into doing this crazy thing that was sure to lead to absolute personal devastation. I felt like bro' rabbit after he'd been outsmarted by the fox.

Over the next few weeks before my departure, my mind was a private hell. I had made the dumbest decision of my life. Now, how was I going to cover myself? What strategy would I use? I figured I'd be living in a dormitory with other high school boys. What if they got wind of my problem? They would ridicule me off the campus. You know how cruel kids can be toward those who have obvious weaknesses or disabilities. I spent more time in prayer during those weeks praying to God that He would eradicate my problem in the nick of time. After all, a miracle was the only thing that could save me now, and I was not too proud to call upon the source of all miracles.

I stayed up late and drank as little water as possible, reasoning with infantile logic that this would bias conditions in my favor against bed-wetting. Hey, what did I have to lose? I was desperate! At that age, I knew nothing about the dangers of dehydration, nor did I care! As far as I was concerned, I was already in a life or death battle. The certain humiliation that lay before me could very well kill me. I figured if I only slept about five hours a night, maybe I wouldn't have a chance to wet the bed. Unfortunately, my plan didn't work and I became even more of a basket case.

During the long bus ride to Norfolk, I developed a strategy for ensuring that I would be assigned to a private dormitory room. If there were only a limited number of singles, I wasn't going to sit back and pray that chance would be kind. I would be aggressive, even obnoxious if need be, to push my way to the front of the line and get one of those rooms. All I had to do was get myself a single room, and that would buy me time. With my acumen, I would figure out a way to hide the evidence. At the time there was no way for me to be aware of the one gaping hole in my strategy. So in the interim, I relaxed under the illusion of having a solution.

Despite it all, there was one absolutely positive outcome to this strange debacle which eluded me at the time, of course, but would come to light many years later. There would be many occasions later on in life when I would need to know the meaning of faith. There would be tight spots when I would consciously turn to God in faith after all else will have failed me. It would be then that I would look back on my Norfolk State summer experience and realize that I had indeed learned the meaning of faith in the most dramatic way. The mere act of going to Norfolk at that time in my life represented nothing if not a pure act of faith.

Now for the shocker. When I arrived at Norfolk State College in the summer of 1965, I discovered what everybody else must have already known: There were no dorms for male students! At that time Norfolk State was a small Black college of modest means. Instead of dorms, they relied upon the sympathetic citizenry of the surrounding community to provide rooms for many of the male students. I was one of five boys assigned to live in the home of an elderly couple. As it turned out, there were two two-person rooms and one single. You don't even have to ask who got the single. As already alluded to, I would have killed for it. The fact that I didn't have to proved beyond a shadow of doubt that there had to be a God. Without even a struggle, it just sort of fell into my hands.

Still, I wasn't out of the woods yet. I had to rethink my plan. If I had messed up in a dorm by ruining the linen or mattress, it would have been an impersonal act. In a private home, any such infraction becomes personal. Given this added twist, I really had to overcome my problem!

The first night I hardly slept at all. I didn't want to sleep for fear of what might happen, but no one can stay awake forever. The second night I could no longer hold back the tide of nature. I slept like a log and indeed I wet the bed. It wasn't that severe, but still I could have died. I was about ready to go AWOL and return to Georgia. Really! I thought of just running away and disappearing, and I probably would have if the following surprise had not occurred. For some strange reason after that first night, *I never wet the bed again*! It's true, and to this day I have remained dry. An adage that I have found to be true proved itself once again: **THE THING THAT I MOST FEARED WAS THE THING THAT I MOST NEEDED TO FACE. ONCE I STEPPED OUT ON FAITH AND FACED THE DRAGON, I WAS HEALED.**

It was years before I fully understood the higher spiritual and mental principles underlying my healing. Of course, some Divine Power had masterminded the whole thing and that's all that matters ultimately. It worked through Mr. Dawson, the administrators at Norfolk State and the elderly couple that housed me. As it is written: All things work together for good for those who love God. I had called upon this Power in a time of great despair and It answered by working out all of the minute details.

On the human level, I can now see why I had the problem in the first place. My home was like a battle ground. My father was an alcoholic during those years, who used to get sloppy drunk and raise hell all night, every night. There was no peace in the household. He would rant and curse at my mother, accusing her of unmentionable vices and threatening to engage in all kinds of violence against her in the presence of us kids. To us she appeared to be a bundle of raw nerves walking around, screaming and crying all the time. She was chronically depressed and sick. She would send me running to the store two or three times a day to get her a B.C. or Goody aspirin powder to calm her nerves.

Our house was not a home; neither was it a pleasant place to be. All of us kids were sympathetically depressed, as well as nervous and angry. We were in accord at that time in hating our father for being so evil, but in this case there was no strength in numbers. There was nothing we could do. I stayed away from home as much as possible during the day and tried to do all of my homework at the school library during the recess period. There was no guarantee that I would be able to concentrate on anything scholastic once I returned home to that hell hole.

When I went to Norfolk, it was the first time in my 15-year life that I had slept in a home where there was peace. For the first time, I witnessed a married couple acting civilized toward each other, and to be honest, I couldn't quite fathom what was taking place. It just didn't compute. Once I accepted that it was real, that they weren't pretending and that people actually lived like that, something immediately began to change within me. The effect was so calming that after a summer of such nights I never wet the bed again.

This was my first healing. The second one would come seven years later when I would be healed of osteomyelitis, an "incurable" bone infection. No matter what happens to me now, I have witnessed the invisible power of Spirit work miracles in my life. Thus I will never again doubt what Spirit can do.

OSTEOMYELITIS

It was at the age of 14 that I was mysteriously afflicted with osteomyelitis, a severe case of bone marrow infection in my left arm. Fortunately, I was right-handed. Even so, for the next eight years, I lived with continuous, excruciating pain, because all of the medical opinions had delivered the same verdict: *incurable*! Thus HS2 was not the first incurable disease that I contracted.

When medical emergencies arose, my mother had only one recourse, and that was to take us to the poor people's clinic, which was free. To say that they badly botched the medical treatment of my badly swollen and infected arm would be a major understatement. Such a statement would imply that I had been treated at all. In fact, what actually happened was more akin to neglect. You know, the old "take two aspirin and call me in the morning" shtick. And when that didn't work, they began to mumble something about amputation, which cured me of all desire to seek further opinions. I terminated my visits to the free clinic abruptly.

For many months thereafter, I wore a full length cast on my left arm all the way up to the shoulder. Even as a teenager, I figured that it was better to live with the great pain than to entertain any further discussion about amputation. And since I had to wear the cast, I went on and played basketball and football daily on the local playground. Nobody had ever told me about the metaphysical concepts of visualization and positive thinking in those days. All I knew was that I wanted to do exactly what the other boys did, and that's exactly what I did. There was no discussion about it and everyone accepted "the Fugitive," as I was instantly renamed in the image of the then famous television hero, Richard Kimble.

Eventually, when I became employed as an engineer in Cambridge, Massachusetts at the age of 22, I found myself in one of the first group practice medical plans (known as HMO's today) in Boston, the Harvard Community Health Plan. It was then that I was introduced to an affable, enterprising young Harvard-trained orthopedic who was interested in trying a radical experimental approach for treating my diseased bone. He took me on as a Harvard Medical School study case. I still have vivid memories of being wheeled before the theatre of studious young med students as exhibit "A," as my case was discussed in the third person. Have you ever been exhibit "A"? I know that my doctors meant well, but it's the eeriest of all possible human experiences being dissected, exposed and talked about as if you weren't even present. After an operation, a month in the hospital having my system flooded with potent broad spectrum antibiotics, and another 11 months as an outpatient taking strong antibiotics, to everyone's surprise I found myself effectively cured. Why? Nobody was ever able to explain it. After all, osteomyelitis is still considered to be incurable.

To be sure, I still have pain in that arm from time-to-time, but it's not even close to the intensity that existed before the treatment. Though the bone in my left arm was permanently deformed by the disease, I continued to be an avid basketball player for years thereafter.

I've often thought that taking powerful antibiotics for a year could have wiped out some of my natural resistance to disease. My propensity for readily acquiring infections throughout my history would certainly support this postulate. Regardless, I learned a long time ago that there is absolutely no percentage in complaining about the quality of life that has been granted us. In the great card game of life, we are dealt only one hand for starters. Even if that hand comes up HS2 or osteomyelitis, it is up to us to figure out how to make that hand pay off. I figured out a long time ago: **YOU GET NO POINTS FOR WHINING.** There simply is no room for sympathy or self-pity in the successful enjoyment of life. **WHEN WE SUCCEED DESPITE ALL ODDS, IT IS THEN — AND ONLY THEN — THAT WE GLORIFY GOD.**

As I was saying earlier, there just aren't any accidents in life. The more you explore into the core of any element of life, the less it seems like an accident. Whether it be a plant, a fruit, a bird, a flower, a muscle, a rock, a molecule, an atom or a newborn babe, if you probe deeply enough you will be forced to acknowledge an underlying divine pattern — i.e., a pattern of perfection — with renewed appreciation.

By the time I got out of college, I was ready to pursue the life of pleasure with abandon. What could have possibly stopped me or turned me around? I was arrogant, cocky, self assured, and equipped with a college degree and a good job to boot. Oh, I was young and even erudite, I thought. At 22 I was a boy-man with a promising future. I had places to go and things to do. There is no question in my heart but that I would have continued to slide down the slippery slope to certain doom if something like HS2 hadn't forced me to stop and reflect. It's not too far-fetched to surmise that I may have even been dead by now.

When a man is on top of the world, he doesn't reflect and he doesn't examine himself, his motives or actions. Why should he? He thinks he's already in heaven. He has money and influence, lots of friends, a fine car, and women enough to keep his ego stoked.

There are few down moments and little time for self-reflection or boredom. Like a modern day celebrity, everybody is telling him exactly what he wants to hear, which is how wonderful and brilliant and unique he is, and there is absolutely no motivation for going within to search for answers.

Fortunately for all of us, the spiritual universe is constructed so that the forces of life push us towards Truth. Something will always go awry when we are spiritually out of alignment, and here's the rub: to the uninitiated, it will always seem like an accident.

CHAPTER 3: THOSE DEVIL-MAY-CARE YEARS

THE WILD YEARS

During those wild post-college years from about 22 to 26, I darn near burned myself out. I hung out in bars and blues clubs, smoking marijuana and drinking "what-have-you's" every night. I had "friends" in Boston, Georgia, Florida, Chicago and Montana, "friends" meaning women whom I could hook up with when I was in town, but I didn't have a steady girlfriend anywhere. Why bother? In a world of no-strings attached sex on demand, many boy-men in their 20's wouldn't think of tying themselves down to just one woman. Without knowing it, I had boxed myself into a corner. I was afraid of intimacy or commitment; therefore, it seemed that I couldn't bribe a woman to love me — I mean truly love me. Yet I was active all the time; frantically so. There was no shortage of women, and there was no shortage of bodies. But real love — that feeling of comfort, of security, of belonging — could not be found.

Bear in mind that the time was early '70s, right on the tail of the sexual revolution, just before HS2 and AIDS became realities. We young people thought we had the world in our hands, and that we could have all the sex and pleasure that our hearts desired — with no consequences.

Of course, I needed to examine myself. Since I wasn't willing to risk loving anybody, it is axiomatic by the laws of Spirit that I was only receiving just compensation. Sex was available; it always is.

But what I needed most was to experience genuine love. The thing that I cherished most, freedom, I had. Still, I was the loneliest bar-hopper in town, a type of urbane, modern day Prodigal Son.

Professionally, I was an engineer working for a prestigious consulting firm, Arthur D. Little, Inc., out of the Boston area. As such, I travelled extensively, which explains why I had friends in so many cities. Psychology tells us that one of man's greatest needs is the need to belong. That must have been what I was seeking. During all of those years of poverty before and during college, I thought that when the day finally arrived that I would have money, drive fine cars and escort attractive women, I would be happy. I really believed that. I guess that's what makes learning so awfully difficult. You just can't tell a young person who has been denied all of his life that money won't make him happy.

As a young, single engineer, I never managed to accumulate a whole lot of money, but I was light-years ahead of where I had been before. I know this story is an old one, but what surprised me was that within a short period of time, I became less happy than I had previously ever been, and not just for fleeting moments or days, but permanently. I found myself day-dreaming all the time about those bygone, idyllic days in Georgia when I was dirt poor. All of a sudden, those were the good ol' days. I finally realized that I had possessed something back then that had since been lost. Indeed, I had been happy.

Upon taking inventory in my mid-20's, I realized that I had lost that simplicity and that purity, seemingly for good. I came to know a new, generic type of boredom, which I reluctantly accepted as something that just happened to you as you entered into adulthood. But just what marks the advent of adulthood? At 25 we still don't tend to think of ourselves as being full-fledged adults yet. When we're fresh out of college or at the beginning of a career, we may be totally focused on trying to have a few of the things we missed out on earlier. We may be trying to fit in with the crowd and hold onto whatever peer status we have earned. We may be still trying to retard the day when our old friends who aren't yet wrapped up in corporate ascension, business accounts, and credit cards will accuse us of having changed. Yet secretly inside, we suspect that we have become one of that dreaded group called "them," the very characters we never wanted to become like. That youthful spunk and innocence has been lost. At 25 we know we're not yet fully adult, because we're still wondering what it will feel like when we become adults. It's the same thing we went through in high school when we anguished needlessly over what it was going to feel like to be in college, or enter the service, or get married. Then, taking college as an example, as soon as we became bona fide freshman, we realized that we had graduated to that level only to become acutely aware that we were not yet upperclassman. And so the mystery and the angst and the impatience associated with life's progression continues. It seems that we never quite arrive to the world's satisfaction. And if we have, we don't know it because nobody has told us yet. So what's the difference? Meanwhile, it always seems that whatever group we're not a part of is having all the fun.

As a growing young man, I anticipated each new level in the upward spiral with eagerness and excitement − at least, up to a certain point. Beyond that, I wanted to retard the hands of time and go back to a simpler time, which, granted, is not a healthy desire. Such a retrogressive desire is motivated by fear of the future coupled with over-romanticization of the past. At that point we become like salmons swimming against the natural current of life, depleting ourselves of all of our healing vitality in the process.

Man in his naturally-aligned state is spontaneously healed of all his diseases. It's only when he allows his fears and neuroses to pile up and reinforce themselves that dysfunction is created and sustained in his body. Healing takes place naturally when Truth is revealed. If you feel that you have become like the salmon swimming upstream, it is instructive to recall that at the end of the salmon's journey, it dies.

At 26 I was a very old body. I had been hanging out, predominantly, in blues clubs. I had seen a number of my favorite blues singers die from one drug or another − usually heroin, sometimes alcohol. Back in the late '60s through the mid-'70s in the Boston area, I recall weeks and weeks on end going to my favorite club over in Cambridge to see a favorite, not-yet-discovered blues singer. Every night, those in attendance would experience something special. How I recall sitting in those clubs night after night high as a kite. Some of greatest blues artists of all time would often appear in those little joints around Boston for as little as three to five bucks cover. The commercial world didn't even care that some of these artists existed. It would be another year before I would pick up and move to Los Angeles. There were little nooks and crannies hidden away from the main drag in Boston that gave time the illusion of standing still. When I'd go back the next week in hopes of seeing the same blues singer, I'd often find that he (and ocassionally she) wasn't playing there anymore. He would have moved on. I was never able to adjust to the way the beat played on while nobody seemed to care, but I guess that's show business.

Eventually, you manage to corner one of the waitresses, nonchalantly, of course. If you're too eager to get information, they'll know that you don't fit in; that you're not one of the regulars. They may even guess that you're an infiltrator from the corporate world — an engineer or something — which would be curtains as far as picking up chicks was concerned. You ask the waitress, "Hey, where is ol' Luther Georgia-Boy Snaky Shake Johnson tonight? Is he gonna play?" You're thinking that maybe he's just late. The waitress looks at you through sort of a startled, drug-induced stupor that you come to instantly recognize after years of hanging out in places like that, and says, "Oh, Luther died last night. Ya want another beer?"

That just about sums up that entire life. You hear varying accounts of his death. You even meet some ardent Lutherites who don't believe that he's dead, and proceed to spread new rumors to that effect, but invariably the verdict that prevails verifies that indeed another outstanding artist has succumbed to the dirty needle. I guess I must be overly sentimental, but I was never able to adjust to the prevailing appearance which indicated that nobody seemed to care. It was definitely *un*cool to care.

Today, I realize that there was no way that I could have even approximated being happy while maintaining such a lifestyle. We all want to discover for ourselves what it means to be in natural alignment with the spiritual order of the universe. The lifestyle that I used to live was not in natural alignment. Just pick any block of blues lyrics and analyze it. You'll find such enlightened messages as, "It's thirty below zero, and my woman done put me down..."; "Whisky and women done wrecked my life..."; and other lessons in song about hard times, heartaches, booze, drugs and women — or drugs and men if the singer happens to be a woman.

Those of us who considered ourselves to be ardent blues followers would go into those clubs and get ourselves fully immersed in the pain as if it was some type of perverse elixir. Those itinerant, drug-fueled blues singers were our ministers, their messages our religion, and the joints where they played and shot up, our churches. In the smoky caverns of our minds, those singers were the only people who really knew how rotten, unfair and painful the outer world was. We turned to them as our philosophers. They were the only ones who were honest enough to talk about it. They were our therapists. They weren't helping me to get better, but they were showing me that they understood, and at the time, that was better than what I was receiving from the rest of the world.

Ironically, those blues clubs provided the first step in my journey towards personal healing. For the first time in life, I admitted to feeling pain. Before, I had denied any recognition of pain. It would be some years before I would learn that there was no universal necessity for pain. All I knew was that one day I was going to move away from Boston and start anew in California. It was a most intransigent vision, one which had been with me since I was a teen-ager. I didn't know then why the urge was so strong to take up permanent residency somewhere that I had never been before. By the age of 27, I would make the trek to California; by the age of 31, I would make the connections that would lead me to give up the negative life, blues and all, forever.

During the blues club years, a typical night would involve getting drunk and high, and if I was lucky, laid. We called it "getting lucky," but what a misnomer. Little did I know then that the life I had chosen was leading me down a one-way alley, along a steady descent into hell. Actually, if the truth be told, I was not very proficient at "getting lucky." I was clearly a man out of control during those rambling years. Spiritually aligned, I was not.

The most important thing that I learned during that period was that without something higher on which to set my sights, there just wasn't any way in creation to find the elusive formula for lasting happiness. This was a surprising revelation to me, one that I did not admit readily. I put up a real good fight at first, because I wanted to believe, like 99 percent of the world, that I could find happiness without turning to God. The "something higher" that I needed turned out not to be booze, drugs, women, sex, fancy cars, money, college degrees or a secure career. I'm not exaggerating when I say that the more of these things I acquired, the more my life went downhill. I'm sure this cannot be solely attributed to the acquisition of things as much as it can to the lack of balance and the complete absence of any recognition of the spiritual dimension of life.

In retrospect, I can't believe some of the things that I did during my lost years. I can't believe some of the ladies that I picked up — or was picked up by — or some of the disgusting, embarrassing situations I got myself into. Looking back with some degree of objectivity, I guess I have to conclude that I must have been bent on self destruction. I must have been an accident waiting to happen. I can't believe that I hated myself that much, to subject myself to some of the situations that I did. While everybody seemed to be telling me that I was better than I thought I was, I realized that my consciousness was filled with self-hatred. It used to embarrass me when somebody would compliment me. I wanted to be average so badly that I over-reacted by acting out subhumanly. "See there! Look at me now," I seemed to be saying. "I'm not anything close to what you thought I was, am I?"

On some level, I felt inferior. I felt that it was inevitable that I would disappoint those who believed in me sooner or later. Why not take control and get it out of the way by being as disgusting as possible from square one? Subconsciously, I thought it was a dandy idea.

When I worked for Arthur D. Little in Cambridge, Massachusetts, at first I was received as one of the shining young lights in the Chemical and Metallurgical Engineering Department. I wasn't exactly a conformist in dress or style, but somehow they thought that I was smart enough, hard-working enough, and worthy enough of their investment. But the honeymoon didn't last long. My whole attitude evoked feelings of inferiority. I downgraded myself by acting so nonconformist and fiercely iconoclastic when in fact I was simply an obnoxious bore. In truth, I harbored a deep fear, a fear that I wasn't good enough, a fear that I couldn't cut it, a fear that they wouldn't like me, a fear that I would disappoint the company and my boss who had taken such a risk to bring me on board, a fear of failure. Most of the time my fear manifested as hostility and defensiveness.

Looking back, I can't believe how much of a basket case I was. They weren't going to get the first shot at hating me. It's sort of meaningless to hate somebody who already hates himself. At best, I elicited pity. I pulled a coup. I pulled the rug right out from under them. In fact, I pulled so hard that they remained standing while I fell down. And when I cried foul, they didn't even know that the rug was gone.

My problems weren't only with the people at work. I had fought with my family, too, especially my brothers and sisters. For many years, I tried to compensate by doing many things for the family and making frequent trips home to show my parents what a good adult I had turned out to be. But after visiting my parents in Georgia, or my brother's family in New York, I would inevitably start a fight and get defensive and sullen over some petty incident and wind up getting run out of town. I felt like a man without a home, a veritable *bête noire*. From the beginning I had never accepted Boston as my home, and due to the experiences that my life course had taken me through, I no longer felt at home upon returning to my parents' house either. It was time to move to California and change my act.

There must be an existent God. Considering how obnoxious I was to my respective employers, there just is no way that I could have maintained jobs and paid the rent throughout all those years if there hadn't been some omniscient force or a power for good looking out for me. There is just no way. I tried everything that I could to defeat myself, but, nonetheless, I kept getting breaks. Not rewards, mind you — just breaks. The difference is that the higher laws of the universe never reward us for being wayward, even though we may err out of ignorance. If we are earnest in our search for Truth, it is consistent with the nature of life to promote us. After all, the nature of life is toward onward and upward progression. Conversely, if we take a negative approach to life, this promotion will transpire through pain. In my case the price was tremendous pain.

If I had awakened dead one of those mornings, I wouldn't have been a bit surprised. I was sure that I had been worse off than dead many times. I had gone through a period of about a year at the age of 20 when I thought I was dying for sure. Having been diagnosed as having gonorrhea and syphilis, simultaneously, with no logical idea of when and how the prerequisite exposures could have taken place, I almost went crazy. Literally! That was long before my wayward, blues club years. At the time I was still in college and could only find dates on rare occasions. Upon discovering that I had syphilis, I just knew that my brain had been irreversibly infected and that my heart was diseased and inflamed, just like the medical encyclopedia says. Every organ seemed to hurt; every area of my body seemed to attack me. I was afraid to close my eyes to go to sleep or to be alone. I lived in constant fear of death. There were occasional bouts of paralysis, which reinforced my suspicion that I was as good as a goner. Eventually I gave up my preoccupation with death, but it would be almost 10 years before I would discover higher truth and real peace.

No aspect of our lives is incidental. Everything that we have done and thought, and continue to do and think, has bearing on what's happening to us today. From a metaphysical perspective, there is no doubt about this. The nature of God is such that It supports only what is the best and highest for each of us, but this same God cannot and will not intervene in our lives and usurp individual free will to force a certain notion of "good" upon us. When we go against the grain of natural, spiritual law, the experience which follows will normally be construed as "bad." This experience will tend to be bad, painful or horrible, but paradoxically, it is also good. There is no substitute for a horrible experience in leading us inexorably toward Truth. The Higher Intelligence that is God knows this. The only way It can bring us into alliance with the perfect life is by allowing, through Law, for the possibility of our having horrible, uncomfortable and embarrassing experiences that masquerade under the names of gonorrhea, HS2 or what have you, until that glorious day arrives when *we* decide to change.

Now, God is not willing these things upon us any more than He wills bankruptcy upon a gambler. He can only allow for the *possibility* of all of these choices. In every case I made the decision to engage in the act with the individual of my choice which eventually led to disease, the same as when you drop a coin into a slot machine, you don't know if you're going to get 7-7-7, three cherries, or just the pits. But if you come up with pits often enough, you will learn to leave that machine alone. Then if you're really smart, you'll see that the problem is not just with that particular machine, but with the whole *idea* of slot machines and gambling. We can see here how there can be various levels of lessons through one simple act. It usually turns out that a prerequisite for understanding the higher lessons is further losses, pain and embarrassment.

Though these negative possibilities exist, it is important to understand that there is no mental or spiritual law in life which says that we have to first experience gonorrhea or HS2, say, before we can begin emulating the perfect life. Therefore, on some level, whichever experience we find ourselves in must be the result of choice. My degenerate experiences are no different than those of many other guys and gals, but few will ever admit it. We're all too caught up in projecting images of innocence and playing victim. I'm not proud of how I've lived, but I know that we have to tell the truth. Healing can only come through truth. I figure that if I go into enough personal history, all who read this account will surely discover parts of themselves and, perhaps, sense how they can begin to turn their lives around. The singular point that I continue to attempt to drive home is this: At some point we all have to totally own up to everything that we have done and are doing (so-called sins of commission).

And if we haven't done anything, then we have to own up to what kind of negative thoughts we have been thinking and continue to think. **THERE REALLY IS NO DIFFERENCE BETWEEN OUTER EFFECTS AND INNER THOUGHTS.** They intersect at the crossroads of our minds and appear as the fabric of our lives.

It is said that everybody wants to go to heaven but nobody wants to die. Well, the same can be said about healing: **EVERYBODY WANTS TO BE HEALED, BUT NOBODY WANTS TO CHANGE.** Think about it. Who really wants to change? I know I don't — but I also know that I must! The universe requires that we change or die. The catch which keeps so many bound in sickness and disease is that nobody *can* change unless she first takes inventory of what has really taken place in her life and then takes ownership for all of that drama that shields her from truth.

As an avid fan of talk shows, I know how their guests, many of whom have written autobiographies, tend to deal with the tough issues concerning their private indiscretions and embarrassing peccadilloes. With few exceptions, the authors of most autobiographies tend to tell just enough to titillate without making themselves look too bad. This is human nature. Though they seek the fame of authorship, few are ready to grow in the public arena. They know that to do so first involves great pain. Wherever there is growth, you can take it on faith that pain has already run interference.

OTHER SKELETONS IN THE CLOSET

A lot has been written in the print media and shared in HS2 support groups, I'm sure, about the touchy, sensitive and embarrassing issue of how to tell others that you have HS2. For years, this issue was ultra-sensitive to me. Sure, I can expound for days on what you *should* do. Like anybody who has experience in this area and is reasonably intelligent, I can produce a neat little list of do's and don'ts, but let's face it: None of us are as disciplined as we present ourselves to be. None of us quite live up to the lofty standards that we often impose on others. We're talking about an Embodiment

Gap of the nth order here, which is the difference between what we believe and what we do. We're also talking about an "honesty gap," so let's face up.

Why do some doctors smoke cigarettes and others take drugs? We know that many of them do. Surely they know better, don't they? It must be rough for them having to live up to the images of their profession. Oh sure, they're responsible. They bought into it just as surely as I have sold myself as a serious, no-nonsense, studious, intelligent, positive, right-thinking, God-loving, nice guy — the kind average parents would like to introduce to their daughter. But I'm not that.

Eventually I realized that there was only one way that I was going to be able to deal with relationships and that was to defrock myself of the wishful thinking that had occupied so much of my mental energy. Things were NOT as I wished they could be, and that was that. What it finally came down to was this: I wanted a solid one-on-one relationship in the worst way. This was a realization that I had denied for so long until I had convinced myself that it wasn't true. I had even weaved a self righteous cocoon around myself to render my state of chronic singlehood noble. The truth was that, with HS2, I figured my prospects of finding a genuine, committed relationship was near hopeless, if not nil. This is the raw truth. After everything else failed — all the clever rationalizations, claims of spiritual healing and having been called to a higher purpose above the temptations of the flesh (ha, ha) — it became crystal clear to me that it was time to stop running and turn around and face the wind, as cold as it was. Come hell or high water, it was time to recoup some semblance of self worth and chance to be whatever it was that I really was beneath that bogus facade. If you can relate to what I'm talking about, shout: "Hallelujah!"

Now it has become my obligation to tell the truth about me to whoever will listen. Nobody else can do it for me, and nobody else can do it for you. No longer do I enjoy living behind a mask, being set up this way. I would much rather the world think that I was scum, so long as it meant that I could be free. To be free! free! free! — that's what I crave.

This discussion brings to mind an event that took place one summer during my college years when I worked for the Atlantic-Richfield Research Center (ARCO) in Harvey, Illinois, a suburb located south of Chicago. It was 1970 right after my junior year.

It turns out that during the semester before I went to Chicago I had been treated for the "clap" back at MIT's medical center before leaving for Chicago. Those who know anything about life at MIT in ancient days will wonder how in heaven's name did I manage to catch the "clap" at MIT, of all places? It is well known that there weren't any women there to speak of. Take my word for it, it wasn't easy. For good reason, my memory is quite fuzzy about that episode of my life.

My theory was that the GI's brought all that stuff back from Vietnam, because the war was still going on in those days. Of course, I now know that that was not entirely true. Indeed there was a strain of gonorrhea that was imported from Vietnam which confounded a lot of people, including doctors, because it did not produce the common symptoms that had always been associated with gonorrhea. Later, I would get a dose of that strain, as well. As you can see, I was smart, but not too awfully bright during those days. Thus to my great chagrin, I became an expert on sexual maladies at a rather young age.

The problem with that new form of clap was that it did not result in a discharge or the signature pain in men that became legendary with the old form. This was a relief for men, but it wreaked havoc on women's internal plumbing. With no early warning mechanism, many of them eventually wound up sterile.

Well, you would think that this was bad enough, right? Well, there's more. Before going to Chicago, I had tested negatively and been released by my doctor at MIT as A-OK. When I arrived in Harvey for my pre-employment physical, the doctor called me into his office for consultation and told me that I had — you won't believe this — SYPHILIS! I could have died! Whereas the clap was not considered to be a big thing among my macho cronies, syphilis was a horse of an entirely different color. There were no bragging rights associated with having this.

Naturally, I didn't believe that doctor for one minute. It simply could not have been true. I was not just in denial. I was incredulous! I was livid! I was beside myself! I did not believe that the doctor was on top of his craft, so I requested — no, DEMANDED! — a second Wassermann Test. How could I have the Big "S" when I'd just been cured of the clap and hadn't even shaken hands with a woman since? It had been months. I may not have been the brightest guy in the world, but I knew that I couldn't have caught syphilis from studying, and that's all I could remember having done.

Maybe it was the toilet seat. Well...maybe. I was ready to revive that lame old theory. At that point I was pulling straws. I mean, I was about ready to believe in Satan, or enroll in a Bible college in the deep South or anything. My only question was, "Do I really have to go through this? Is it really necessary?" At the time I'd have just as soon died than have the Big "S." If somebody could have stopped the world, I certainly would have gotten off.

All I could think of was brain damage. Why is it that we always think of brain damage when we think of syphilis? Remember those sensational, high school sex education films of the '50s and '60s? Well, they are obviously still playing in some part of our collective mind. I'm referring to the ones that paint the most graphically-repulsive images of sexual diseases. I guess they were more potent than I previously thought. We used to laugh at them, you know. If you're old enough, you may remember when they used to show parts of people's bodies falling — or worse, *rotting* — off after having engaged in adolescent sex? And considering how they depicted diseased organs, you could have only concluded that having your organ fall off was the lesser of available options.

Of course, syphilis is nothing to sneeze at under any circumstances. By no means do I wish to trivialize it. Without proper treatment — medical and mental — it will definitely reduce your IQ and render you a basket case, no question about it. But over the next few months I nearly induced instant death as a result of my fear. And as you should know, fear can be as lethal as the natural consequence of any disease.

The second test results eventually came back from the laboratory, and indeed it was confirmed: I did have the big "S." Not only that, but the disease was in the second stage!

If you think I was upset the first time they told me the news, this time I was totally schizoid. Though I didn't completely check out, as far as getting any productive work out of me, I was fairly well kaput for that summer at ARCO. I went totally nonlinear after that. So they put me in the hospital, where I flipped out for 10 straight days. Actually, I was just waiting to die. I just knew that about three-fourths of my brain had already been eaten away before they diagnosed this thing and that I would never be able to graduate from college or hold down a steady job after that. Nobody could have convinced me otherwise − not that anybody was trying. Death was imminent, I was sure, and it would be a slow, convulsive descent into dementia. Anxiety stemmed from the fact that I just didn't know when.

What's important to realize was that I was a 100 percent intellectual human being. The thing that I was most proud of − perhaps, my only laudable attribute at the time − was my intellect. By all measurement systems, I was smart − I mean, pure head. I could think, figure, compute. My forte was simple and straightforward: I possessed the gift of making A's. I hadn't been born rich, White or good-looking, but I could breeze through hairy mathematical equations with the greatest of ease. And now, my most valuable asset, my brain, was rotting away. The verdict was finally in: Life was indeed unfair and there was nothing worth living for any further.

Was I ever seething in anger! Naturally, the target of my anger was the doctor who had treated me at MIT's infirmary. I had a major problem coming to grips with my discovery that an educated man of medicine could apparently be so incompetent. I still looked up to doctors at that time as being omniscient administers of health. All summer long I seethed over that man's incompetence. The practice of suing doctors for malpractice was not in vogue yet, so I never considered that as an option. I doubt if I would have, anyway, for suing has never been in my nature. However, beating the hell out of stupid doctors was.

I worked the angles, looking for a way to take one last flight back to Boston to challenge my doctor face-to-face, knowing that I could not be responsible for what my anger might lead me to do. The only reason I didn't do it was...well, I was broke.

I was angry with my doctor at MIT for telling me so glibly that I was fine and releasing me from his care. As I mentioned, I had been treated by him for the clap a few months prior. It was obvious that he had not adhered to the best follow-up procedure because once he had diagnosed me as having gonorrhea, which requires a culture test, he did not check me for syphilis, which requires a special blood test, known as a Wassermann. In 1970 I was still unawakened, and thus, possessed by a wicked temperament. I guess I'm lucky I didn't induce a heart attack or apoplexy, because I remained furious for a long, long time.

Perhaps I needed somebody to blame. Well, I *know* I did. I just wasn't equipped psychologically, socially, or mentally to work through such a devastating blow. Neither could I think of any other avenues of support to call upon in a strange city. Being in Chicago for the first time, I had no connections. Not only that, but all of my time was spent going from doctor to doctor and hospital to hospital doing what had to be done. It was a long time afterwards before I realized that as far as negative sexual experiences and diseases were concerned, I was just getting orientated for things to come. HS2 was still five years down the road, lying in wait.

I was 20 then. Ten additional years had to pass before I realized that the doctor at MIT was not my problem. GI's returning from the war were not my problem. Bad luck women were not my problem. The clap was not my problem, and neither was syphilis. I looked in the mirror and, lo and behold, there was my problem! In living color, staring right back at me. My problem was five-eleven, weighed 165 pounds, was Black, had a goatee and passed under the initials *B.J.* By golly, I had found my problem and it was I!

Specifically, my problem was associated with the way I lived my life, the way I thought, the way I viewed the world, the way I looked at women and the way I used them. My problem was that I didn't have any idea what love was, yet I was out there trying to make it in life based on some incredibly screwed up notions. There I was giving life my best shot, but not realizing that, in terms of effectiveness, I could just as well have been peeing in the wind.

The synapses in my brain were badly misfiring. My thoughts weren't clear, and neither were they consistent or coherent. Why shouldn't my own brain join in this conspiracy against me? The old central processor was misfiring like a piston engine with crossed wires. I was in need of some new thoughts, new notions, new ideas. A tuneup wouldn't get it; I needed the mental equivalent of a major overhaul.

There were other amusing facets (in retrospect) to my bout with this couplet of STD's. Many people wonder how it feels to have the clap. I believe it is especially important for ladies to know, because they are always talking about how much pain they endure while having babies. Now I realize that it is criminal to compare these two experiences. One is a very positive passage which — I agree with women — men will never experience firsthand, at least not on this plane. We just have to accept that. The other one is nothing but pure hell with no redeeming features.

I know women who are very shy and soft-spoken, and, perhaps, even classy and demure, who have confided to me that they shouted horrible, vile epithets at their doctors during labor. You talk about locker room profanity, I can't believe some of the invectives women told me they shouted during labor. One friend of mine, who is a devout Catholic and model of the gentle, sensitive female, told me that she called her doctor every "sonofabitch" and "bastard" in the book during her first labor. To see her, you just wouldn't believe she's capable.

Human beings are both complex and *private* beings. We are all capable of doing things that appear to be totally out of character, so far as our public personas are concerned. The part of a person that we see is only a small part — trivial in fact — of who the person really is. All the cockamania, inflated images that we put so much energy into projecting are nothing but a decoy at best.

Besides my Catholic friend, another woman swore that she begged her doctor to go ahead and kill them both so as to take her out of her misery. Admittedly, this may be hard for some to imagine, but it's not hard for me. You see, I've had the clap.

I've told you about labor; now let me tell you about the clap. Let's say that you are male and you have the clap. You could be watching the funniest sitcom in the world — Bill Cosby or Louie Anderson or somebody — but it wouldn't make any difference at all; you wouldn't laugh. I guarantee it. You wouldn't laugh because you would be aware that sooner or later nature was going to require that you go to the bathroom to urinate — or should I say *try* to urinate.

Now make no mistake about it, you most definitely will *want* to urinate. There won't be a question concerning your desire. Your bladder will be exerting so much pressure on the door to your urethra that you will know something is about to be forcefully ejected, somehow, through some orifice. That much, you are willing to accept. What you are not willing to accept is that you are going to allow this hot, high pressure, burning ammonia and uric acid to spurt freely out of your male member. It's impossible to imagine at that point how such a ridiculous little protrusion of elastic flesh could have once been the pivotal point for so much pleasure — which, at the time, seemed worth it.

There are times when it seem that the universe has a perverse sense of humor. Though life is not ultimately cruel, it contains many absurd ironies. It is interesting that the woman's focal point of pleasure also becomes the center of pain during childbirth.

Before I proceed further in my description of this dance of agony, let me suggest that a guy with the clap would probably do anything to avoid going through the simple ritual of urination in a public rest room. Let's face it. The general public is not used to hearing a grown man cry, no less scream. And fainting is not out of the question. I don't care how brawny or brave he may be, there are three things that no man can take gracefully: to admit that he's lost, to be drawn and quartered, or to urinate when he has the clap. Given a choice, he'd probably chose to be drawn and quartered.

Maybe that's why they named it the clap, because after every successful urinary performance, you deserve applause.

So there he is in the john and he's trying his best to maintain a positive outlook on life. A safe bet would be that he is NOT thinking about the next time he's going to have sex. In fact, it's like the morning after an all-night drunken bout when one finds the very smell of booze repugnant. When he's in that john, he is absolutely convinced that he never wants to have sex again. Furthermore, he's beginning to question the advisability of even dating! Why even risk getting that close.

So there he is. Maintaining a positive outlook means that he is reciting positive statements to himself such as, "I am not going to die. I am simply going to pee. My bladder is not going to explode. Once I get started, this is not going to hur-r-r-t...owwwwwwww!!!" No, he did not finish. He simply forced about two cc's through — that's only four drops. Without being aware of it, he just ripped a couple of tiles off the bathroom wall with his bare hands — and that's the good news.

Now, you may be thinking, "Hey, this guy is really exaggerating. How could it hurt that bad?" Let me explain. If you have ever played with a free-flowing water hose, one without a nozzle on the end, you know that the water just sort of gushes out in a lazy, solid stream. Surely, you found it difficult to wash your car with such a stream. To increase the pressure of the water jet, you had to slide your finger over the end, partially cutting off the area for flow so that water was forced out through a restricted opening. This it did with great violence. Then the water would scream out of the opening in a directed jet at high velocity and literally blow the dirt off the car.

It's the same thing when a man has the clap, except that, internally, his "water hose" has become inflamed and raw, and the end of it has just collapsed on itself and closed off. Obviously, I haven't been to medical school, but I guess it would be safe to suggest that the body is trying to heal itself. If I didn't know better, I'd say the body is trying to *kill* itself!

Okay, let's assume that it's trying to heal itself. I say that's fine and dandy, except for one thing: it needs to open up for business. The experience can best be likened to trying to pee fire. A guy's mind plays a lot of games during the experience. Like it is with most things unpleasant, he simply wants to hurry up and get it over with, but he also wants to slow it down so that it doesn't hurt so bad. All in all the whole thing takes about two hours. No, really, it just *seems* like two hours.

The problem is that he knows that he is going to have to go through this entire experience every time he gets the urge to go. For the next three weeks, the time it normally takes to become cured, he will be keenly aware of all things diuretic. He will not drink any beer or coffee or soda, and he'll avoid all water that isn't absolutely essential. To heck with what doctors say about drinking lots of water during an illness, given the choices he'd rather dehydrate.

It's amazing how those of us with addictions can't seem to control our appetites for sex, cigarettes, or alcohol under normal conditions. However, let something horrible befall us, such as a devastating disease, and all of a sudden we become willing – *and able* – to stop drinking, smoking, and having sex for however long it takes. Man may be bent on evil, but he's not a complete fool.

Isn't it strange? Maybe – just maybe – this is why the Ultimate Power that controls our universe has made it possible for us to suffer these debilitating and embarrassing episodes of disease. It's during such times of heightened awareness that we become the best darned people that we can ever be – sensitive, moral, caring, empathic, contemplative, thoughtful, prayerful, AND spiritual. Glory be!

IF I HAD A SECOND CHANCE

I often think of my childhood and high school days when I didn't quite know what sex was all about. Nonetheless, I was preoccupied with sex. In those days, I was so uncomfortable with strange new sensations of touch, newly-emerging body hair, and that characteristic heavy breathing brought on by proximity to the opposite sex. It was a time of innocence, a time before terms like the "clap," the Big "S," or HS2 had any meaning to me, and before the experience of innumerable other infections, ointments, antibiotics, injections and embarrassments. It's comforting even now to harken back to that time and bask in the feeling of naïve innocence. For some reason I need to know that there was once a "before" that I can still remember so vividly and occasionally imagine myself immersed in.

Even the hectic and frightfully insecure first couple of years of college were "pure" in that sense, though by that time I was nearly a decade less innocent. I was a frustrated young lad my entire first year because of the cultural shock of living and adjusting in a foreign land (Boston) — at least, for this Georgian — and the competing priorities of academic survival versus the fulfillment of social and physical needs. In other words, hormones were overflowing from my very ears like superfluous energy from a runaway nuclear reaction, locked up jelly tight in a physical house that didn't seem to have any use for them...or so it seemed.

Do you know how it is when you're virile and male and 18? I made it through my entire freshman year of college "celibate" by default. It certainly was not my choice! I'll never forget that year. Sure, I was only 18 years old then, but I had long before sampled the nectar of human ecstasy. And like the human animal that I was, I was never going to settle for sour milk again.

We all know that rock cocaine is highly addictive. Though I've never had it, it can't be more overpowering than sex to the normal male teenager. Maybe sexual preoccupation is different for some male teens. I hope it is. I can suppose that those who are reached early and taught about love, responsibility, sensitivity and things like that, or those who are socialized differently will have an entirely different experience than I had. Given that we don't all have the same life mission, other guys must certainly have different lessons to learn during their life cycles. There's no doubt but that everybody came here — or was sent here — for different purposes, and clearly one of my major ones has been to learn the true meaning of love. That includes learning about the proper roles of these related human aspects: the physical, sensuality, sexuality, and discipline. At every turn in my life, the lesson has consistently come back to me in undeniable ways: **LOVE EVERYONE. LOVE YOURSELF. LOVE GOD.**

This seemingly simple lesson has been so difficult for me. In fact, before I learned to recognize who I am in Truth, it was impossible. Before, I would always be trying to determine whether the person at whom I was peering through these all-too-human eyes was worthy of love. If that person appeared to be despicable, then I was unable to love him or her. Even after I learned that such failure on my part was limiting my own growth, it didn't make any difference. I was spiritually retarded. As such, I was simply unable to control my feelings, reactions, or behavior. I wasn't sure that I deserved to be loved. Therefore, when I went to the fount of my soul to fill my cup with unconditional love, I found that it was dry. I was forced to keep hating others for being so imperfect, even though my condemnation of them was the mental equivalent of dragging a heavy weight suspended from a harness around my neck.

I was caught in a vicious cycle of conditionally judging myself due to my inability to unconditionally love others. I judged them based on who I thought I was. I thought I was who I appeared to be. There was no way out. I was like a rat caught in a maze with no roads leading out. Without some new input, I was doomed to continually live the senseless life of self-inflicted bondage. I accepted as normal that my relationships always ended with me smelling like a rat.

But oh yes, Martha, there is a God. The day did arrive when I received that fresh infusion of spiritual manna from heaven, and by the grace of God I was awakened from my deep sleep. I ate from the tree of life and dipped my cup in the fountain of unconditional love. And like fairy tale magic, when I looked into the mirror of life I could see that the rat was only a mask which had at last cracked and fallen away. By Jove, there was a real person inside. No longer was I merely a phantom of a man. What had seemed like an endless maze to the rat was now littered with distinctly marked exits to the spiritual man. At last, I realized that who I was in Truth had little to do with the criteria by which I had been judging myself. Excitement followed. Great possibilities were emerging from behind the cobwebs of my mind: If I could love myself, could the love of others be far behind? Oh, this new consciousness is exciting! I couldn't wait to explore its implications.

I finally realized that even though I was a "bad boy" there was a pattern of perfection at my center and core, which was suddenly allowing me to exercise right choices just as it had previously allowed me to exercise wrong choices. When the verdict was announced, I discovered that I had been the only judge all the time and didn't even know it. By recognizing that perfect something at the core, I realized that I could summon it to the surface and take control of the choices in my life.

At that point, it began to dawn on me that I was beginning to truly like myself — that is, the only self of me that mattered. Could love be far away? It was frightening at first, such awesome power. And at times it still is. I realized that I had to stand alone much of the time, independent of family and friends and the advice of many that I used to listen to. It seemed so cold and uncomfortable, by comparison, to the safe, self-deprecating mode of the past. I hadn't realized that to truly grow I would have to learn not to listen to anyone but my real self, i.e., the self that is rooted in God. Indeed, such selective listening is not learned. It must be consciously cultivated.

I don't mean to suggest that I never listened to another person. I did, but there was a subtle shift, a change. I just reached a point where I didn't worry about what they thought. No longer did I feel obligated to take anyone's advice. To be concerned with keeping everyone happy depletes the vital energy. Everything was heard, but I only obeyed that which aligned itself with what seemed to ring true with my inner voice. No apologies.

Finally, I was beginning to love myself — not in vanity, but in divinity. True enough, it wasn't the love that I had always thought was love. At last I was responsible for whatever happened to me. Now, I could see a relationship between what I believed, the choices I was making, and the results that were taking shape in my life. No longer did I have to worry about whether a certain thing was happening to me because of what somebody else did or said. Finally, I realized that there was nobody else as far as my decisions were concerned. Once I got clear, and once I decided to decide, it didn't make any difference what anybody else was doing anymore.

I could accept them for who they were, along with whatever choices they might have made. Finally I knew what I wish I could have known all along: Their choices simply did not, and could not, affect my life.

Getting back to my macho teen-age years, I successfully emulated the errant ways of my adult role models. In the small southern town of my birth, teachers were at the top of the order as role models. As I grew up, I learned that even some of our most respected, married teachers were doing it to and with each other. It was shocking to my young mind to discover that they were that human — so common in spite of their lofty, authoritarian positions. I saw so many cases where marriage was not being observed as something sacred. How could this be happening in the Bible Belt, and yet people didn't even seem to be outraged? We think we're living through an "anything goes" sexual revolution today, but people are no different. The same old tired games have always been played. As I emerged from innocence, I was as shocked to discover which adults had known about these shenanigans as I was to discover which ones were doing it. It was as if there was a conspiracy of adults. They taught us to be uncompromisingly moral and virtuous, standards that so many of their ilk didn't even seem to be interested in. Was I living in some kind of strange black comedy, or was this real? Maybe we were all players in a prolonged nightmare, and I was just the last one to be told.

In my high school girls were still being tossed out of school for committing the dreadful error of — now get this — becoming pregnant! It didn't matter why. There were *no* extenuating circumstances. There was an old hag — I mean teacher — whose job it was to go around and survey the waistlines of girls rumored to be pregnant. Boys, if fingered and found to be fathers, were tossed out too, even if they were the wrong boys. I know. I was about two seconds from being tossed out of my high school within two weeks of graduation because I was reported to have been a willing participant in the pregnancy of a certain young lady who just happened to be my girlfriend at the time. This was despite the fact that I was slated to give the valedictory address for my graduating class and had earned an unblemished, exemplary record throughout my school years! To say that our principal was insensitive to students' needs would be putting it mildly. I found out later from adult friends in high places that I wasn't even going to be consulted before being tossed out by the principal. As hypocritical as it turned out to be, the upholding of moral standards in the deep South in those days was such that circumstantial evidence was good enough.

As it turned out, I wasn't even the guilty party. To indicate how naïve I was in those days, I was the last one to find out that my girlfriend was pregnant, long after all of the teachers and a number of assorted students knew. That she had been sick and had missed a number of days from school was not news to me, but what I didn't know was that she had undergone an abortion. It turned out that she hadn't told me because she didn't want me to know that she had been surreptitiously seeing this older guy, an ex-boyfriend who was 23 years old. Of course, I was quite intimidated and jealous of him. To a high school kid, 23 was very old. I was aware that he was part of her history, but I had been told that he was not on the scene anymore. Oh, how I long for the good ol' days of naïveté.

It could be questioned how I knew that the pregnancy was not, in fact, mine. Actually, I didn't really know. My girlfriend and I were sexually active at the time, but, as it turned out, the math obviously didn't add up. Though I earned straight A's in math, but it wouldn't have taken an Einstein to compute that a fetus of that age could not have been mine. Figuring forward from the day that I first "knew" her in the biblical sense, there was no way that I could have qualified. That's why my sweet and innocent-acting little girlfriend didn't let me in on the secret at the time. I'll say this: If she had told me that it was mine, I'm sure I would have believed her. Beyond that, it's conceivable that we would have been married, and the course of my life would have taken an entirely different course. Perhaps, I wouldn't have had to write this book.

Of course, I don't believe in chance, fate, accidents or looking backward with regret. The experience that actually transpired was the only possible one for me, and I gladly accept it. There are no experiences in my history that I would have preferred to avoid. I made it through by the grace of God. Now that I know better, my only concern is to apply present wisdom to create the kind of tomorrow of my desire. It would be the height of recidivistic ignorance if I should repeat the mistakes of the past. Mistakes during one's youth are necessary, for they are learning experiences. However, once we understand the truth about our relationship with Infinite Spirit, that we are created out of a perfect pattern, and that through Spirit we have unlimited choice, we have to realize that there is no reason to cooperate any longer in our own self destruction.

Lest I give someone the impression that I can create any reality that I choose independently of Infinite Spirit, let me clarify my position right away. I cannot. My role is that of sub-creator, governed by the Laws of Spirit, which are immutable. In this sense I have free will to make life-supporting choices in my life, but with these caveats: (1) I must understand that I of myself can do nothing, and that it is only Infinite Spirit that has the power to carry out the dictates of my thought. (2) This must be a *conscious* process. (3) I must learn, understand and embody the truth about the relationship between man and the Absolute. (4) Then I must work daily to conform to that higher truth by aligning all of my thinking and my actions, even in the simplest matters, with the divine laws of life.

There can be no ego in this kind of approach to life. I must never give the impression that I know something that others do not know, that I can do something that others cannot do, or that I have some kind of mystical power that others do not have. All that I am talking about is surrendering. This does not insinuate that we don't have ego, only that we understand that there is no place for it in the spiritually-aligned life. Everyone has an ego, but we must also learn to stop yielding to the ego. We are spirit and physical, celestial and terrestrial, and we have a calling to consciously strive towards the higher choices. While you must choose what is best for your life, I am working to let go of those modes of thinking and actions in my life that are ego-driven — gradually...gradually...more and more with each passing day. Though I may never completely transcend my ego, I have learned to be acutely aware of it. I now know its power and its nature, it range and its modus operandi. I can recognize it when it crops up and make the choice concerning whether to yield to it or yield to Spirit in any situation.

There are those who say that it's good to have an ego. Granted, since it exists it must serve a useful purpose. Even so, we don't have to become self satisfied in this respect. The statement that it's good to have an ego is common enough to be platitudinous, but the truth remains that ego is associated with human ambition and competition. Ego plays its role well in sports and in business, and quite successfully so. However, what is successful is not necessarily good. It helps people to land lucrative contracts and powerful positions; of this, there is no doubt. But all of this is just more of the all-too-common garbage that is associated with the world and its mores, none of which has the slightest thing to do with spiritual or surrendered living. In fact, it is the antithesis of spiritual living. Where ego is consciously courted and submitted to, no one will ever find fulfillment or happiness in a significant way. Just read history.

In high school, it was the uncanniest thing how our teachers and adult role models thought that we students didn't know who was messing around with whom. On the contrary, it was all that the students talked about — which teacher was seen where with whom. Sex education was something that most of the teachers had not been taught themselves! In our taboo, hush-hush, society, so many of them were caught up in the paradox of having to be role models, professionally and morally, although they hadn't really worked out their own sexual identities.

When I look back on that scene, I realize now as if it was the most startling of revelations that many of those teachers were very young, inexperienced, provincial — even country — people. Many were in their 20's and 30's, younger by far than I am now! Looking at my life and the many years of confusion through which I evolved, I now understand the paradoxes that confronted our teachers. At 30 I certainly hadn't worked out who I was sexually. The only difference was that they fell into the category of the omnipotent professional known as "TEACHER!" To 15- or 16-year-old students, superiors who are 25 or 30 years old and have that much power over their lives are omnipotent. They could just as well be gods.

We didn't realize that they, too, didn't have all the answers. The world of the adult is a mysterious thing to a kid. We figured that they surely must have held all of the answers to human sexuality. Teachers, by definition, are established as role models and authority figures. Upon taking the job, without necessarily knowing it, they bought into a game called "Let's Play Omniscient Role Model," and we all paid the price — teachers and students alike.

It was a tough job for a teacher back in those moralistic, Bible Belt days of yesteryear. They were charged with upholding a set of moral standards that many of them obviously did not believe in, yet the way the game was played, they were never to show vulnerability in front of their students. In other words, they couldn't humanize themselves by admitting, "Hey, I'm just like you. I'm not really om-niscient or omnipotent. I have the same feelings and emotions as you kids, and to boot, I don't have all the answers any more than you do."

If I had it to do over again...? I guess I'd make the same mistakes anew. Fortunately, I can't go backward in time. I shall, nevertheless, have another chance. This is the promise that the Creative Live Force has given to all of us, that we can renew our thinking, become transformed and choose again. Thus I am doing it all over again *now*! Indeed these are the best years of my life — tomorrow's good old days, as it were. Thank God that I've grown enough in wisdom, hunger and perseverance to put these new ideas into practice. So no, no, Nanette, I would never go back. I am in my right place, and at last, I am even in my right mind.

CHAPTER 4: SEARCHING FOR LOVE IN ALL THE WRONG PLACES

THE "IMAGE" OF HAPPINESS

After surviving the wild years of my immediate post-collegiate existence, the time finally arrived when I consciously decided to make a change toward a more meaningful, committed relationship. At least that's what I thought, but as it turned out, the mind was willing but the heart just wasn't mature enough. Oh, I had lived with a lady on and off over a span of two years while in college, which had the form but none of the substance of commitment. Simply stated, it was a relationship of convenience. In retrospect, I have to admit that I used that lady — or, more likely, we used each other. Back then, my primary commitment was to my books, which left little time to either maintain or pursue a relationship. Still, I was 20 and male and the hormones were raging. I wasn't that conscious. My actions could best be described as more programmed than reasoned. As far as love and dating were concerned, I was driven simply by hormones and lust. There wasn't that much more to it. Though I wasn't in touch with deeper feelings and motives, I suppose I must have known all along that I wasn't interested in the highest good of my live-in girlfriend. Nevertheless, I encouraged her to hang around until my graduation.

Why do young men so often behave like this? I guess it's just one of those rudimentary stages of life that Shakespeare described in his "Seven Ages of Man," which helps you discover who you are, what you feel and how the laws of life impact you. Before that relationship was over, I learned the meaning of heartbreak, rejection and pain. When she left me and dove straight into a heavy affair with another man, I was forced to deal with feelings that I hadn't even known existed. I learned in a hurry that the universe exacts compensation and that you never really get away with anything.

I didn't have another respectable relationship until I made 26. Her name was "Sophia." Life is strange. After all of those years of social wandering and loneliness in Cambridge, it turned our that as soon as I committed to move to Los Angeles, I met someone decent in Boston. I had just landed the perfect job in Los Angeles, but they wouldn't be needing me for six months. I left Cambridge on the 4th of July, 1976, the highly-celebrated day of the our nation's bicentennial, and for the next year and a half, Sophia and I maintained a long distance romance. Finally, she packed up everything she owned and we U-Hauled it cross country to live happily ever after in Los Angeles. She would swear later on that I had promised to marry her upon her arrival in L.A. That's not how I remember it. Anyway, I never got the chance. Only a week after arriving in L.A., she was critically stricken with a mysterious, degenerative disease. After only four months in L.A., the relationship was dissolved tragically and bitterly.

Sophia met all of my then listed criteria. You know the personality wish list that single people make up when they're interviewing for the perfect mate: "She has to be intelligent, independent, cute..." Well, Sophia was modern, classy, feminine, gentle, professional, open-minded, beautiful...she was everything that I thought I wanted at the time, and yet the relationship still didn't work. Hmm, could it be that a good relationship is more than the sum of the parts? As I mentioned earlier, though I had made the choice to stop fishing in the gutter of life and dating whatever the tide washed ashore, I still was not interested in Spirit or Truth or ultimate purpose. Well, that was my problem, though I had no hint of it at the time. It was later revealed to me that I had left out the most important element. I had undergone a drastic improvement, but I was still coming up short. I had achieved about 99 percent of everything that I wanted, but the one percent that I neglected contained the Truth. No matter how good a recipe is, if you leave out the main ingredient it still won't work.

What made my relationship with Sophia so memorable was that it marked the first time that I risked telling a mate the truth up front about my having HS2. The spread of HS2 was in its infancy back in 1976. I didn't know much about it and neither did my doctors. So just as I'm sure that I understated the seriousness of my condition, I'm equally sure that Sophia didn't fully understand the implications of her pledge to hang in there with me. As it turned out, she was stricken with a weird case of pancreatitis within a week of her arrival in L.A. and our new start together never had a chance. She became ill almost to death, and so did the relationship.

It may seem cold to state, but I know that illness serves a purpose in the higher meaning of life. If there is anything hidden that needs to come to light, we would be wise to bite the bullet and face it voluntarily. If not, life in its divine wisdom has created this perfect tool called illness, which, during its natural course, will flush everything out into the open. Sophia and my relationship certainly was no exception.

Prior to her illness, I saw Sophia as a pure angel. I couldn't have imagined her lying to me or taking on the cloak of bitter anger to the point of unforgiveness. Due to her incapacitation at my hands, so much doubt and confusion trickled to the surface that it sent us fleeing in opposite directions. We didn't even know the two people that evolved from the confusion. All of a sudden I was forced into the role of guardian, nurse and caretaker, while simultaneously trying to launch a new career in California. I signed up to live with her, but I wasn't ready for any of that "for better or for worse" business. Somehow, I hadn't understood that all of these issues fell under the same umbrella as total commitment. Thus I was an unconscious liar, having declared that I was ready for commitment without understanding all of the implications of my words.

Under the duress of sickness, I learned that my fiancée wasn't the age that she had claimed. Her true age was prominently displayed on the clipboard at the foot of her hospital bed. She was a year older than I, but she had given her age as a year younger than mine. I also learned that her hair wasn't the color that she had claimed. Being stricken the way she was, those roots started growing out and there was nothing that she could do about it. At the time, of course, I was embarrassed for her, and I quickly forgave her little peccadilloes. It didn't matter to me that she was older than I or that her hair wasn't blond. It was years later before I was able to put the whole picture together, however. As it turned out, we were merely two young, unevolved people who did not know themselves or understand the higher laws of life.

Here again, it seemed that I had been the victim of the worst possible luck. It's amazing how life oftentimes forces us to deal with the very thing we scheme so craftily to avoid. I was beginning to wonder if, perhaps, God hadn't placed some kind of curse upon me. Of course, I have never believed in a devil or satanic force, so the cause had to be either me, God, or some unknown third party exerting mental control over me.

Under the duress of illness, we were forced to examine other previously-ignored differences, for example, the fact that she was White and I was Black. You see, we had already agreed that her Whiteness and my Blackness were of no consequence. Again, we were wrong. Our personal agreements are not the same as universal laws. We had also merrily glossed over the fact that she was Catholic and I was Christian (at the time). Like millions, we were religious in name only. It had no practical impact on our lives. When the chips were down and there she was lying flat on her back, wasting away in that hospital, she found herself overcome by massive guilt. I had to ask myself, where did the guilt stem from? Then I realized that it derived from her Catholic upbringing. We learned in a hurry to respect the fact that we are products of our pasts. We didn't want to be, but we were. Now I'm not against interracial relationships. My experience does not prove that people can't change their attitudes or successfully marry interracially, but it does substantiate how important it is to face up to the realities of every facet of a relationship, no matter how minor. We can declare that certain problems don't exist but that doesn't make them go away. With

Sophia and me, our religious and cultural programming had been lying dormant all the time, just waiting for the right moment to wedge their way to the forefront of our awareness. Still, I am not making a case for being religious, because I think there is something higher. But we mustn't ignore the impact of early religious training — or even indoctrination — on our lives.

It gets worse. After Sophia had been ill for a couple of months, her mother flew out to "help" during her daughter's time of need. Well, I had always thought of mothers and daughters from civilized families as being loving and harmonious towards each other, but these two got along like two pit bulls. I was seeing another side of my "angel" that left me reeling in incredulity. All of this couldn't be attributed to Sophia's illness, either. Instead of bringing forth harmony, my home became a veritable war zone. I had never heard a mother and daughter go at each other with so little respect in all my days. Oh boy, was I growing up! The truth is they loved each other, but they just couldn't stand to be in each other's presence for too long. There are many who can relate to this.

If you think the rest of this story is fiction, I won't blame you. But it really happened. I am a witness that life is stranger than fiction. Sophia's mother developed serious heart irregularities while she was visiting us, and before I could catch my breath, she, too, became hospitalized. All of a sudden I had a demanding 8-to-5-plus job plus two deathly ill women in the hospital to look after. The doctors wanted to perform triple bypass surgery on the mother's heart immediately, if not sooner, as they were afraid she might die at any minute.

I felt sorry for Sophia. Not only was she forced to grapple with rapid weight loss and the unbearable pain of pancreatitis, but also she suddenly had to begin worrying about whether her mother was going to die and leave her alone.

I don't understand all of the reasons for events. Maybe the sequence of events forced Sophia to reexamine her attitude and come to a higher appreciation for her mother. Sophia came from a broken home. In fact, her mother had been abandoned by a gaming, philandering husband. Thus there was no father on the scene or money in the household at the time. Consequently, I went broke during the whole ordeal. Cold though the decision was, we decided to fly Sophia's mother back East to her own home for her heart surgery. It was clear to me that I was in no position to take care of her during the long post-operative recuperation period, but I still felt guilty about my decision. Shortly thereafter, I sent Sophia back to live with her mother, where both of them had to face the twin struggles of surviving and recuperating at the same time.

Though I kept sending her money, Sophia grew angrier and angrier with me for screwing up her life and leaving her down and out and unmarried. She felt that if I had married her as I supposedly had promised, she would have been better protected. Granted, she had a point, but on the other hand she never accepted any responsibility at all for the way things turned out. We were in our late 20's. Indeed I intended to marry her, but neither one of us had ever broached the subject of dates, terms or particulars. I was led to believe that she felt the same way that I did about it — that the formality just wasn't that big a deal. As usual, I was wrong.

Sophia's untimely illness totally dominated the course of our relationship. I think I understand now. On the tail end of the Vietnam war and the Free Love era, we weren't into formalities, conventions and morals. Be that as it may, as sickness ensued and Sophia's Catholic-laced true feelings emerged, she began to feel dirty and sinful and used. The only way that she knew to redeem herself was to plead innocent. There is another factor that came into play. As she lay emaciated in the hospital bed, there was this roving group of Bible-toting Christian volunteers who came by periodically to "pray" for her. It should come as no surprise that they were none too approving of me or of our relationship, a fact that they didn't even try to hide. Catholic guilt is a deeply embedded phenomenon, which I would admonish others never to ignore. In later years, I would court two more ex-Catholic women who ended up spending years to free themselves from similar residual guilt.

Again, I believe that what transpired was not accidental. Divine Law stepped in once again and forced me to deal with the folly of my ways. The truth I was forced to face was that I didn't really feel comfortable with the prospect of marrying Sophia, and I have reason to believe that the feeling was mutual. God is merciful, indeed, even though spiritual Laws cause us to reap much pain. Spirit has provided the universe with powerful means to awaken us from our deep sleep and shock us into awareness.

There is no doubt but that I loved everything Sophia stood for. I'm just not sure that I loved her. I couldn't have loved her because at that point in my life I didn't have the slightest idea what love was. I had no idea what life was all about. I was sleepwalking through life, totally unaware of what was transpiring. Not only did I not know who she was, but neither did I know who I was. Not only wasn't I receiving the right answer, but I wasn't even asking the right questions. I was intelligent enough to know that I was *supposed* to be more responsible, but I just wasn't there yet in consciousness. There was so much confusion and pain and things were awfully screwed up.

Sophia represented a symbol that I wore around my neck. The only thing that I was sure about was that I didn't want any more of the degrading relationships that were so reminiscent of my past, so I arbitrarily opted for the symbols of a successful relationship: looks, class, style, sophistication and salary potential. True to the plan, I acquired the form, but that did not turn out to be enough. The universe was screaming at me: "No, no, that just won't do. You've got to acquire Truth!"

Sophia left and things continued to go downhill from there. It was May of 1978; I remember it well, for after liquidating all of my assets I was forced to move out of my luxury townhouse apartment and sell the new car that I had bought for her. Of course, I gave her all of the money. From a borderline hefty 130, she had dropped to 83 pounds and was steadily declining. She could barely walk, no less drive. Special arrangements had to be made with the airlines to fly her back East in her condition. To raise the rest of the money that I needed to help her survive this ordeal, I made the aforementioned changes, rented a small house and took on a roommate. After having shared accommodations with some 30 different roommates during my college years, I had sworn that I'd never take another roommate in this life, no matter the cost. I lied.

There is no doubt in my mind today but that Sophia's strange, sudden disease was brought on by the burdensome weight of her repressed emotions and guilt. In other words, no physical or organic cause was ever found for her condition. There simply was no material cause. I literally went broke shuffling her around from specialist to specialist, but not one was able to diagnose the cause of her malady. They tagged it pancreatitis, but could not comprehend its origin in one so young and clean-living. They kept trying to force her to confess to alcoholism, a neat diagnosis that would have made the puzzle fit, but such was not the case. Sophia was one straight arrow.

SEARCHING FOR MS. GOODBAR

After Sophia, the ensuing six years saw me slide steadily downhill into a succession of lousy relationships. Just when I didn't think that life could get any worse, it did — progressively worse.

It's rough out there on the sexual battlefield. The soldiers of opposition can be brazenly calculating and callous during those young adult years, leaving many scarred carcasses in their wake. I was one of those scarred carcasses. Oh, I was intelligent enough and, at least on paper, it seemed that I might have a promising future. But the women I encountered during my 20's seldom cast their lots on potential, and that pained me.

The irreducible fact was that I was still struggling financially. I did not possess the sort of material accouterments that might impress a lady. My style of dress and choice of wheels were strictly second, or even thrid, class. Though I was 28 and had been out of college six years, I had been busted by the devastating experience with Sophia. This is no veiled plea for pity; I'm simply telling it the way it is. I empathize with those who are still out there and who are still seeking. Though I have found my life mate, by no means am I smug. I haven't forgotten what it's like. Furthermore, I have it on good authority that the scene is no different today. When I watch dating programs on television such as "Love Connection," it is clear that the preponderance of quests in their 20's and early 30's still place superficial accouterments like physical characteristics and occupation above all else. This is not to criticize them — after all, I did the same thing — but to simply point out that some things never change.

After graduating from college, indeed I did land a good job and was finally in a position to purchase some of the longed-for trappings of success, but the wound had already been set. I was determined not to become yet another fickle dissident who couldn't wait to buy my way into acceptability. You know how it is. As soon as a young person pulls down some decent cash and thinks he (or she) can move up in class, he attempts to rush out and buy his way into the world. It's the old nouveau riche syndrome, or in this case, nouveau just-barely-able-to-fake-it syndrome.

Someone once said of humans that we are always buying things that we don't want to impress people that we don't even like. Years earlier, I had wished and hoped that I could have bought the things that would have impressed the type of ladies that wouldn't give me the time of day. Take any man with a modicum of pride, and he'll seize every opportunity to wholly and completely deny in the class of woman that he cannot have. He will go so far as to badmouth her (or her type) and put her down in front of his peers. Yet at the same time, there is something in him that knows it's all a lie. Give him an opportunity where it becomes realistic for him to impress such a woman, and he won't be able to sleep until he has at least given it the ol' college try. I've seen this pitiful scene played out many times. Unless a man is exceptionally advanced on the scale of wisdom, it's a sure bet that he will go for it. It's stupid — I don't claim to understand it — but this is man. I wish I could say that I was an exception, but I'd be lying. Many were the times that I made a total fool of myself over a woman. "Am I good enough," such a man will ask, "to make a woman like that fawn over me?" There have been buddies whom I've warned about getting involved with certain women because I knew they didn't know what they were getting into. Plus I knew these guys' values and I feared that they couldn't handle it, but it didn't make a bit of difference. Mind you,

I'm not suggesting that I was right for trying to deter them. I'm just being honest. Clearly, it was their prerogative to go ahead and get involved. Conversely, there have been buddies, as well as family members, who have warned me. The worst relationship of my life, which I'll be discussing in the next section of this chapter, is the most painful example. Obviously, I didn't heed their advice. The woman in question represented everything that I thought would make me whole and I wasn't about to forfeit my chance to conquer her. Yes, *conquer*! This is painful to admit, but I maintain that we can't get healed unless we are willing to take full responsibility for our part in the creation of the problems of our past. There are no accidents in the universe.

It had always been important to me to remain true to my grass roots, or even plebeian, values. Whatever good fortune might become my lot, there was no way that I was going to allow myself to be enticed by some good-looking temptress, the type who would have surely rejected me previously. At least, this is what I told myself.

Moving to Los Angeles was a pivotal juncture in my life. Along with the outer change in location, there was a corresponding inner transition which began to take place. Gradually, I began to let go of past anger and hurt. This took place in spite of a couple of major setbacks. Consequently, my self image, along with my understanding, began to improve. Los Angeles softened me and provided me the space to develop a new outlook on life. After a few years of basking in the mellow lifestyle of southern California, I arrived at a point where I no longer had a need to reject anyone. Instead, I learned to use my energy in a more positive, attractive way. Instead of using valuable energy to reject, I learned to focus my energy on attracting whatever it was that I wanted.

Los Angeles afforded me that opportunity to change. Of course, I was conscious that the move would do me good. For years, I had been dreaming of moving to California. Ever since leaving high school a decade before, I had been circulating within the insular academic circles of Cambridge and Boston. As a result, I had allowed myself to become socially skewed. There is a certain comfort which comes from embedding oneself in academia. When you chance to lay it on the table and examine it, it looks an awfully lot like fear. There was something special —but not good — about academia. I got caught up in all that stuff to the point where I really believed with my friends that we were superior to the working classes, the heartland and most of the rest of the nation. There is no need to point out the inherent hypocrisy. It's not uncommon for college kids to get caught up is elitist beliefs. To illustrate the point, I found myself having to apologize to my friends when I "deigned" to move to Los Angeles. One just wasn't supposed to move out of northeastern academia to southern California unless he was some kind of mindless surfer dude, or sun-worshipper, or crew cut warmonger or R.O.T.C. graduate. San Francisco, okay. But L.A., never! This is the way we thought.

Though I didn't know it at the time, this was the beginning of my blossoming into radical independence. Southern California it was, and I never looked back. I found that there were so many healthy women in L.A. — mentally, that is — that it completely turned my thinking around. As one comedian quipped: I wouldn't leave L.A. for heaven!

To be honest, there is superficiality and plasticity in L.A. — buckets of it. Everyone knows that. However, there is another side to L.A. that is all charm and conviviality. And best of all, there is a healthy quest for spiritual expansion in L.A., an openness and freedom and tolerance — religious tolerance, even. It's a city where the prevailing atmosphere is mellow, loving and accepting, plus the sun is always shining, which makes it semi-impossible for people to hold a grudge, even people who are as angry as I was.

Why did I bring this part of my history into a story that's ostensibly about HS2? That's just the point; it's all one interconnected picture. The reason we seldom understand why so-called bad things happen to so-called nice people is that (1) we seldom investigate the case far back enough in history, and (2) we seldom tell the whole story concerning our undergirding roles and thinking which may have led to our reportedly unlucky fates. Everyone looks innocent until the whole picture is revealed, and then all of a sudden we find that no one is innocent.

Events are not fortuitous, for there are no accidents. We *always* play a role in our downfall, whether it's a disease, a lawsuit, investment gone sour, automobile collision, a lay-off or failed relationship that eventually brings us down.

There is a special case that does not follow from my thesis, which is when apparent tragedies befall infants and children. I am excluding that special category here. It can, however, be understood, but only after a committed investment in the study of the fundamentals of universal spiritual philosophy, New Thought or metaphysics. These fundamental studies are beyond the scope of this book.

There were lessons that I had to learn. For starters, I had to learn, somehow, that there was no future in pursuing women just for the sake of contest; that all people, White, Black or otherwise, are God's children, and I had to learn to recognize, accept and love them in Spirit. I had to learn that education could not make me a better person; that I had to cease from my pleasure-seeking ways if I was ever going to find real contentment; that not only did I have to stop avoiding Truth and seeking answers in the world, but I also had to learn to rely *only* on the Infinite as Source.

How else could I have learned these lessons had it not been for HS2? It is obvious to me that it would have had to have been HS2 or something equivalent. Viewed in this way, I am forced to conclude that there is just no way HS2 could have been an accident. If anything, it was a blessing.

My devastating experience with Sophia should have ushered me out of my 20's into some kind of better life, but, unfortunately, it didn't. It was no time after I sent Sophia back east to recover — less than six months — when I ran into a hurricane that I'll call "Marsha." All universal truth philosophies promise that we will someday reap everything that we have sown. Rightly understood, this law does not represent a curse or a punishment. It's just the axiomatic outcome of pure Law (capitalization implies that it is a Universal Law or Law of God). You might call it karma. I had spent most of my 20's dilly-dallying in the lives of a variety of women, some young and some not so young. Sophia's near fatal illness and my subsequent financial ruination should have been a warning that a change was in order. I didn't take any time to process what had gone wrong with Sophia. It was with all of that baggage that I plowed straight ahead into my next moribund relationship.

MARSHA

It is important to note that my perception at the time was that I had completed my relationship with Sophia. It is only through the wisdom of hindsight that I could objectively assess my previous perception for what it was: dense, male-oriented obtuseness, inability to truly feel or be close, and the desire to insulate my pain by delving into another relationship post haste. Such behavior is not uniquely male; women do it too.

Human desire blinds us to so many of the higher truths. At that point in my development, I couldn't have heard God's warning if it had been at the decibel level of a jackhammer. I was too young, too ignorant, too immature, too bull-headed, too arrogant, too self-righteous, too intellectual, too hedonistic, too selfish, too carnal and too needy. And as the punch line goes, those were just my good qualities. Despite these shortcomings, I somehow managed to fool enough people into believing that I was a fairly good guy.

Geez, don't ever believe in images. Human beings, being intelligent, are capable of projecting almost any image whatsoever it they really want to. It's all a matter of how much energy they want to put into it. White collar criminals prove this everyday.

Continuing to explore how I managed to attract the most negative relationship of my life — I'll just call her "Marsha" — it all began after I graduated from college years before. I had needs. Oh, how many times I wished that I didn't, but my miserable life was driven by my needs. As preposterous as it seems in retrospect, deluded by youth, I thought that I was God's gift to women. Well...perhaps, not exactly God's gift, but a pretty good catch nonetheless. Clearly, I never thought that I had the physical attributes, but I was sure that I had the intellectual one — at least that's what I thought at the time. You might say that I had delusions of grandiosity. Of course, the women had no idea that I was this great gift, which was the problem. They couldn't have known because the whole play was taking place in my head. It was a play staged by a fool for an audience of one. Obviously, I was frustrated.

It seemed that the world just didn't place much value on intellectual qualities. A guy could be as dumb as a doorknob, but if he was tall and brawny with a couple of well-placed dimples, women would die for his attention. Or so it seemed. Women represented a way of proving something for me, a way of proving something that I felt I had been denied. It was a love-hate attraction of the worst kind. Even though I was in desperate pursuit of feminine validation, at the same time I could not imagine being committed to any lady past Saturday night.

I am not judging anyone here. There was nothing wrong with either the women or their doltish Don Juans. It was I who was not balanced. I refused to let go and accept life the way it was.

I am aware of other men who are perfect gentlemen, verifiable "nice" guys, who regularly engage in 10 times more degeneracy and deceit than I ever did, yet they are exemplars of the community, church leaders, officers even, perennial teachers' pets, or guys who married the minister's daughter, the doctor's daughter or the high school prom queen. Nobody would ever guess that these smooth operators, real G.Q. clones, could be so lowdown and untrustworthy. I used to envy guys like that — you know the kind who do all the devilish stuff and get away with it — but now I wonder if, perhaps, they aren't secretly living in a private hell much worse than I experienced. Today, they may be worse off than I, because they've painted themselves into a corner and can't tell anybody. You see, they have images to uphold.

Today, I refrain from condemning guys who fit this model. Maybe they haven't grown up yet, but I realize that I must strive to see the Christ potential in everyone, especially those who are most selfish, despicable and destructive among us. If I can't do this for them, then truly there is no hope. Not only that, but then I am no better than they.

My experience with Sophia left me living far below my means, but I figured I deserved it. In my own secular way, I thought I was paying penance by living humbly. Suddenly, my financial status was dismal as I found myself living from loan to loan and paycheck to paycheck. I was convinced that my experience had been a once in a lifetime freak occurrence which could never be topped during the rest of my natural life, even if I lived to be a hundred.

Enter Marsha.

Compared to what Marsha had in store for me, my relationship with Sophia had been a day at the beach. Our relationship comprised the most stressful and bizarre and unhappy three years of my life. Kafkaesque, even. In every respect it was truly a relationship from hell. There I was living with a woman who obviously did not love me, and who, if the truth be told, blatantly despised me. This is not just my opinion; she didn't miss a day telling me as much. Yet I stayed with her for a number of reasons, none of which had any bearing on truth. It should surprise no one to hear that I had zero self esteem. Marsha knew that. She was a psychologist!

At the time Marsha was the most intelligent AND physically attractive lady that I had ever thought myself lucky enough to win the affections of. For the earthly, material man, this is a dream come true: beauty and brains in one package. In this context, I'm speaking of scholarly intelligence. As a Ph.D. candidate in the field of behavioristic psychology, Marsha made it perfectly clear to me that it was my obligation as a man to continue to support her while she was pursuing this worthy goal. One thing was certain. As a behaviorist she was able to get lots of practice using her manipulative, mind control techniques on me. I admit that, at the time, I had a weak mind. I knew nothing about metaphysics or mental science. I was her human guinea pig.

Behaviorism in the hands of the wrong person can be quite a nefarious weapon. It can be used to control people who have personality weaknesses or weak minds and to get them to do what you want them to do. Of course, locked up in the confines of such a relationship, being controlled and manipulated by the extremes of sweetness and harshness, sexual stimulation and long periods of deprivation, I lost all sense of objectivity and personal respect. Due to my ignorance concerning my true identity at the time, this woman led me to believe that I was worthless, an utter sexual disappointment and failure, who on top of it all was cursed by having HS2. She was the first woman among those in whom I confided about HS2 to turn this information against me, and I want to tell you it hurt. Of course, in those macho days, I never admitted that it hurt. Being the male stoic that I was, my range of emotions were neither broad nor sophisticated. I just went around angry and bitter all of the time.

Clearly, Marsha wasn't a balanced woman, but neither was I a balanced man. It took many years for me to realize and admit how I had masterminded my own undoing...how I had tricked Marsha into entering that ill-fated relationship with me. At the time that I met her, I felt extremely lucky. I had finally met the woman of my dreams. She had the looks — and I was after looks in those days. She was Black; I was Black. She was a high achiever; I was a high achiever. She presented herself as one with high income potential (what a joke that turned out to be!); I was hungrily in pursuit of the good life — you know, the best that money could buy. Though I eventually told her that I had HS2, I did it in a devious way. There was no way at all that I was going to risk losing her during the initial infatuation stage by telling her that I had HS2, and that's where I made my mistake. **I SHOULD HAVE TOLD HER THE TRUTH RIGHT AWAY!** I blew it. You talk about pouring water on the fires of passion, I was convinced that the admission of HS2 would be the world's quickest passion quencher. I just couldn't bring myself to do it at that time in my life.

How I tricked her — and it was deliberate — was by feeding her only the picture of the rosy side of romance until *after* intimacy. I was from the streets, and it has always been held as sacred lore among men in the streets that if a man could get a woman in bed first and really satisfy her, he could confess anything afterwards and she would still cling to him. It's disgusting once you understand the larger picture of life, but at the time it made sense. Even so, I eventually bit the bullet and told her the whole scoop long before we decided to buy a house and live together — but by then it was too late. She was already hooked.

I was all of 29 years old and incredibly stupid when I met Marsha. She was 28. To be sure, neither one of us was a candidate for sainthood. What we were were master manipulators. We were both impressed with what we thought the other person could do for our social status, so we pretended to ignore the glaring problems. This brings to mind witty statements that are often voiced about relationships: "Last time I married for love, but this time I'm marrying for money." "If a man (or woman) has enough money, I can learn to love him (or her)." Well, it ain't so.

Marsha was visibly upset upon learning that I wasn't the candy-coated sugar daddy that she'd originally assumed, but she rationalized that at her advanced age (really!) she'd gain more by sticking it out with me than by starting over. From that day forward, she never let me forget what a great sacrifice she had made for my sake.

Marsha held one job or another during most of the time that we were together, but she tended to lose jobs quite frequently. It is important to understand the subtle emotional issues in this part of my story so that we can see how people with HS2 can unwittingly allow themselves to be exploited. This is a clear case of emotional blackmail, an insidious aspect of the HS2 experience with which I'm sure many have dealt. When you're already convinced that your life is worthless, it doesn't take much for someone whose life is equally screwed up to step in and manipulate you as if you were a dog. What's a little more punishment?

The biggest problem for me then was that we had conjointly purchased a home without the legality of marriage. Ouch! Like I said, my lessons have always tended to be hard ones. Yielding to her constant nagging to upgrade ourselves materially, I had sunk a lot of money into that house. Every time I threatened to leave, Marsha would put on an Oscar caliber performance, threatening suicide and all kinds of life-or-death illnesses. It was frightening.

For awhile, that ploy was effective in bringing me to my knees. I had always been broken by a woman's tears. After I got wise to it, she escalated warfare to another level: a homicidal threat! This woman was not about to risk losing that house by any means. It was the sole purpose for her agreeing to enter into the relationship with me, an agreement which was broken immediately after I signed on the dotted line. Despite the fact that we weren't even sleeping together or dating each other any longer, she had me believing that I would be responsible for her death if I left her holding "the bag." The bag in this case was the mortgage. It was no small wonder that during the time that Marsha and I were together, I was constantly besieged by HS2 outbreaks. In 1980 I was a long ways from being healed.

I might add that Marsha did not have HS2. Although unbeknown to me at the time, she also had a low self image problem, but she was able to camouflage hers by pretending to be superior to everyone else. She took full advantage of her status as a clinical psychologist. Plus she was a super intellectual, impressive in group discussions, able and willing to sling the crap with the best of them. She knew all of the recondite technical jargon of her trade, which she used with the cutting precision of a surgeon's knife. There was no one that she was not willing to put in his or her place by the selective use of her sharp tongue. It was difficult for me to believe as a young man, still caught up in hedonistic values, that such a physically beautiful, publicly sweet, shy and even, demure, woman could privately be such a conniving, screaming virago. What an education she was.

Our situation was complicated. She couldn't afford to keep the house by herself, for I was the majority owner and majority contributor to the mortgage and other monthly bills. I was her verifiable sugar daddy. On the other hand, I could afford to keep the house by myself, but she was determined not to move out no matter how sweet an offer I made. And I did make offers. At first, I, too, wanted to hold onto the house at any cost. We gave meaning to the concept of the irresistible object and the immovable force. I was driven by the factual real estate wisdom that we hadn't lived in the fated house long enough to recoup our costs. It was the first time that I had owned any part of a house, and I didn't see any way that I was going to be able to afford another one soon. Besides, I was over-extended creditwise, being hog-tied by the pressure of being in the heaviest debt of my life, thanks largely to my attempts to satisfy Miss Marsha.

Anyone who has ever been caught up in a bad relationship knows that the biggest problem is determining when to cut your losses. You keep thinking that your luck's going to turn and the nightmare will end. Marsha, for all her faults, had been absolutely charming at the beginning of our relationship. (Isn't it always that way?) I kept thinking, "Please her. Do what she says and make her happy. Pretty soon, she's going to see the light and love me the way I deserve to be loved." Wrong! I gambled, but this time the dealer won.

In the beginning it was Marsha who demanded that we purchase a house. Perhaps, you've never met anyone like Marsha, but she was the type who, when she wanted something, wouldn't allow any peace in Gotham until she got it. You can be street savvy and well-experienced, but the first time you meet someone of this ilk, you just aren't ready to handle the situation. After I yielded to Marsh's cease-less whining and pleading and agreed to use my good credit rating and income to go in with her on a house, I was forced to borrow money from a number of friends so that I could come up with the majority share of the closing costs. So not only did I begin this relationship saddled by huge side loans, but I also had to deal with a rather hefty mortgage payment every month.

Like most first-time buyers during the initial years, I was strapped to the max. But did this cause Miss Marsha to have any empathy for me? No way! After we got the house, she simply took on another material obsession. She had to have a car. And, of course, since she was status conscious beyond all reasonableness, it couldn't just be any car. It had to be something that her friends considered to be "classy." Her friends, no less! I don't think she ever recovered from the revelation that I couldn't afford to buy her a Mercedes.

For the record, all of this took place in the late '70s and early '80s before words like *Yuppie* were ever coined.

So all I heard for the next few months nonstop was "car, car, car, car, car..." I mean, for God's sake, I was only a man. God just hadn't equipped me to deal with this. Marsha was like one of those fast-paced commercials for a wind-up doll: "It whines, it feigns sickness, it pouts, it nags, it becomes seriously depressed, it cries real tears." All of this got to me in the expected manner, rendering me willing to do almost anything to end the ceaseless barrage. I didn't know that people even existed who were like this. I extended my credit once again to obtain for her what was a very expensive car by 1980 standards. My once elastic credit line was extended to the snapping point.

After awhile, I was even willing to sell the house at a loss. Though I wasn't too swift in getting wise, I finally came to my senses. I finally realized that my sanity was the only thing that was important. What I found out then was that my mate was not going to budge in any way that could even be faintly construed as cooperation. She figured that I wouldn't do anything to jeopardize losing my stake in the property. However, this time she was wrong.

Adding to my insecurity and fear at the time, Marsha, in her constant search for new ways to manipulate me, continually threatened to expose me by telling the world about my secret scourge, HS2. As previously mentioned, she was a professional behaviorist. During her training she must have taken a course in emotional surgery because she knew exactly where to insert the knife, where to cut and how much to twist. She knew exactly where all of the vital lifelines ran. That was a major factor in my decision to stay with her for three long years, two-and-a-half of which were well past the point of hope. I believed that she was going to expose me. I lived in fear, the fear of being blackmailed. If I should snatch the carpet of financial support from under her, then, by Jove, she was going to pull the carpet out from under me and threaten mine. We were locked in a sparring match that was pure tit for tat.

Her arsenal included the ultimate offensive of calling my parents, sisters, brothers and friends, if necessary, to tell the world the truth about me. Eventually, when I decided to leave, she did just that. I don't know what she told them. None of them has ever told me the entire story of what was said in those private conversations. If she did tell them, they probably would have been too embarrassed to question me about it since I had never publicly admitted that it was true. Ahh — it's so good to grow into spiritual maturity. No one could ever blackmail me again into being afraid of the truth.

Near the end of our sordid relationship, when it became clear that she was losing her control over me, Marsha went hysterical in an attempt to convince me that I had given her HS2. Though I tried with great sincerity, I was never able to verify this one way or another, but I doubt if it was true. After two years of living together, I knew she had not contracted it. During the last year of our relationship, sexual activity between us was about as frequent as snow in Georgia. Not only that, but for years during my "captivity," she had openly flaunted the fact that she had outside boyfriends. They constantly called the house, and she dressed up regularly and went out to clubs and bars late at night, particularly when she was on one of her hate campaigns. I protested vehemently against this, but to no avail. She knew that I was possessive and jealous during those days, and she was right in thinking that it would break me for her to go out with another man.

Obviously, I'm not proud of my past chauvinism, but this is the truth. As I said, Marsha wasn't a woman to be taken advantage of. She knew exactly where the jugular ran.

When she told me that she had contracted HS2 from me, I initially believed her. I have always been meticulously responsible. There was no way that I could walk off and leave a helpless, tearful, broken woman. She knew this. It bothered me so much until I eventually went to a renown spiritual counselor for consultation. After listening to the story and meditating deeply, something told her right away that Marsha was lying. At least, that was her intuitive belief. Up to that point, such a possibility had never occurred to me. I had thought it would be heartless to even ponder such a thing. But gradually, I was beginning to see the light. Something good had to come out of that relationship. It was becoming clear that I wasn't going to be able to reform her, so I concluded that I might as well save myself.

Some may question how I could have lived with a woman without knowing if she had HS2. Easy. That woman was the most secretive person that I've ever known in life. She made sure that every aspect of her life was kept mysterious and complicated. Every little thing was such a big secret with her. She was insecure about everything, especially her body. If anybody was more uncomfortable with her body than I, it was she. You couldn't have thought it to look at her, for she was gorgeous! Nevertheless, she was continuously trying to remake every part of herself, when she could afford it, through cosmetic surgery. She had recently had her jaw broken and reset to improve the esthetics of her face and cheekbones, and she was considering having her knees broken and reset to correct what she considered to be unattractive legs. Because of her knees, which protruded a little and caused her legs to be slightly bowed, she would never undress in front of me. Not only that, but she never wore dresses *anywhere*! Though she really was very attractive, she would only wear pants.

The spiritual principle that kept coming back to me was: **LIKE ATTRACTS LIKE**, as least so far as consciousness is concerned. I can see clearly now why I attracted a lady like Marsha into my life. Heck, it was perfect. We had the same hang-ups! She had her own private closet, private bathroom and private bedroom. She didn't even let me drive her car, despite the fact that I was paying the monthly note. I'm talking about a private individual. Whatever I knew about her was what she told me. She even tried to hide from me the fact that she had a period!

So when she told me in the waning days of our "arrangement" that she had contracted HS2 from me, as far as I was ever able to determine, that was just another behavioristic ploy of hers to control me. If I am wrong, may God forgive me. If that was in fact what she was doing, then there had to be a motive unless the woman was just stark crazy. I do believe with all my heart that this woman was close to psychotic – yes, psychotic! Little did I know at the time that my very life was in danger. But I also found out that there was indeed a motive behind her madness.

Now she didn't just meekly inform me that I had given her HS2. She came at me like some kind of screaming lunatic. She held this thing over my head day and night, about how I had ruined her life, how no one would ever want her again, and how I did it on purpose, and so on ad nauseam. The thing she wouldn't do was allow me to take her to the hospital or accompany her there or to see any of her hospital forms which could verify what she said.

She even took to wearing dark shades, accusing me of having given her the disease in one of her eyes and causing her to go partially blind. This thing nearly devastated me at the time, as I was fairly naïve and I honestly believed that I had destroyed another person's life. But she would never let me see behind those dark glasses.

Sure, I was suspicious. Our history together had taught me not to believe anything that she said on face value, yet she would never present me with any evidence. In the meantime, she had been begging me to go to conjoint therapy with her so that I could get help for what she diagnosed as a severe case of paranoia. She constantly told me, as well as her friends, that I was paranoid. At that point, I nearly believed it myself.

Her thesis all along had been that I had been imagining things about her because of certain male weaknesses and personality defects that I possessed. She would often look upon me in disgust and ask rhetorically, "Why are you so defective? Of all the fine men I could have chosen, why in the world did I have to wind up with you?"

Now I was a man who was always nervous and jittery, because I never knew what that woman was going to do next. I had the sneaky suspicion that Marsha might have been doing her Ph.D. thesis on me.

Later, after I finally surprised her and agreed to enter conjoint therapy with her, we wound up in the office of a certain psychiatrist hurling invectives at each other like a couple of idiots. Of all the old issues that were dredged up to make a case, she never brought up the one about HS2.

Now for the motive. I had discovered shortly after I began living with Marsha early in 1979 that she was having affairs with other men. It wasn't a great secret. In fact, she seemed to take pleasure in flaunting it in my face. After a certain point, we were living together only to keep up a front. She regularly taunted me with the sordid and graphic details of her various affairs. Since she continued to dress up and go out "partying" long after the time when she claimed that she had gotten HS2, I figured that she conjured up this claim about having HS2 to keep me emotionally enslaved. Her greatest fear at the time was that I would leave and force her to lose some of her creature comforts. Since she was still pursuing her Ph.D., she needed me to hang around a little longer.

That was the nature of the confusing psychological battle that constituted my life during those years. There really were no protagonists in our story. We were both conniving, scheming idiots. I am not trying to establish who was right, or to justify the way that I felt. As my story has already revealed, by no means was I an angel during those days.

Given that Marsha and I had not yet learned what real love was all about, there were lots of games being played on both sides. I was unreasonably jealous and given to fits of extreme anger. During that most negative phase of my life, the more she tried to make me conform to her picture of how a man should act, the more I resisted and retaliated by withdrawing, getting angry, screaming, fussing, calling her names and sleuthing on her. My friends who know me today can't believe that I did those things when I tell them about the old me, but, yes, I used to pry into Marsha's private affairs to sleuth out what I could find. It didn't start out that way, but began only after she began to stay out late, sometimes all night and sometimes for weeks. Today I realize that her actions did not justify what I did. I was wrong. My only other alternative was to leave, but I didn't have the backbone to do that. Remember, with HS2 I didn't think I could attract another relationship.

Our relationship was a lot more decadent than what I have described here. Decadence has no limit in its creativeness. I won't get any more descriptive, because it would not be germane to the uplifting spirit of my current story. The closest thing that I can relate it to is a scene out of *Marquis de Sade*. By the final months of our relationship, we both slept in separate rooms, behind closed doors with guns by our sides – yes, loaded pieces. Obviously, I didn't sleep too soundly during those years. I slept with one eye open. She didn't trust me and I didn't trust her. Some of you know exactly what I'm talking about from your own crazy experiences. A number of my respectable buddies have told me stories that are equally as bizarre as mine, or worse.

But why did I suggest earlier that Marsha was psychotic? Many a night I awoke and found her standing over me with a loaded gun to my head. Believe it or not, though, it didn't really bother me. Somehow, I didn't regard her as dangerous, but just a bit wild and somewhat of a bully. However, once when she was under lots of pressure from school and was forced to stay home on Saturday night to study, I got dressed up and went out to cruise. It didn't seem like that big of a deal to me. Unbeknown to her, I didn't have an outside girlfriend, or even any friends. To my great dismay, I didn't have anywhere to go. After cruising around for a couple of hours, I came back home.

The moment I entered the house, she just cracked. She had that look in her eye and she went straight for the gun, which fortunately was in another room. All the while she was uttering obscenities about what she'd visualized me doing with another woman during my absence, and she made it utterly clear that she was going to blow me away. This time I knew she meant it. I immediately grabbed her and consoled her in every way that I could, while striving to gain control of the gun.

I lied my butt off that night, telling her I loved her, I wouldn't do anything to hurt her and that I was never going to leave her. It took a long time to calm her down and bring her back to herself. She had that unmistakable look in her eyes that night that people sometimes get when they have nothing to lose. She had clearly blown a fuse. I don't know what was going on in that vivid imagination of hers, but whatever it was it had taken her to the brink. I knew right then and there that if I survived through the night, I would move out the next day no matter the cost. (Brilliant thinking, huh?) And that's exactly what I did. She suspected as much and doubled back from work the next morning and caught me in the act of moving. She locked me out before I was able to remove half of my belonging, and to avoid a certain shootout, I just left.

For the next few years, everything was worked out with an intermediary, usually a lawyer. I had finally come to my senses.

How often in relationships we all stay too long and sink into the pit of sickening and dangerous games because we don't want to give up anything. We're unable to be logical when we are all wrapped up in it. I realize now that no matter how much evidence I may have found during my sleuthing, there was no way that that particular woman and I should have remained together. I didn't want her back. I was just locked into a desperate, destructive game, which robbed me of all energy and vital enthusiasm. It was like being in a dream where I was on a treadmill and couldn't get off. The truth was that I knew how. I just wasn't willing to jump off, that's all.

How did I ever get myself wrapped up in such an incredible nightmare? I have often asked myself this question since the moment I eventually walked away from house, lawyers and endless round-robin arguments back in 1981. Time sometimes distorts facts; however, one thing is clear: **I DESERVED EVERY BIT OF WHAT HAPPENED TO ME!** If I haven't learned this one fact, then I haven't learned a thing from that whole sordid experience. In such a case, I believe that I would be destined to repeat the experience. As a seeker of spiritual truth, I would only be another sad hypocrite.

I barely escaped from my relationship with Marsha by the skin of my chinny-chin-chin. Whew! I had many nightmares in which I thought that I'd been doomed to live out my fate with that mad woman. If I had remained there by reason of marriage or children or some perverse sense of duty or obligation, I'm sure I would have committed suicide by now. Or else, she would have killed me. Or mercifully, my subconscious mind would have conspired to create within me a fatal disease. This is the way it works, you know. I shall forever be grateful to the Divine, for I know that It saved my life. It gave me eyes to see what was going on and provided the strength that I needed to walk out of that relationship. I count the entire saga a blessing because I know that it could have been cancer or some other rare, degenerative disease that could have been summoned to reveal my lessons about life.

There was no harmony in my home, day or night, for three long years. Somebody seemed to be always upset or screaming, or conniving, or cheating, or sulking or retaliating, or fighting, or malingering in a ploy to evoke pity. There was never any straightforward, honest interaction. Considering how unfulfilled I had been with Sophia during much of the two years prior to meeting Marsha, and unhappy the four post-college years prior to that, and the four-and-a-half years during college, two things are clear. First, I had been consistently unhappy in my social life since high school. Secondly, my life had gotten progressively worse. In fact, I had hit rock bottom in self esteem, health, energy, faith, optimism and finances. After escaping from Marsha, my next home was a cheap motel in Hawthorne, California, with all of my clothes stuffed into a single room.

I remember thinking how absurd my life had become. There I was, 32 years old, a working professional with an advanced degree from MIT, living out of a $22 a night motel room in Hawthorne with no telephone or direct address. The motel was so cheap that there wasn't even a dead bolt on my door. I lived with the fear of returning "home" any day and finding myself cleaned out. Considering the course that my life had taken, I wouldn't have been a bit surprised.

CHAPTER 5: FACTS AND FIGURES

HS2 VERSUS HS1

Although it's not widely known, the majority of people in the general population have recurring oral herpes, which is known as herpes simplex type I (HS1). This condition has been known for eons as fever blisters or cold sores. Ask any doctor. And in case you think there is a drastic difference between HS1 and HS2...well, there isn't. In fact, the viral molecules are so similar that it takes a skilled laboratory technician using highly-sophisticated equipment to tell them apart.

In the old days before the rampant proliferation of HS2, HS1 was confined to the mouth, and HS2, whenever it appeared, to the genital area. Then gradually, HS2 began to show up in and around the mouth, while HS1 began to appear genitally. This most enlightened migration began to take place during the sexual revolution of the '70s, undoubtedly due to the indiscriminate practice of forms of sexual activity such as fellatio, cunnilingus and "69," acts that became standard badges of qualification for those who would boast of being good lovers. Let's not pull any punches here. I'm not trying to be lascivious, but I have to tell it like it is.

All of the popular erotic magazines pushed these practices as being mentally and physically healthy during those experimental years from the late '60s to the early '80s. To question these new mores was to be labeled an old fuddy-duddy, a square, or some type of uptight, medieval, sexually-repressed individual, perhaps from Victorian times. I know because I was so labeled by more than one woman. There were many who weren't into committed, one-on-one relationships during those days. Or maybe it was just the young women that I socialized with. Every man was put on notice that unless he proved to be a good performer, he was likely to be replaced post haste. This is something lots of young men worry about, being replaced by another man who is a better lover. Out of this fear is borne that irrational, destructive, persistent form of jealousy that is so common to young men (and the women who try to love them).

As we all know — and it's seldom acknowledged publicly — men, as a group, will do anything to win the favors of women. And I mean ANYTHING! If women declare that long hair is sexy, they'll go for that. By the same token, moustaches, beards, earrings, and now the ubiquitous but horribly *un*-masculine pony tail have found favor among men trying to please women. You may recall in the late '60s how even rednecks took to wearing long hair, and military men on leave donned wigs to win favor with the opposite sex. You just couldn't convince my friends and me when we were in our 20's and early 30's that we would be attractive to women if we didn't at least pretend to be "cool" or "hip." I can vouch for the fact that almost every sexy, cosmopolitan sophisticate that I met during my gaming years expected her man to engage in uninhibited sexual practices, preferences which they made known in chillingly frank terms. That's what they thought it meant to be liberated.

To be frank, I suffered greatly during those years for being an uptight Southern Black man, a group that is well-known for playing it straight when it comes to sex. My breed was often put down for being selfish, backwards and sexually unenlightened. And don't believe that it didn't bother me aplenty! It certainly did. But as soon as I came into an understanding of my right relationship with God and became crystal clear about who I was sexually, the entire issue vanished. Miraculously, I began to attract committed one-on-one women who completely accepted me as I was. ONCE I STOPPED READING *PLAYBOY* AND TRYING TO LIVE UP TO ITS STANDARD, AND STOPPED APOLOGIZING FOR THE WAY

I WAS, WONDERFUL THINGS BEGAN TO HAPPEN FOR ME...and are continuing to happen to this day.

What this whole debacle points out is just how selfish hordes of young people can be under the guise of sophistication. We place so many demands on each other in courtship; then we wonder why there are 30 million people with HS2 and a rapidly growing number with AIDS. It is time for us to admit that we at least know why. I'm not sexually-retarded or square, and I'm all for people having fun and enjoying themselves. Neither do I care what consenting adults do in privacy behind closed doors. But — as part of my attempt at an objective assessment of how 30 million intelligent people (like myself) in a modern, sophisticated nation ended up with HS2 — certain things have to be said. As these words roll off my tongue (or pen), I realize that they are not easy to digest or liberal or politically-correct, but still, they have to be said.

It's easy for me to attack some of the mistakes made by men, for they are so obvious. To attack men is to attack myself, which, I suppose, makes it all right. But the truth is that men and women are in this life together, and both have contributed equally to the mistakes of the past. In this same vein of searching for truth and trying to expose error, I hope I can say a few things about women, too. Though it hasn't always been acceptable to admit it, women can be brazen pleasure-seekers just like us men. Though men are often viewed as aggressors, our female counterparts are increasingly using us to satisfy their pleasure needs. The way the sexual power equation is tilted in the singles world, if women say lick, men respond by asking where and for how long. Like Pavlov's dog, single men know what is required to make that bell ring. And those who don't know are paying big money to find out. Why else did rednecks, hard hats and hippies alike grow long hair during the hippie era? Because it was also called the *free love* era, that's why. There's no difference between races, politics or nationalities when it comes to man's preoccupation with pleasures of the flesh.

By no means am I attempting to exonerate men for their part in the love games of the past. Women were not responsible for what men did then, and they are not responsible for what men are doing now. We men are. A woman cannot lure a man unless he is willing, but the unfortunate fact is that he usually is. And if he's willing, it can only be because he wants to use her as much as she wants to use him. Of course, I didn't realize all of this back then. I, along with all of my "running buddies," played the game of sexual conquest to the max during the '60s and '70s. We had no loyalties except to our next conquest."

If this seems crude, just know that we have to begin our investigation into the metaphysical meaning of disease and suffering by admitting the raw truth before we can go to God with a clean slate. I'm not going to sugar coat important issues. Through this process, perhaps we can stop being hypocrites and move into a position to receive our true healing.

The best that I can determine from research indicates that HS2 has been a medical issue in this country for only about 18 years. (This does not mean that HS2 did not exist before 1975. It did. Indeed I contracted HS2 in 1974.) A medical paperback that I purchased, entitled *What Every Patient Wants To Know*, written by Robert Rothenberg, M.D., and copyrighted in 1975 doesn't even mention herpes once. This was one of those "Everything You Ever Wanted to Know" books that was so popular in the '70s. Yet the subject was neither listed in the index nor under chapters on infections, contagious diseases, sex, or female disorders. This is not to denigrate Dr. Rothenberg's book. Instead, it illustrates just how little of a problem herpes was considered to be in 1975. Even so, consider this: The medical literature states that, even back then, over 80 percent of the American population would have tested as positive for herpes simplex antibodies. When you think about it, this is truly amazing. It casts doubt on our ability to ever really claim to know anything for sure.

As I mentioned before, people have had fever blisters and cold sores on their lips for as long as any of us can remember, and some of these sores can look rather horrible. Medically, these things are caused by herpesviruses, yet nobody in the past ever referred to them as herpes. People just said, "I have a fever blister or a cold sore." In fact, what they had was only by chance related to a fever or a cold. However, these rather innocuous terms are effective and practical euphemisms.

Nobody has ever winced at having to admit that he or she has a cold sore, except for the discomfort of having it. Certainly, people don't get down on themselves because of it, concluding that they are no good, their lives are in ruin and that a vow of celibacy is the only option available as a result. Neither do such people feel forced to go and maintain a code of silence, swearing never to enter into marriage, have children or ever attempt to have any semblance of a normal life. On the other hand, hordes of people have sworn off sex, marriage, dating and many other normal pleasures just because they have HS2.

I doubt if anyone ever committed suicide as a result of contracting a cold sore, or lapsed into totally destructive, relentless anger due to it. Yet I've read of many cases where such extreme and inappropriate behavior has characterized those who've acquired HS2. It's difficult to imagine how anyone could react that way, yet at one time I fell into the exact same category.

ASYMPTOMATIC TRANSMISSION

Many of those who have the HS2 virus never, or almost never, suffer any effects at all — so they report. They are completely asymptomatic. Furthermore, it has been medically documented that many of the donor partners of HS2 subjects have either always been asymptomatic, or were asymptomatic at the time of transmission. A leading medical researcher reported in the Spring 1992 edition of *THE helper*, an ASHA publication on herpes, that about one-third of all source partners (those who were believed to have transmitted HS2) were found to be truly asymptomatic at all times. Asymptomatic transmission of HS2 by a method known as viral shedding is quite a complex issue, one that is not fully understood by anyone at this time. However, it is gaining more attention as we proceed into the '90s, the third decade of HS2 prevalence in this country. Naturally, there is a lot of anxiety among HS2 subjects, uninfected partners of HS2 subjects and aware, uninfected singles in general. The questions are many; the answers are few.

I have two comments to make concerning this subject. First, the subject of asymptomatic transmission is still an extremely gray area in the world of medical research on herpesviruses. There is no consensus at this point on exactly what is going on. Secondly, much of the information that has been reported was obtained from interviews with HS2 patients. As will be substantiated later in Chapter 7, where I discuss my experience in an HS2 experimental drug program, it is not very difficult for seemingly sincere, articulate people like me to fool our doctors. Any aspect of one's sexual identity is an extremely complicated subject. Even when our intentions are honorable, it is difficult to be perfectly straightforward about our sexual behavior.

Do I believe asymptomatic transmission occurs? It is certainly possible, but I'm also convinced that you can't get reliable information by interviewing people about their sexual histories. This is especially true when it comes that carries as much stigma as HS2 in the average person's mind. All I know for certain is my own experience. The evidence indicated that I did not contract HS2 asymptomatically, and I certainly haven't passed it on asymptomatically. Surely, as an educated individual of privilege, it would help me to save face by saying that I received this disease asymptomatically. Or, maybe I should say, it would help my donor partner save face. That way, nobody's at fault and we both get to be innocent victims. That way, neither of us has to accept any responsibility because it was something that could have happened to anybody. It had nothing to do with my behavior or my lack of sexual mores.

The other fact that I know for sure, based on my own experience, is that I haven't passed HS2 on to either my wife or either of my previous two girlfriends dating back to 1983. Nineteen eighty-three was an important marker because it was then that I cleaned up my act and took a vow before God to become 100 percent responsible for my actions.

Again, let me state that I believe asymptomatic transmission occurs — maybe not as frequently as reported, but it occurs. Even so, from a higher spiritual perspective that doesn't get anyone off the hook. The spiritual universe is governed by cause and effect. Though everybody is not ready to look at this yet, things happen for reasons. Thus no matter how we contracted a particular disease, there is something in it for us. No mistakes have been made. Armed with this understanding today, I couldn't care less *how* I contracted HS2. But I do want to know *why*. That is what this book is about — the process of looking into our own souls to understand, accept and heal the reasons why the particulars of this experience were necessary for those of us who have been so affected. Though I'm not against the progress and discoveries wrought by medical science, individual HS2 subjects can miss the whole point of having HS2 if they put too much emphasis on a rationale that impersonalizes their plight or deflects responsibility for their condition.

Modern life seems to be rife with so many social threats. The news that HS2 can possibly be spread asymptomatically just represents another risk to add to the list. For those who are still at risk, their reaction upon hearing something like this must be: "Oh God, another thing to worry about." Asymptomatic transmission can be very frightening to someone who already has HS2 and is sincerely trying to be responsible concerning his or her sexual behavior. The news that HS2 can now be transmitted even when there are no symptoms present (prodromal tingling, redness, rash, itching, vesicles or sores, scabs) can be nothing short of devastating for most sexually-active HS2 subjects whose partners are HS2-free. And if they are single and have not yet hooked up with committed partners, it's even worse. For that minority who have chosen celibacy, the possibility of asymptomatic transmission would not increase their level of anxiety, but most HS2 subjects are not celibate. And a certain percentage of those who are will not remain so forever. At least, it is reasonable to expect that they would like to have the option of resuming normal sexual activity once they've become mentally healthy again. At least that was true for me after I went through my self-imposed period of abstinence.

For the HS2 subject, asymptomatic transmission can only be

viewed as yet another personal assault. Yes, it is personal. Very personal. Asymptomatic transmission represents yet another devastating setback to the sincere soul who has been struggling to deal with one of the most insidious attacks to his or her sexual esteem imaginable. If you don't have HS2, take my word for it. If I were Webster, under the word *devastating*, I would list HS2 among its list of synonyms.

Certainly there are worse assaults than HS2 in this world. Everything is so relative and so subjective, but not to the one afflicted. Pain is pain. In a comparative or objective sense, a stumped toe is preferable to brain cancer, but try telling that to the fellow with a stumped toe.

One of the lessons we were sent to this planet to learn is compassion. We must never underestimate the impact of any assault on another person's life, no matter how trivial. BUT HE OR SHE MUST! While we must learn to have compassion for those with HS2, stumped toes, brain cancer, etc., their task on this planet is to learn ways of diminishing the effects of these various assaults. This is what successful spiritual living is all about. Our prayer might be: "Infinite Spirit, I don't care what experience I attract out of this life, with your strength and your guidance, I know that I will overcome it."

It is this knowledge that keeps me sane. Once we understand this, we will realize that there is no reason to fear asymptomatic transmission of HS2, HS2, brain cancer or anything else. Everyone must eventually face the fact that there is no such thing as risk-free living. Although we don't know what's going to happen next, we must learn to approach tomorrow with the faith that, whatever happens, it's going to be all right. With the love of God, we will be able to overcome it. This is what life is all about, and personally, I wouldn't have it any other way.

HS2 STATISTICS

I grew so weary of hearing the "expert" projections of dreary HS2 statistics during the genesis of this problem in the United States.

Every time I heard one of those reports, it caused my mouth to dry out and my heart to skip a beat. All the so-called experts seemed to be selling was fear, fear and more fear. This provided the major motivation for me to get serious about writing my own story. As early as 1980, I found a number of published articles supporting numbers of between 20 and 50 million people in this country alone who supposedly had HS2. Today's most reliable sources seem to have settled upon the figure of 30 million. Obviously, nobody knows for sure how many people have HS2, and I doubt if anybody's going to conduct a telephone poll. I'm convinced from my personal contacts, conversations, and interviews with a wide range of people that the majority of those who have the condition would not admit it if asked.

This shy strangeness about sex is still perplexing to me. People aren't ashamed to admit that they have a cold or a fever blister. In another vein, it's not as strange as it is revealing, considering how people in our society are so negatively programmed concerning anything dealing with sex. We prefer to relegate all public treatments of sex to prurient interests. Given that sex sells — and at a premium price — it would be costly to demystify it, would it not?

Dealing in round numbers, there are about 250 million people in the United States. If 30 million of these people have HS2, that amounts to 12 percent of all people in the United States, or roughly one out of every eight people.

Just think about it. How many people do you know? I maintain a mailing list of about 400 relatives and personal friends on my personal computer. If 12 percent of the people on my mailing list have HS2, that's 48 of my personal friends. Now I am only aware of one or two whom I know to have HS2, and maybe three or four more who have thrown out hints in that direction. That still leaves a gap of about 42 people who are either dealing with the same thing that I've been dealing with for so many years or else they represent a subset of incredible statistical oddities. Or perhaps, they just aren't telling. There are other possibilities not yet considered, one of which is that there are NOT 30 million people in the United States with HS2.

Okay, let's suppose that there are only 20 million cases, which is the lowest estimate that I have seen reported. In that case, only eight percent of the people are affected and only 33 of my close, personal friends and relatives are in the same boat that I'm in. Again, if only six of them have admitted to or hinted at having HS2, that leaves 27 who must be residing in the undercover of the twilight zone, instead of the 42 that I calculated based upon the higher initial estimate. Even 27 is a whopping lot of folks in one's personal circle.

Many sources have estimated that as many as 50 million people may be affected nationwide. At that level of incidence, it is possible that as many as 80 of my personal friends have HS2. Being human, naturally, they would never talk about it due to the shame and embarrassment they would feel. If you have never been forced to deal with anything like this, you'd be hard-pressed to understand the all-pervasive, deep-rooted, psychological devastation that the experience of HS2 visits upon one's consciousness. It's not an easy thing to shake. It's like taking a hit from a 30 megaton nuclear warhead on one's self esteem. Of all human qualities, it may be true that the way people feel about themselves is more closely tied to their sexuality than any other attribute. It's nearly impossible to find a good defense against the initial onslaught of HS2 or to deal with the fallout afterwards. By no means should anyone ever assume that dealing with HS2 is a trivial matter.

Now that we have examined the upper and lower limits of reported HS2 estimates, for the sake of consistency in the ensuing analysis I'm going to assume that the normative figure of 30 MILLION CASES is correct. Remember where I suggested that there may be other factors in assessing HS2 statistics which have not yet been considered? Well, I believe that there exists at least one additional, significant factor, a factor which supports my contention that there may be as many as 48 in my personal circle who have HS2.

First of all, it should be stated that it's a medical fact that about 80 percent of all the people tested in this country test positively for herpesvirus. This includes type 1 and type 2. It should also be noted that there are a large variety of herpesviruses, such as the types that reportedly cause chicken pox and shingles, as well as the

Epstein-Barr virus, which seems to be creeping up on the horizon lately in certain parts of the country. Much is available in libraries and bookstores on the subject for those who are interested in pursuing knowledge on that level.

Eighty percent is a very large number. That's about 200,000,000 inhabitants of the United States, or about 320 of my personal friends. If we assume again that 30 million (12%) have the type 2 virus, that leaves 68 percent (80% minus 12%) of the entire population that have types of herpes other than type 2. My friends, that's a whole lot of folks! I'm not saying that you should stake your life on these numbers. Mark Twain was known to have stated, "There are three kinds of lies: lies, damned lies and statistics." My aim is simply to put some meaningful boundaries around the great fear and ignorance that is still dominant in discourses on HS2.

Now the truth is that these herpesviruses are not affecting all of these hundreds of millions of people. Heck, the overwhelming majority of them don't even know that they have it. Medically, they are referred to as being asymptomatic. It's just one of those conditions that lots of people test positively for. This is not to understate the seriousness of HS2 for those who have active, recurrent infections. There are medical risks which have to be addressed by qualified physicians.

The fact that some people with herpesviruses are asymptomatic may seem a wee bit perplexing, but life is literally loaded with paradoxes such as this. The reason it may be perplexing is two-fold. First, we are programmed, by and large, to think negatively and to expect the worst. Secondly, because of the way that education and the social order are structured in our society, we are not normally led to explore abstract ideas about life in this manner. In spite of how objective we think we are, we still carry around many sacred cows. Too many concepts are promoted as indisputable facts, which the mass populace often accepts uncritically.

Regarding our tendency to think negatively, we tend to extrapolate a little bit of data into the worst case scenarios. Look at the gloomy predictions being echoed by so many "experts" on any subject of sociological significance. Whether it be AIDS, drought, predictions of earthquakes in California, the greenhouse effect or the Japanese business invasion, the ominous sound of the warning bell is all too familiar.

Concerning all calamities, I will concede this: It is totally consistent — and necessary — to the perfect and completely dynamic life that God has designed for us on Earth for all possibilities to co-exist. There must be total choice at all times, including the possibilities of manifesting AIDS or HS2, as well as suffering from hurricanes, drought or wars at all times. As strange as it may seem, the universe wouldn't be perfect if this were not so. Paradoxically, this is proof of the perfection of the universe, as diametrically opposed to our normal way of reckoning as it may seem. If this doesn't make sense to you at this point, continue to contemplate these issues.

Despite what you might be led to deduce, the acceptance of this concept of the universe doesn't strip us of having control over our destinies. All we need to understand about this system of perfect order is this:

ALL NEGATIVE CONDITIONS ARE COMPLETELY REVERSIBLE.

Don't try to find proof for this scientifically. Though a given individual may or may not possess the key, the same Universal Intelligence that knew how to create the Earth, the sun, your plants and your body has provided the means through impersonal Law for the creation of HS2 or AIDS. The beauty of this is that the same Universal Intelligence contains the means, which humankind can tap into through Spiritual Laws, to reverse or completely annihilate these conditions.

Now this is something that everyone can understand. As yet, everyone may not possess the key, but they can understand it. The first step is understanding. Once it is understood and accepted, each one can choose to take the next step, which is to approach life with the desire to tap into that Infinite Intelligence. Instead of continuing to wring our hands in despair, this is how we must learn to expend our energy. Up to now, many of us have been working in a manner that is totally counterproductive to our good. If you are new to this way of thinking and haven't yet had the prerequisite years to investigate these concepts on your own, I beg you to just keep the door of possibilities open and hang in there for now. If you are sincere in your desire to understand, by the Laws of Spirit that understanding will surely come.

This reminds me of a story that I heard in a metaphysical setting. There was this baseball umpire who was officiating a certain baseball game. A play was on and one of the players rounded third base and proceeded to try and steal his way home. Anticipating that it was going to be close, the player realized that his only chance was to slide hard into home plate. So he hit the dirt, and dust flew everywhere as the catcher stood there and attempted to put the tag on him. As the dust settled, people stood up in the stands and began shouting and screaming for the umpire to give a sign: "What is it, ump? Is he safe or is he out?"

But the umpire was not intimidated. He calmly stared back at all of them and said, "It ain't nothing 'til I call it!"

I think this succinctly epitomizes the way the universe works. Also, where so-called disease statistics are concerned, we, too, can assert: It ain't nothing 'til we call it. Unfortunately, because of the prevalence of race consciousness (the prevailing negative consciousness of the entire human race) we are predominantly inclined to think negatively as a society. Immediately upon entering this life, we become programmed that way. What does it really mean that a certain number of people test positively for HIV, or that almost everybody tests positively for herpesviruses? This is the question that we must answer before we can truly be healed.

It's part of the perfect order of things on this earth plane that the possibilities for all of these conditions exist. This fact, we cannot control. However, the thing that we can control is this: What are you and I calling it? Perhaps, we aren't doing such a good job managing the causality that lies within our control. Why not join me in using the power that is vested in you by Universal Spirit to make all grim predictions concerning your health false? Why not begin calling it the way *you* want it to be, and not the way the "experts" and predominantly negative news media report that it has to be. Stop repeating negative predictions. Use your creative imagination and unlimited intelligence to think of new, life-enhancing possibilities. Then go and spread *that* news.

Now I have already established that somewhere between eight and 20 percent of the entire population have HS2. Then I showed how this could easily translate to between 33 and 80 of my 400 personal friends. These numbers were based on straight, across the board averages, taking all Americans into account. It was assumed that every person was equally likely to acquire HS2, young or old, child or adult, big city dweller or rural denizen, single or married. In fact, there is reason to believe that the percentages may be significantly higher among young to middle age adults in big city areas where moral standards tend to be a lot more *laissez faire*. Let's take a look at the effects these considerations might be expected to have on the numbers.

Clearly, if there are 30 million people in the United States with HS2, it is plausible to postulate that they must be in greater concentrations in the 16- to 50-year-old age group than among those less than 16 years old or older than 50. Now, this is not what one would call a scientific study. Though I was trained in science, I don't do scientific studies anymore. I write for the masses, not for the elite. Furthermore, I have no desire to prove anything here. I only want to promote some new ideas for interested readers to ponder. This is a scoping exercise in which my aim is to define the lower and upper limits of the problem. It is no more than a plausible, educated analysis of available data based on what is known and what is not known.

If we take this argument a little farther, I have already established that the spread of HS2 in the United States was not an issue before about 1975. Surveys have shown that a small percentage of people had HS2 as early as 1970; however, I know from experience that there were very few doctors in 1975 who were familiar with actual cases of HS2. That's just how rare it was then. Thus, effectively, we have roughly 18 to 19 years that this condition has been spreading.

The results of a detailed survey of 3,148 people with HS2 was published in June of 1981 by HELP/ASHA. Although theirs was not a scientific survey, it did indicate that less than one percent of the study group were under 20 years old. Since the survey was completed nearly a decade ago, and considering the trend of sexual behavior in this country, it is possible that the percentage of young people with HS2 is higher today than it was then.

Another important finding in the cited study was that slightly more than half (50 + percent) of the respondents were either married or cohabiting in a committed relationship, with 12 percent reporting that they contracted it from their spouses. So clearly, this puts the lie to any belief that HS2 is exclusively a condition of single people. Although the problem may be more grave among single people than married, those 12 percent who were married represent an important bit of information which tends to support one of my main points:

VERY FEW PEOPLE GET REJECTED IN RELATIONSHIPS BECAUSE OF HS2.

This belies the fact that for many people there is tremendous emotional trauma associated with having HS2, especially during the first few years.

Okay, let's go a little deeper into the stats. There are about 91 million households or 65 million families in the United States, including about 56 million children under the age of 16. Thus I can exclude those 56 million children from my baseline group of people who could possibly show a significant incidence of HS2. What I am trying to determine here is just who are the people who could possibly have HS2? How many people are there out there who are vulnerable?

Let's assume that kids under 16 are not likely to get it. The same can be postulated for married people who are faithful and have been with the same person for a long period of time. Similarly, people who are celibate, invalid, or nuns are probably quite safe — again, assuming that they don't already have it. A number of recent surveys have indicated that about 10 percent of all adults are celibate.

If the truth were told, we would probably find that a sizeable percentage of those who are celibate or are on spiritual quests have HS2. After all, something drove them to God. This is not a cynical or malicious attack on piety. It really doesn't matter which road leads us to Truth or Ultimate Reality, as long as we find it.

The aforementioned HELP/ASHA survey found that 10 percent of the respondents had ceased all sexual activity as a result of having contracted HS2. My experience suggests that a large percentage of these celibates became very "spiritual" after HS2. It is only natural. If this statistic is extrapolated to the entire HS2 population, there would be three million HS2-related celibates out there today. That's a whole lot of folks and, possibly, a whole lot of frustration.

Though I have included the over-60 population in my analysis, I will treat children under 16 and adults over 60 differently. In other words, my estimates for these populations would be inflated if I assumed that each member of the American population was equally likely to contract HS2.

About 16 percent of the population, or 40 million people, are over the age of 60 in the U.S. Again, to be conservative, let's assume that none of these 40 million people have HS2, which is the same assumption made about the 56 million kids under 16. There is no reason to believe that the percentagewise contributions of these populations would be significant at this time. Of course, some children are born with HS2, but I am also excluding this population as statistically insignificant. So now we have a total excluded population of 96 million, or 39 percent. By deduction it's safe to say that the remaining population, 150 million people, or 61 percent, is currently susceptible to HS2. Now this figure lumps everyone between the ages of 16 and 60 together, including sexually-active and promiscuous adults along with those who have chosen lives as virgins, celibates, the married-but-faithful's, and those who happen to be physically disabled.

Notice that I am not excluding the disabled or the predicted 7.5 million celibates from this population. By no means am I suggesting that celibates could not have HS2, or physically disabled people cannot have sex. As will be apparent soon, it won't significantly affect my final predictions.

The current population between the ages of 61 and 75 would have been between 42 and 56 nineteen years ago when HS2 first began to surface. Clearly, by considering only those between 16 and 60 today, I am excluding for now that population between 61 and 75 that may have contracted HS2 when they were younger. The effect of this exclusion will serve to make the numbers that I am going to derive lower limit figures, which is fine. In other words, the actual numbers will be worse than my derived predictions. Regardless, we will gain a personal feel for what commonly-reported statistics mean, or more important, imply.

Many studies indicate that the most sexually active population is between 18 and 34, with the most torrid and indiscriminate activity tending to be during the 20's. These assertions are also totally consistent with my own observations and experience. If we zero in on this group, we'll be talking about 67 million young adults, or 28 percent of the total population. For the sake of argument, if we assume that three-fourths (75 percent) of the estimated 30 million HS2 cases in this country fall within this group, we would find that 33 percent, or one out of every three young adults between 18 and 34, must have HS2! This is an astonishing statistic, and yet it is highly credible.

By corollary, the remaining 25 percent of HS2 cases would be spread among those between 16 to 17, and 35 to 60, a group consisting of a combined 80 million people (33 percent of the population). If I treat these groups identically, the expected incidence among each faction would be 9.3 percent, or nearly one out of every 10 people.

To summarize what we have just deduced, assuming 30 million cases of HS2 in this country, the following risk levels can be expected:

Ages 0-15:   Very low statistical risk[*]
Ages 16-17:   1 out of every 10
Ages 18-34:   1 out of every 3
Ages 35-60:   1 out of every 10
Ages 61 +:   Very low statistical risk[*]

Basically, what these informed "guesstimates" indicate is that for fun-loving, party-going, nightclub hopping, actively-dating young adults, it is reasonable to assume that anywhere between one out of 10 and one out of three (10 to 33 percent) of your closest same-lifestyle friends can be expected to have HS2. The numbers may be affected by the city in which you live, as well as the type of friends with whom you hang out.

Although there are no numbers to support this, I would wager that those who live in major melting pots like Los Angeles, New York City, Chicago, Boston, Dallas, Miami or Atlanta, to name a few, can expect to be at maximum risk. Sexual mores tend to be more lax in larger cities, which also tend to attract more drifters, runaways and transients. The same is true on college campuses. During my travels over the years to numerous small, medium and large towns as an engineering consultant, it became quite evident that there were more sexual opportunities in the largest cities and on college campuses. Peers of mine hated to spend long stints in small towns for that very reason. People in small towns tend to have roots and rather traditional values. They belong to neighborhoods and families, which tends to normalize individual behavior and make one's activities accountable. Though it's not often voiced in just these words, every guy knows that seduction is much easier if he meets someone who is detached from her family and its values.

However, there is another side of the ledger. Despite possible geographic variations, there are probably no cities left in America where the risk of contracting HS2 is low. This is true for two reasons. First, the sheer number of people with HS2 today is extremely high. The second reason derives from pure mathematics and can be explained by modeling the spread of HS2 as a transient geometric

---

*Note: Very low statistical risk does not mean that individual risk is necessarily low. For the sake of this cursory analysis, the statistical risk for those 15 and younger or above 60 is assumed to be low. Regardless, a 14- or 15-year-old who is sexually active will greatly increase his or her risk, especially if the relationship is with an older person who is in a higher risk group. It is probably fair to assume that the over-60 group is generally more mutually monogamous, conservatively single or even celibate. Plus, its members were at least 44 years old, and thus more settled, when the HS2 epidemic began to spread.

progression. To put it simply, HS2 was injected into American society some 18 or 19 years ago and has been spreading ever since. With this kind of head start, I would venture to say that sexually-active teen-agers and adults in American cities and on college campuses of any size share a fairly high risk today. In any group of 100, it is reasonable to expect that from 10 to 33 have HS2.

To offer some quasi-statistical support to my speculation about large cities, a recent study conducted by the city of Los Angeles shows that 55 percent of its households do not consist of the conventional family, which is structured around a married couple. Thus there are a lot of people in this trend-setting metropolis who are either living together with or without kids, sharing accommodations, raising children as single parents, or being reared as children without the traditional parental couplet. Thus it's easy to surmise how the rate of incidence for HS2 and other STD's would have ample opportunities to spread in trendy melting pots like L.A.

I certainly don't wish to forbode doom by these conclusions, and neither am I making a value judgment about what kind of household is better or worse. Some may not even have a choice. Everyone has to have to figure out which is better for himself or herself. For instance, I've had three live-in relationships in my premarital past, but as I began to study and practice a consistent spiritual philosophy, I was naturally led to seek out a totally-committed, monogamous relationship. As a result, I finally entered into marriage a few years ago at the rather mature age of 38 — and happily so, I should add. This works for me at this time in my life, but no one should assume that I believe that everyone would be better off it they did the same. My only advice to anyone is to go with God, be true to your own heart, and allow yourself to be guided from within. Spirit will direct you properly and you will end up in your right place, just as I know that I am in mine.

In interpreting any statistics, we should remain aware that numbers don't mean anything if *you* happen to be the one who, for whatever reasons, has acquired HS2. You can be a near saint, 12 or 92, but if you have it, that's what you have to deal with. Statistics might tell you that the odds are 100 million-to-1 against your acquiring it, but if you have it your probability is now 100 percent. In that case you can forget about statistics.

Whether there are one out of every three or one out of every 10 people in your circle and age group with HS2, the only clear conclusion from these estimates is that the numbers are high. They are probably higher than you may have previously assumed. The prevalence of HS2 is certainly higher than you would be led to believe from open discussions on the subject — if there are open discussions on the subject. Strangely enough, nobody's talking about this situation publicly, which only goes to prove one point: There's a whole lot of suppression going on. This is the real HS2 tragedy.

I have met more than a few women during the past 18 or so years, and I can say this for a fact: Not a single one that I have dated has ever admitted to having HS2, including the one who passed it to me. Why, I ask you? I have known a lot of guys, too, over this same period, and I haven't ever heard one of them come straight out and admit it either. A few have let me know indirectly, either by hinting, or telling a mutual third party, or trivializing the seriousness of the condition, or making a joke out of the whole thing. Not a single guy has come straight out and stated: "I have HS2." Conversely, I have admitted as much to a few male and (platonic) female friends of mine, and a few of my female friends have confided the same to me.

Another statistic that has been making the rounds is one predicting that from 200,000 to 500,000 new cases of HS2 can be expected to occur each year. Some sources were reporting the higher figure as early as 1980; others were still reporting the same figure in 1986. Hmmm...strange! In the absence of a medical cure, one would think that as the number of total cases has increased over the years, the incidence of new cases would have also increased. Though plausible, such a linear argument is not necessarily true. Sexual practices could have changed. The incidence rate could conceivably have remained constant or even decreased. Ameliorative drugs are now available which can reportedly shorten the duration of outbreaks under certain conditions. If it weren't for these factors, perhaps the rate of contagion today would be a million or more new cases per year. Who knows? Some would even suggest that the fear of HS2 has led more people to practice safer sex, but I'm not one of their camp. This is more a case of wishful thinking than fact supported by data. It's awfully difficult to make people appreciate risk who have never been burned, and everyone knows that the one universal impulse which will not be denied is the libido. People *talk* about safer sex but then they go right ahead and do what they have always done. Recent surveys bear this out.

Based on a set of realistic assumptions, I have ventured to calculate what the ballpark rate of contagion might be. I realize that my assumptions may be quite different from the data used by medical researchers. Be that as it may, I am using publicly available data from various articles and relying on my years of formal training in science.

By assuming that a hypothetical HS2 subject has one flare-up every two months lasting an average of 10 days (seven days of infection plus an extra three-day margin for extra safety), I can compute that that individual is contagious 16 percent of the time, or an average of one out of every six days. This assumes, of course, that all sores have completely dried up and healed within the 10-day period such that the subject is not contagious after that interval. Please bear in mind that this is not a medical opinion. What I am setting out to do is a rough, scoping analysis. By not taking into account possible asymptomatic transmission, which still falls within a medical gray area, my predictions may be more conservative than inflated. All I'm doing is postulating a set of reasonable assumptions about the course of this condition, which I will than use to calculate some reasonable boundaries for certain HS2-related statistics. I'm sure that anybody with HS2 will find this information interesting. To be sure, what I am doing is all very hypothetical, maybe to the point of being ridiculous. Anything that can be done to assist others in breaking through their clouds of heaviness or seriousness about this condition is worthwhile in my opinion.

Continuing on, if I assume that my hypothetical subject is single and has sex on the average of once a week, or a frequency of once every seven days, his or her pure mathematical odds for random transmission of HS2 is one out of every 42 days, or 2.4 percent of the time. Mind you, this is not the probability of contracting HS2; it is only the probability of transmitting it, because everyone who is exposed to HS2 will not actually develop the condition. Not only that, but a reasonable percentage of partners will already have HS2. This factor will be ignored for now in deriving a first order estimate. The 2.4 percent figure also assumes no discrimination regarding when sex occurs — i.e., total randomness. Total randomness assumes the subject is as likely to engage in sex when he (or she) is contagious as when he is not. From experience, I can tell you that when one is young and single, despite sound and reasonable logic, the libido wins out over the intellect most of the time (if not *every* time).

I am absolutely convinced that the lady from whom I assume I acquired HS2 didn't want to subject me to this risk on that particular night. How clearly I remember — but she was extremely...well, horny! There's no other way to put it. She simply wasn't spiritually mature enough, nor had she developed the discipline, to know how to deal with this most powerful of inner conflicts. When you're young and the libido speaks, male or female, you are prone to rationalize anything. Nod if you know what I'm talking about.

One could argue that if a person was contagious for only 10 days every other month, he (or she) might be able to decrease the odds of transmitting it to zero by only having sex during the safe weeks. Sure! This ideal solution is too simplistic.

First of all, I have already mentioned that this is a hypothetical case. In actuality, flare-ups don't occur exactly once every other month and last for exactly 10 days. Based on studies, and my own experience, there is no regularity to the occurrence. A person has to be extremely well-disciplined to be certain of never subjecting a mate to risk. Mind has to be stronger than libido. Not only must such subjects avoid sex when they are certain that they are experiencing a flare-up, but they must also be steadfast in refusing to have sex during a designated "grace" period before and after each flare-up, as well as during periods when they aren't sure but suspect that they *might* be having a new outbreak. Clearly, it takes a lot of discipline, maturity and patience to practice the safest possible sex. And if you believe in the theory of asymptomatic transmission, there is still a finite, though small, probability of contracting HS2 even if all of the rules of safe sex are obeyed. I am purposely not discussing birth control methods here (e.g., condoms) because I don't know of any that make the transmission of HS2 risk-free. We should not deal in delusions here. The only absolutely safe sex is no sex.

I wouldn't expect a large percentage of the population to have the kind of discipline that is required to significantly decrease the spread of HS2, and the numbers bear me out. Perhaps one percent or less. That percentage would consist mostly of nuns or Olympic athletes in training — and I wouldn't wager too much on the latter. It may seem that I'm selling people short, but in practice sexual discipline is an impossible ideal for the average sexually-active person. Anyone who shucks off this issue and underestimates the power of the libido is akin to a sitting duck, just waiting to be felled. In truth, mind can never overpower the libido. The brute force of will power is no match for this challenger. But all is not hopeless. We must condition our minds to respect the awesome power of the libido so that we can stop tempting the hand of fate.

Admittedly, everyone has the potential to develop the discipline that is necessary to avoid passing on HS2, but potential is not enough. There must be a personal awakening. Good intentions are not enough. The world is full of people with good intentions, but it is forever in need of performance. The first step in mastering any behavior is to first admit what is true. Those individuals who scoff at their limitations, thinking that they will always be able to control their libido, will not advance until they go through Step 1. This is especially applicable to those who are young and those who are in their first years with HS2. Sometimes, it can take a year before subjects get over the depression and accept the most elemental realities — that, yes, they really do have HS2, and no, there really isn't a medical cure. The average middle class American may not be well-equipped for dealing with something of this nature.

Continuing with my hypothetical case, if we assume that about 50 percent of those who are married, legally or common law, are sleeping around, that translates to about 55 million individuals. Next, if I assume that 80 percent of the 40 million unmarried singles are sexually active (32 million), and that 75 percent of those are still playing the field (i.e., not in a committed relationship involving mutual fidelity), that yields a total of some 24 million singles who can be reasonably assumed to represent the highest risk group to spread HS2. If we add this figure to the 55 million probable donors from the married group, I now derive a total of 79 million people who could possibly — and I emphasize POSSIBLY — pass on an STD (including HS2) to someone else.

This is quite a significant realization, because 79 million unfaithful seducers represent 32 percent of the entire population! Now based on my early statistics, it is reasonable to assume that at least 25 percent of those 79 million uncommitted or unfaithful seducers has HS2. This yields at least 20 million seducers who could be subjecting their partners to risk. If transmission or infection of a new subject is assumed to occur during only 50 percent of risky sexual encounters, then the incidence rate will be one-half of the 2.4 percent rate that I computed earlier. Remember, 2.4 percent is the percentage of time, on the average, that our hypothetical HS2 subject, having sex on the average of once a week, is capable of infecting a partner.

Based on all of the assumptions so far, the transmission rate will be one-half of 2.4 percent of 20 million, or 240,000 new cases each year. This is reasonably close to recent estimated incidence rates as reported by disease control experts, although some sources still give estimates as high as 500,000 new cases a year. Within the scope of my underlying assumptions, it is easy to see how the real incidence rate can be as low as 100,000, or soar as high as 500,000. Of the 30 million people who are reported to have HS2, I assumed that only 20 million are actively engaging in behavior that could put another person at risk. There is no reason to argue about these numbers, because I certainly am not going to defend them. This is no more than a plausibility analysis, designed to exercise one's mind so that one can surmise how the spead of diseases like HS2 can occur.

Though these are only rough, order-of-magnitude estimates, they still indicate that no matter how you juggle the numbers the real incidence rate is going to be high. But there is an optimistic side to these findings. By practicing more discipline in the sexual arena, we should be able to reduce the incidence 10-fold within the next five years (by 1998 or so) to about 20,000 to 50,000 new cases a year. This is a totally realistic expectation if we can get people talking and owning up to their roles in the spread and control of this condition.

For my hypothetical case, I could have assumed more than one outbreak bimonthly, or a frequency of sexual activity of more than once a week. Of course, the resultant estimates will be shifted up or down accordingly as the initial assumptions are changed. There's nothing sacred about the assumptions that I used, but at least they give us an idea of the breadth and prevalence of what we're talking about. Since no one knows what the true norms are for sexual behavior, HS2 incidence and frequency of outbreaks, my estimates are as good as any.

CHAPTER 6: CONFRONTING PARALYZING FEARS

FEAR AND OTHER MIND TRIPS

If you (or somebody that you know) are like the estimated 30 million people in this country who have HS2, it is likely that your life is filled with, and maybe even governed by, fear. It wouldn't be unusual. Chances are that your self image has suffered greatly and you liken yourself to those who were called lepers in Biblical days.

If you are still single and have normal sexual desires, you may have torn yourself to pieces whining and crying — for the most part alone, isolated and in the closet — because of what you consider to be your own private secret, or perhaps, your personal cross to bear. It would be perfectly normal for you to be scared to death of dating someone new, or of becoming intimate. Consequently, you may have developed some kind of weird, but compensating and protective pattern of behavior, and the necessary contentiousness and lifestyle to go with it. I know the pattern well. The weirdness is the mask that prevents anyone from ever suspecting you of having anything to hide.

If you are male, the chance that you have developed such aberrant behavior patterns is even greater. Most men just don't know how to deal honestly with anything about their lives that just isn't perfect — as they perceive perfection to be, of course. I can certainly vouch for that.

Chances are, regardless of your faith or lack thereof, since contracting HS2 you have thought about God more than a few times,
as in the question "What is my relationship to this elusive Being, be
it a Him or Her or It?" It wouldn't surprise me to learn that you
have even blamed It, whoever or whatever you conceive God to be.
And I'd wager that God isn't the only entity you've blamed. If you
happen to think you know from whom you contracted HS2, assuming
you aren't Mother Teresa or the Pope, odds are that you have cursed,
screamed at, harangued, intimidated, or tormented that person's life
as well. This assumes, of course, that you have not killed that person.
I am not trying to be funny. This is the reality of normal people
upon first contracting HS2. No one likes for his or her life to be
inconvenienced or altered, none the less their sexual life.

There probably have been a few killings resulting from HS2,
whether homicides or suicides. Certainly there have been lawsuits.
According to the tabloids, a number of stars from the sports and
entertainment industries have been publicly accused of giving HS2
to various of their lovers.

If you are one who believes that you know who you "caught"
HS2 from, chances are you've taken every stance against that person
except one – forgiveness. Then maybe you have. If so, I applaud
you; you're well on your way.

If you were married when you contracted HS2, you may very
well be divorced by now. There are no statistics on this, but I strongly
suspect that the incidence of HS2 during unfaithful trysts has led to
a plethora of modern divorces. If there have been cases where *you*
were the perpetrator (after all, everyone is not the innocent victim)
and divorce ensued, I would bet that your spouse never stopped
loving you, assuming he or she loved you in the first place. More
likely, it was your own guilt, self-flagellation, tears, projections,
dishonesty and inability to come clean and confess the whole story
that drove your spouse away. The irreducible, root cause may very
well have been your inability to believe that anyone could love you
or accept you again after this "horrible" malfeasance you committed.

While I'm betting, I would also wager that you have gone through
a phase of enuring yourself to the entire world in anger so deep that

you have questioned whether you really want to live. Even if you have chosen to live, chances are you haven't quite figured out what for. It probably has something to do with your kids who need you, or your parents who you are afraid wouldn't understand, not that you have been very nice to your kids, or your parents, or anyone for that matter since you got "it."

Besides loathing the person who you think gave "it" to you, you may have grown so accustomed to anger that you find it difficult to NOT hate yourself. Of course, nobody else loves you either, which just compounds the problem and proves your self-fulfilling prophesy that nobody could, should or ever *will* love you again as long as you have HS2. To say the least, the person that I've just described is not very well adjusted. It may not fit you, but I was once that person.

If you fit this pattern, you are living in an unreal world, dominated by fear. Worse yet, your secret solution approach is modeled upon the impossible. More than likely you are obsessed with finding a way to extricate yourself from HS2, the dreaded scourge. Your mistake is this:

YOU THINK THAT YOUR LIFE IS AS
HORRIBLE AS IT IS BECAUSE OF HS2.

The truth is exactly the opposite:

YOU ARE AFFLICTED BY HS2 BECAUSE
YOUR LIFE IS AS HORRIBLE AS IT IS.

Think about this for a moment. My claim is — and I have proven this in my own life —

IF YOU IMPROVE YOUR LIFE, YOU WILL
NO LONGER BE AFFLICTED BY HS2.

Now I know that what I am suggesting is a tall order. You might be wondering: How can this be? What is the mechanism? What do I have to do?

Please, please, I beg you, be patient. We must systematically plow through the steps towards overcoming these HS2-related fears. If you are presently far adrift from the understanding necessary to overcome the spirit-squelching effects of HS2, don't feel ashamed. Just whisper to yourself, "Okay, perhaps — just perhaps — it's possible," and remain calm, open and patient.

If you have any other elixirs in the hat, try them first. I do not expect the average HS2 subject to attune himself or herself to this wavelength until long after he or she has exhausted all other channels. What we have to do may at first seem tedious. First, we have to establish a foundation for truth, i.e., a new philosophy of life, or perhaps, a *modified* philosophy. Then we have to systematically build our lives around it by going back and re-examining every facet of our lives — and our thinking — in terms of this new philosophy. Some of our old approaches will be kept; some will be modified; others will be tossed out altogether. In all cases we must fuse a consistency between our beliefs, thoughts and actions. We will no longer be able to think one way and act another. Such destructive and conflictive living is no longer an option. As of this moment, I declare it passé.

Before you panic, let me add another criterion. You must remain the critical examiner during this entire process, accepting no truths that are handed to you on a silver platter. No one has *your* answer. If you discover some general answers here, they will only become yours after you've sifted through both the precious metals and the dross in your own consciousness, and applied only the part that is required to uniquely fulfill your needs.

No matter where you go or what you do, you probably can't shake that monkey loose that's clinging to your back, that monkey called HS2. Indeed you do have HS2 and you've got it bad. You've got it in your mind, you've got it in your heart, and you've got it in your soul! It's bad enough to have it in the body, but what you must learn is that you don't need to have it in your mind. I'd bet that there are few activities or events that can get your mind off what you have accepted for so long as "your special problem." You've worked it over and over in your mind to where it has become so deeply ingrained — pathologically so. After all, it's your cross to bear, isn't it? Unfortunately, unless a major detour is taken, you're going to become overburdened by it.

Oh yeah, there's one other character trait by which a certain percentage of HS2 subjects may be identified. They are the ones who have become super-religious — self-righteously so. What a perfect solution to their problem! What a perfect defense mechanism.

You may have read an article in *Readers' Digest, Newsweek* or some other magazine about some chronic victim of paralysis or cancer, or whatever, who experienced what doctors call "spontaneous remission," which means that they were inexplicably and spontaneous healed. You may have read about the discovery of some new miracle cure in the medical laboratory such as interferon or acyclovir. Remember interferon? In the early '80s, it was touted as the new cure-all miracle drug. As a result, believing yourself to be a positive-minded person, and an intelligent one at that, chances are you eventually came to the conclusion that "they" are going to discover a cure sooner or later, "they" being the powers that be: the government with all of its billions, those archetypal, bulbous-headed research physicians in sterile white lab jackets who receive funds from Big Brother and convert $$$ into cures and hope and stories of happiness-ever-after for people like you and me.

Thus between outbreaks, when your positive energy was at peak (i.e., when you were not totally depressed), you probably have gone to libraries and researched everything you could find on HS2, poring through medical journals and arcane terminology that made you wonder: "If this thing is that complex, and if people have to be that smart in order to find a cure, then may God have mercy on us all." Of course, I did all of those things. I admit it. Try to locate a book on HS2 at your public library. They are all missing from the shelves! Permanently, too. Pilfered, I suppose.

I understand your plight. Being a college-bred engineer, I got wind of all the hottest folklore about promising cures on the horizon. There were always the alleged miracle drugs in Europe or other faraway places which were not yet approved by the FDA. I don't know which is the biggest lie ever told, accounts of UFO landings in places like Siberia or Wyoming or the existence of miracle drugs in Mexico. There are two stories that will forever play: UFO's always land in totally uninhabitable places and the most effective drugs have not yet been approved by the FDA. And furthermore, they always add, the FDA doesn't want us to have them!

It never ceases to amaze me how the most "intelligent" people, confronted with a personal assualt like HS2 or cancer, can be frequently suckered into this illogic. Remember my earlier challenge to the HS2 subject who would be healed to begin developing a sound, consistent and logical foundation of life? We can be so objective and logical until our sacred little bodies are threatened. This validates for me that so much of what we call human intelligence is nothing more than a farce. That's why in the allegorical story of Job — for those who are familiar with the *Bible* — the so-called devil said to God about his faithful servant Job: Let me rain diseases upon Job's body for a few weeks, and then you'll see how faithful your servant really is.

To be honest, I was not particularly calm during those early days while I was entrenched in my HS2 fears and mind trips. I, too, bought into the lie that there must have existed drugs somewhere which worked, but that the FDA just wasn't moving fast enough to allow the drug companies to put them on the market. Translated: It was, to a large degree, the FDA's fault. So maybe I could go to the library and find out for myself what was being withheld from the common man. What with my degrees in chemical engineering, I could interpret the arcana concerning HS2 in those highly technical medical journals. Maybe I could figure out a way to get some of those miracle drugs for myself, or perhaps get into an experimental program that was not regulated by the FDA. This is all good intellectual logic, right? Who could blame me for trying?

Even so, we need to stop right here and look at how we are always so willing to assign fault to someone else for our dilemma: *It's the government's fault, or it the FDA that's dragging their feet. Why don't "they" do something?*

No, no, no, it's time out for blaming others for our problems. The FDA didn't inflict this problem on me. I did it to myself. Therefore, they are not responsible for curing me. I know this sounds bold and disarming, but it is the truth. It will become clear later why you just can't program your mind to go around believing that someone else is responsible for your dilemma. It's a very convenient and trendy alibi, but, I'm sorry, it just ain't so! Until every person who has HS2 arrives at this point in thinking, he or she will not have a psychological breakthrough.

Plowing through all of that immunological jargon that you'll find in medical journals, one would never guess that most of the major discoveries in life have been serendipitous. It must blow the scientist's mind who has spent all of his or her adult life earning a Ph.D. and doing time-consuming research when some little twerp comes along with hardly any credentials and discovers the big breakthrough. It must blow the doctor's mind when some measly, terminal cancer patient who wouldn't know a milliroentgen from a lymph node all of a sudden undergoes spontaneous remission. How does a doctor explain it when a person is supposed to be dead, yet lives?

If you were brave enough, you may have gone so far as to join a support group such as HELP, and you probably know the meaning of many acronyms, particularly ASHA (American Social Health Association and HRC (Herpes Resource Center, which has replaced HELP). The higher your level of education, the more likely you are to be conversant with a lot of abstruse medical terminology as you have strived almost obsessively to keep abreast of HS2 medical research. What you will find is that most of this knowledge is useless, at least that's what I finally concluded after reading and studying and searching.

What good is it to know about T-lymphocytes, killer cells, and battles between microscopic, physical forces of good and evil in our bodies? That's what I learned from two of the leading available books on the subject, both written by physicians.

To be sure, there were some helpful parts. I realize that it's the nature of the human intellect to desire to delve deep into the how's and why's of anything that is important to its master, and nothing is ever deemed more important than ravages against the physical person. All I'm saying is that the more I learned about the particulars of viral infection, the more it seemed as if the entire world consisted of zillions of invisible viruses threatening my physical well-being. The more I learned about these viruses, the more it seemed that my prospects for victory over them was hopeless. Such knowledge didn't make me better. Ironically, it rendered me worse off as my subconscious mind became literally *obsessed* with possibilities of horror that were much greater than anything previously imaginable in my more ignorant state.

To understand why those technical HS2 books were written in the first place, we have to recall the state of mind that existed before HRC was established, and before HIV was widely known. It was horrible. There was a real need for truth and enlightenment. Just as obsessed as cancer "victims" have been over the years in searching for a cure for cancer, HS2 "victims" were 10 times more anxious for information during the early years.

For cancer patients, some comfort could come from having a documented, well-established pattern to go by. HS2 patients, on the other hand, were left groping in the dark for answers. Nobody seemed to know where the disease came from, how it spread, how to manage it, or how bad it could be expected to get. What I'm describing is the most desperate kind of fear.

I'm not sure it's that much better today. Oh sure, veterans like myself have found a way to be at peace, but as the new generation becomes susceptible, it's probably just as devastating to them to have their long-awaited sexual degrees of freedom ripped from them so arbitrarily and abruptly. Even with the increased information and support systems in place today, there is just no way to prepare for some shocks. That, plus the false sense of invincibility of youth, weakens, if not defeats, the impact of early education.

If the truth be told, many of the long-timers haven't coped very well either. There are many who haven't found peace with their bodies post-HS2. I suspect that there's just not as much talk on the surface about what's going on in people's lives, which gives the illusion that attitudes are better.

Another reason people aren't discussing HS2-related problems as much today is even more convoluted. Some feel embarrassed to be coping so poorly with HS2 when everyone knows that there are much worse diseases at large, particularly AIDS. One tends to feel rather silly for drawing too much attention to himself or herself for having HS2, which usually is not fatal, when so many are suffering from AIDS, which often is. This is one of the strange nonlinearities associated with the inner workings of the mind. Logically, one could argue, "What does one situation have to do with the other?" But let's be real here. Many of our private thoughts are as close to being logical as I am to sprouting wings.

So in the end, after you have read all that there is to read and researched all that there is to research, and still have not found the cure, what are you left with? So much knowledge gathered to enlighten has instead steeped you deeper in fear. As for myself, I began to wonder, "Well geez, if all of these complicated viral processes are going on within my body, what else is possible that neither I nor the doctors know anything about?" Fear proliferated. It seemed that there had to be such a multiplicity of yet unknown, malevolent possibilities, so many, in fact, that it seemed hopeless to expect to ever defeat this slippery bug.

During those early days, the whole thing was just too much for the intellectual mind to accept. I had never before heard of anything being this weird, this insidious, this intractable. And we're supposed to be this technologically advanced civilization. This isn't supposed to be happening to us can-do Americans this late in the evolutionary game.

I can laugh about it now, but I occasionally stumble upon notes, telephone numbers and addresses from the years when I was determined, by will and by might, to materialize a cure out of thin air. Today, with my demeanor so calm and blood pressure so low, it's hard to believe that I could have ever been so desperate.

Back in those days I never stopped to ask myself, "For what end did I want to be 'cured' so fervently?" If I had, I would have been forced to admit that my only interest was in continuing my devil-may-care lifestyle without interruption. Ouch! It was a painful question to face. At that time in my life, there was no way that I was interested in delving to the core of my being and changing into a better man. I didn't want to be a better person. The way I saw it, HS2 had barged into my life and prematurely truncated my fun. It just didn't seem fair. I hadn't sown nearly as many wild oats as I had it in my mind to sow. I was a smart, take-charge young professional with a lot of what the world referred to as "promise." I wanted a cure and I wanted it bad so that I could hurry up and get on with business as usual. There was life to be lived, and I was missing out on my portion. As unflattering as this is to my ego, it is the truth.

To put it more bluntly, **I WAS A HEEL** – plain and simple. All I wanted was to meet fine young women and enjoy them sexually. It wasn't like I pined for the return of perfect health so that I could settle down, marry, have kids and be a model father or citizen. I had no such noble goals. My whole thrust in life was egocentric, macho and selfish. Of course, I didn't see it that way back then.

Like many in similar circumstances, I rationalized that I was this great human specimen who had suffered the unluckiest turn of fate. The reason I mention these perceptions now is because, today, I know beyond all doubt that this is a causal, spiritually-governed universe. Nothing – absolutely nothing – happens unless it has a meaning and a purpose. If you're in a situation similar to where I was, do not make the mistake of stymieing your growth by rationalizing and railing against the tides of fate. It doesn't matter that "everybody is doing it," or that others are doing more than you and getting away with it. Establish your own standards and proceed to be as honest with yourself as you possibly can.

I must have called the Atlanta Center for Disease Control, the HELP Hotline, research centers at the Universities of Washington, Pennsylvania and wherever else research was being carried out, promising cures for the mysterious, elusive HS2 virus. Today, I often marvel at this seemingly intelligent virus. You have to admit that it is a perfect disease. It's the stuff dreams – or rather, nightmares – are made of, i.e., something that you supposedly can't get rid of. It's like something out of one of those campy, late night horror movies – *The Growing Glob*, or *The Gel That Ate New York* – something that as soon as you look for it in one place, it crops up somewhere else. What an experience, huh?

Indeed HS2 would make a good B-grade movie if people didn't take the subject so seriously. The fact that no movies have been made about it tells you something right there. I mean, the movie industry exploits everything that's packageable or promotable, right? Give Hollywood any conceivable angle of mass suffering and tragedy and they will exploit it. The fact that the story of HS2 hasn't been exploited yet as a central storyline in a major movie suggests one thing: This is a subject that hits too close to home. There are undoubtedly many behind the scenes in the movie business who have HS2. They aren't laughing because they don't think it's funny. When a few people have it, it's funny and exploitable. Comedians lived off herpes jokes in the late '70s, but they aren't laughing anymore.

We saw this same trend with AIDS. At first there were numerous office variety jokes about it, most of them highly insensitive and cruel. I remember the period because I became seriously fed up with the guffaws. As it spread to the point where it began to penetrate all lifestyles, all of a sudden it became a serious issue. How convenient it would have been if we could have confined AIDS within the homosexual community or HS2 to only those who are young, single and promiscuous.

Such were the original biases and associations that were connected with these diseases. If you showed up with HS2, you were not treated as much a victim as you were a villain. People assumed you were some kind of low-life for catching HS2. Maybe you were something that crawled out from under a rock.

Even the medical practitioners tended to look at you a wee bit askance, as if to ask: "What kind of person are you, anyhow?" By inference, they seemed to be suggesting that you must be the kind of person who hangs around prostitutes, gets too chummy with Shetland ponies, or engages in group sex and things like that. This remained a popular belief for a long time...until *they*, too, began to show up with it.

As I was saying, cancer is regarded differently than HS2 by the medical profession and by society. With cancer the stigma is much less — at least this was true in the early days of the HS2 epidemic. As a matter of fact, people with cancer usually exact sympathy. Attitudes about diseases are rapidly changing. Cancer is now a "respectable" disease. In most cases it would be unthinkable to blame a cancer patient for getting cancer, except, perhaps, in the case of a smoker who gets lung cancer. Many still feel obliged to stick it to smokers, although, in my opinion, such an attitude is still just as judgmental, and thus unfair.

Though statistics certainly favor the nonsmoker, it's ironic, I suppose, that some of the people who get lung cancer don't smoke, and some of the people who smoke don't get lung cancer. And some physical fitness fanatics have heart attacks while jogging and drop dead in their tracks before reaching the age of 50. Furthermore, if I believe the latest theories about asymptomatic transmission of HS2, some people have this condition — and can transmit it — without having any of its classical physical symptoms. It's a good thing God (i.e., the *Law* of God) permits it to be this way; otherwise, we'd be intolerably self-righteous, would we not?

As I have mentioned, I wore myself out trying to track down the elusive cure. In my defense, I can say that I never allowed myself to become defeated in mind. I really believed that an absolute medical cure would be formulated. I still believe it. In fact, I know it! However, my thinking has changed drastically since those fear-riddled early days. I am well aware that the sought-after remedy is on its way, but today I would rather not have it arrive too quickly. I know this sounds contradictory, self-abnegating and maybe even insane. That it is. I offer no apologies. I'll just say for now that there is much to be gained from the experience of HS2. To search frantically for an external cure, and even to discover one, will not necessarily help someone become a better person. There is a great relief that comes from letting go of outlandish hope and accepting life the way it is.

Despite all the guilt and mind trips that others may have foisted on you, there are a few firm truths that you need to know. Although you may be going through a trying experience, you should know this:

YOU ARE ALREADY PERFECTLY ALL RIGHT!

Ponder this assertion and commit it to memory. Though this may not be true on the physical level, there is a level within your being where it is absolutely true. As for myself, I know that I'm perfectly all right. This is not denial. Don't get seduced into thinking that you are going to be all right *when* you become healed. Either you're already all right or you aren't. As wrong as it may sound, it's just that simple. If you don't feel that you are all right at this moment, I'm here to tell you that it has nothing to do with HS2.

You wouldn't consider yourself to be socially unacceptable if you had a bad cold, would you? No, because you know that it would eventually pass. Well, so it is with HS2. Every episode that crops up will eventually pass. I realize that there are many other considerations, concerns and fears associated with having HS2, and you are right not to trivialize them. Together, we will explore the implications of each of them. If I am qualified at all to help you through this, it is because I have progressed all the way from the near-suicidal state in which no one could have convinced me that I was socially acceptable, to where I am today. Mentally, I can honestly report that I am remarkable healthy and extraordinarily positive. There is so much good in life and so much to be thankful for until oftentimes it is hard for me to contain myself. I just want to jump up and down and shout with joy, exclaiming to the world how happy I am.

Too often we feel that the only person who will accept us is someone who is in our same predicament. Too often we mope through life searching for sympathetic partners, the discovery of which could actually deter our mental healing. I am well aware that this sentiment exists among many who have HS2. Nevertheless, it is not necessary. In fact, I believe it is mentally unstabilizing for someone to view himself or herself in that way. It may take work, but it is of paramount importance to view yourself as being all right and perfectly acceptable just as you presently are! If you have the attitude that you are only acceptable to others who have HS2, you cannot simultaneously maintain the attitude that you are presently all right. Remember the challenge of thinking clearly, consistently and logically. It is logically impossible to be simultaneously okay and not okay. But let's face the truth about the situation:

EVERYONE YOU MEET WON'T ACCEPT YOU, BUT THAT DOES NOT MAKE YOU UNACCEPTABLE.

Good things began to happen to me, but none until AFTER I learned how to be happy and accept myself as being all right. I learned that acceptance must always begin with me. Then others will simply pick up on *my* cue. Granted, it is bizarre how it works, but this is exactly how it works.

There are many unseen snares and subtle fear traps along the HS2 highway. Another fear trap to avoid is the one whereby you find yourself being too grateful. Let's say that you are one with HS2 who is presently in a relationship with someone who is aware of your so-called problem, and, for whatever reasons, this mate of yours is not your true spiritual mate or soul mate. That mate may not be providing the genuine love that you need, but regardless, you may feel forced to stay in the relationship because you are so grateful to have finally found somebody who accepts you with your HS2 condition. Now don't lie to yourself about this. This is a subtle but painful predicament to be in. It is the perfect example of being caught between a rock and a hard place. Unfortunately, I've been there.

One of the women that I lived with (Marsha) turned my trust in her against me. My secret became a wedge that she used to bludgeon me. Because she knew that it would devastate me for the whole world to know my worst secret, she treated me like her private slave. It was blackmail, pure and simple. That particular ex-girlfriend constantly taunted and abused me, figuring there was no way I'd blow her cover and reveal her psychologically abusive ways to family or friends.

There's no pain like being a hostage in your own home, terrorized by your own mate. And it's got to be the depth of spiritual bankruptcy sitting around thinking that you deserve better, while too paralyzed by fear to act in your own best interest. You must be careful not to be *too* grateful. It's easy to get suckered into feeling that you owe eternal gratitude to someone because they accepted you with your "awful condition." **YOU DON'T OWE ANYBODY ANYTHING!** If you let someone blackmail you — as I did — it's just going to take you that much longer to extricate your mind and rebuild that vital self esteem that you need.

Whatever you may do, just don't lie to yourself. Are you hanging onto someone in a compromised relationship because you don't think anyone better will accept you? If you're in that predicament, I can tell you now that you may as well release that mate right away. That person is not your true mate. You don't even know love if you have to compromise your basic self worth in order to have it. Real love is the essence of freedom — total freedom. Of course, not many people ever experience that, including those who *don't* have HS2. But why set your aim as low as theirs? Go for all the gusto. I did.

If what you're experiencing feels like anything else, then believe me, it ain't love; and it certainly ain't freedom. The operative factor in that case is fear.

Think of the plight of the woman who stays in a destructive marriage for the sake of the kids, or because she doesn't feel that she could support herself financially. Talk shows base their survival on such cases, which we know almost never lead to happiness or fulfillment. The same is true when the issue is HS2. You must not let it be a discounting factor when you're negotiating a relationship.

NO PITY, PLEASE

Of all the things that I desire, the one that I want least is for anybody to feel sorry for me. To attempt such would be to miss the whole point of this book. Yet if the past is any indicator, it will surely happen as sure as there is breath in my nostrils. People have to express life from whatever vantage point they happen to see it, and that's the painful truth. Even so, hear ye, hear ye, I neither want nor need sympathy.

There was a time some years ago when I openly courted commiseration, thinking that it was important for my well-being. But now I know that sympathy and pity are totally paralyzing and non-therapeutic. Neither is necessary for my happiness. As far as I am concerned, these twin crippling agents are nothing more than false substitutes for real compassion.

We all know that it's in some people's nature to go around pitying everyone. Indeed, we all know the type who can't be happy unless they can find someone to pity: You might hear them ask, "Did you hear that so-and-so has cancer? Oh, the poor thing. What a pity." Whereas I hate to rebuff anyone's gift, my only wish is that some of my joy will rub off on those who are given to pity and sympathy. Perhaps, if they can feel the joy that I feel in this state of total freedom, they will realize the futility of their pity.

As a practicing spiritual practitioner, I learned about pity from my work with a client, Connie Beebe, a beautiful young spirit who is currently a paraplegic confined to a wheelchair. In the early days after her accident, she wanted to pity herself, but I wouldn't let her. Neither would her husband, although they had been married for only a few years. He was an unusually supportive man who continued to see potential in her beyond the bleak appearance of those first months in the hospital.

At first, Connie's neck was either fractured or broken to the point where she couldn't sit up and support the weight of her own head. She would need a spinal cord operation. In addition, she was not able to use her hands to wash her own face or feed herself. As one might imagine, when I first met her she was extremely distraught. The cheery, optimistic expression that I had been told once characterized her personality had been cruelly wiped from her face. Regardless, I still saw an astounding, underlying beauty in her.

As harsh and unsympathetic as it may sound, after establishing a relationship with her, I immediately told her to get up and stop whining and do something with her beautiful life. It was not difficult for me to convince her that she was a beautiful, exceptional, gifted person whom God would not have created if He did not have something grand and special for her to do. I believed this then, and I continue to believe it now. It took awhile, but once she got the message she did indeed cease from whining and self pity.

There was another important factor in Connie's mental victory. While I was visiting patients in the hospital as part of my volunteer effort to practice the spiritual principles that I had been studying for a number of years, another young man who fashioned himself to be some kind of New Age, hands-on healer was also coming to "help" Connie. Ah, California, the land of fruits and nuts!

Each time I saw her, I had to spend the first hour answering questions raised by this man and allaying the feeling of guilt and confusion that he left her to deal with. Since he couldn't heal her or see any improvement after a few weeks, he became increasingly moralistic and hostile, attacking her faith. In his eyes her problem had to be that she didn't have enough faith. Though I never met him, the story I got from her was that this man became quite angry with her for "not wanting to get well." He began laying all kinds of guilt on Connie about her having some kind of evil spirit in her, and not being willing to accept God, or the light, or whatever he called his own personal elixirs. As a hands-on healer, he created quite a stir among the hospital staff. The nurses were clearly uncomfortable with his presence, but they didn't quite know how to handle him. He became so unwelcome there that I had to be very careful during my visits so that they didn't think that I was also into any kind of weird healing business.

Though I didn't have any special promises to offer Connie, I helped her to re-establish a strong belief in an unconditionally loving God — not the God that she had believed in before, but the true God that loves us all regardless of circumstances, afflictions, and conditions. As a result — and possibly, in spite of me — she continued to make record-breaking progress.

I worked with another client during that same year, a woman of 37 who apparently chose the other fork in the road. She was not healed on this side of the great divide. She passed on instead — ostensibly from diabetes, but it was clear to me that she simply lost the will to live.

Life is purposeful in every respect just the way it is. In fact, life is more than purposeful; it is perfect! Nevertheless, I must temper my enthusiasm at this point, lest I give the impression that I am touting some kind of airy-fairy, pie-in-the-sky healing philosophy. We'll revisit the issue of life's perfection later. It's difficult to see, merely because each of us has been doled out a challenge just different enough from everybody else's to camouflage the sameness in all of them. Who are we to think that somebody else has been dealt an unfair hand just because that's the way *we* see it? Who among us is so objective or possessed with vision so clear that they can believe in what they see? It's time for us all to awaken and get on with the work — and the pleasure — of living.

Before I proceed, let me clarify a potentially misleading phase, the notion that human problems and challenges might be "doled out." There just isn't any power "out there" that is doling out obstacles and curses for humans to suffer. Such an argument would smack of the fire and brimstone brand of orthodoxy to which I do not subscribe. I don't believe in such a judgmental or volitional deity. In reality, although each of us may have a proclivity towards a certain type of challenge, there definitely does not exist any external entity that inflicts suffering upon us.

Each of us has different fears, out of which we create different kinds of challenges through the Law of Mind. It is written that the thing we fear will come upon us. The Law of God works through our subconscious minds. So we say that we create our own negative experiences out of the content of our subconscious minds, since this is where our fears lodge. At any rate, regardless of how we may have gotten into a particular predicament, by focusing our mental energies on the affirmative thing instead of on the negative, we can be liberated. In the final analysis, I would think that this is all that matters.

So no, I don't want anybody to feel sorry for me. There is, however, something that you can do if you are really sincere. You can participate with me in consciousness on behalf of our collective freedom. The potential is absolutely stupendous. Since all minds are connected to the Mind of God, if you think a good thought about me, and if it is sincere and from your heart, I will feel it. The same thing holds true for anyone else that you desire to help. This is one way that you can send me a message without ever having to go to the post office. Think about it.

The world is full of "nice" people who are sending up prayers 24 hours a day to some remote deity to do this, that, or the other for people. I'm sorry, but this isn't the kind of assistance people with HS2 need. I know I'm stepping on some well-manicured toes, but if you want to begin the process of working towards effective healing, you have to cease from actions that *look* good on the surface but have no bearing in spiritual principles. There are many things that look right on the surface, yet are useless.

Those who don't have HS2 but want to be supportive of someone who does may be a bit perplexed by now. They may well be asking themselves, "If I can't express sympathy, then what in the world can I do!" Certainly, there is something of value that you can do. If you are sincere, you can make a tremendous difference, but, perhaps, not in the way that you think. The potential is enormous, but you must exercise great discipline to go beyond doing the kind of perfunctory things that are purely self-serving. The object of this exercise is not to do something quickly on the superficial level which will make *you* feel good. Instead, your first step must be to refuse to pray for anyone with HS2 to get *rid* of anything. If you are sincere about wanting to help a friend, go ahead and pray for him or her, but when you pray, follow this simple guideline. Don't focus on healing. That's neither your business nor mine. That's God's business.

Whosoever rises up to meet the conditions for being healed will be healed. That's as sure as the morning sunrise and the pull of gravity. God would not and COULD NOT deny him or her that. God is already perfect, so what sense is there in asking God to establish what Spirit knows is already there in the life of a certain individual? It is not God who has to do the work. This perfect Mind doesn't know anything about HS2 in the first place — or any other disease. It is only we who do. God doesn't have to come "down" to our level; it is our task to move "up" to God's level. This is not to say that the subject, once ready to rise up in consciousness, mustn't stand up and claim his or her healing. Each one must, but that's a bit different than having someone else attempt to do this for him or her.

GET A LIFE!

YOU - ARE - NOT - A - WALKING - HERPESVIRUS!!!

This may sound funny, but you would be amazed to discover the number of people who go around thinking and acting as if this is what they are. If you recognize yourself as one of those people, then just STOP IT! Replace that errant thought with the following reinforcing thought:

I - AM - AN - OUTSTANDING - PERSON! I - HAVE - VALUE!

Say it out loud. Now repeat it 25 times. Notice how good it feels. If you don't feel that you have value, you are NOT going to find anybody to value you. Not only that, but neither are you going to find anyone to love or to be loved by. You may have relationships, but you will never know a rock steady, effortless, harmonious love until you are convinced of your own value. Think about it. Why should someone love you if you are projecting a message that says, "Hey world, I have no value"? If such is the case, stop searching for love "out there" and do something to increase your sense of value. Go to school. Take a course. Teach a free course yourself, or tutor kids, or give a seminar. Volunteer for some major assignment, or publish an article. I don't care what you have to do to get your mind off yourself and get those positive energies flowing, just don't do nothing! — to turn a very ungrammatical phrase. But do do something.

I did all of the above, much of it gratis. That's right, FREE! Some thought I was a fool for giving away free workshops, seminars and publications, but they simply did not understand. Yes, there were those who thought that they were taking advantage of me, but that would have been impossible. What they didn't understand was that I needed to do those things for me. I wasn't going to let a little hard work and a few bucks stand between me and my blessings. Or not even a lot of bucks.

I have heard some say, "If I could just find a good relationship, I'm sure that I would be healed of HS2." But guess what? They weren't looking for others to give their love to. They were looking for others to love them! And that's a horse of an entirely different color. They had the whole thing backwards, which is why every one of the people who think like this is still searching today. If you feel that love can heal you, then there must be others out there thinking the same way. How are people ever going to connect if everybody's sitting around waiting for somebody to come into their life and love them first? Why not help others to obtain their healing by loving them? Maybe you are the savior. Maybe you are the healer that you've been looking for. If you don't believe that you can do that for another, then obviously you don't believe that anyone else can do that for you. Everything's reciprocal.

We all have value and worth regardless of our conditions and predicaments. Whether you have only a week to live, are in a wheelchair, or was born with great handicaps, you still have value and a purpose in this life. It's up to you to find it. Your challenge may appear to be many times greater than that of others around you, but that doesn't matter. Remember that there are certain conditions in life that you can't do anything about (so far as I've been able to determine). Actually, this is true of most conditions. So don't waste your time worrying about why others seem to have been born with much easier challenges than you. In other words, get a life!

Don't make your life relative to any external standard. A life is a life is a life, and your life is no exception. Your life is whole, perfect, and complete as is, with no regard for what someone else's life is, or more accurately, *appears* to be. So figure out what you can do, what you have to offer, and do it. Before you start, first sit down and get super clear with yourself about where you are with respect to relationships, romance, love, etc., and where you are with respect to your willingness to be committed to anyone that you might attract into your life. What are you willing to give up to have what you desire? Make no mistake about it, you always have to give up something in order to gain something. But I also agree with those who say that once you've gotten there it may not feel as if you're giving up anything. Of course, hindsight is 20-20. Once you've really adjusted to the new change and the new life, unless you keep a journal you'd be hard-pressed to remember how difficult life once was — and I encourage you to keep a journal or diary as you go through these processes.

In truth, you will have given up something, and you will have gained something, but only *you* will be able to say whether it was worth it. As I said, even if you're open there are certain things about your life that only you will ever know. Whatever you do, don't get caught up in subscribing to books and teachings — and there are many — which claim that you can get something without paying a price.

Spiritual and metaphysical people can sometimes be too "enlightened" for their own good. Too often they shy away from teachings which connote that they might have to give up something. There are many who don't like any part of the idea of sacrifice, so they reject it. I can play the game of semantics as well as any metaphysician, but let's not miss the point because of our own sensitivities to certain words or phrases.

Words in themselves don't mean a thing. All they can mean to you or to me as individuals is whatever you and I have agreed that they mean, plus the personal connotations and feelings we impute to them. That's why we must strive to remain open and persevere in our attempts at communication. I don't know what the word *God* or *truth* or *healing* or *cure* means to you unless you tell me. And if you haven't thought about it very deeply, you may not know either. Even in the ideal case where you do know, I had better stay in communication with you, else I'll make the egregious assumption that what I thought these words meant to you yesterday is the same thing that they mean to you today. If you have an open mind, your concept of things is steadily evolving and being refined with each passing day.

Too often, we nouveau spiritualists allow words to trigger limited meanings that predate our conscious pursuit of Truth. Narrowly-defined meanings have no place in the ever-evolving dynamic of spiritual living. Everyday, people are breaking through to deeper and deeper meanings of words and concepts that have been moth-balled for too long in the hope chests of their consciousness, some-times for as long as a lifetime. Sometimes longer. Some will have trouble remembering having had to give up anything to gain the hap-piness that they are experiencing today. We tend to adjust ourselves in life thusly, as if there is some type of automatic normalizing factor at work.

The study of Truth, by definition, is fraught with paradoxes. Sometimes, truth arguments seem to be little more than a play on semantics. Perhaps, this is why so few people master it. I try to be careful in how I use words, but I don't want to be so precise as to unduly complicate a simpler phrasing that may impact someone who is in acute pain and may need to hear the truth in a more compromised form at a particular moment. Such a person may be perching on the precarious brink of awakening, and the tables of his life may be tilted by the particular choice of words and phrases uttered at that moment. After all, unless I can assist such a one in getting through this moment, he or she won't be interested in the deeper kernels of truth. It is for people at this level, as opposed to the puristic spiritual student, that I am writing.

WHAT'S IN A NAME?

Herpes — ugh! Does the mere mention of the word *herpes* cause you to recoil in revulsion? Be honest. If you're like most people with herpes simplex type 2, I expect that it does. After all, this isn't exactly the topic of most dinner conversations.

This leads me to pose the question: What's in a name? For sure, there's more than meets the eye. I read a study a few years ago that discussed the psychology behind the marketing strategy used in naming fish. This study pointed out that the less desirable types of fish tended to have names that connoted "low grade," "undesirability" or "ugliness." I thought, "Hmmm...this is interesting." Certainly no one would argue that names like hake, sea robin or skate occupy a lower rung on the poetic ladder than names like trout or salmon. As any fisherman knows, the former are repulsive, while the latter are the *crême de la mer.* This belies the little known fact that many inhabitants of the repulsive family branches are surprisingly tasty and proteinaceous.

A few years ago, the fish industry contrived a program to change the names of certain types of fish that, up to that time, had not been highly sought after for culinary purposes. Now, people are eating many previously-scorned low grade varieties of fish every day in fine sea food restaurants across the nation, and it's simply because someone was smart enough to adorn them with more appealing names.

They are even marketing and serving shark these days! Excuse me, but when I was growing up, no self-respecting person in the United States would dare eat shark. A shark was supposed to be something that ate you! Nowadays, many "new" names are showing up in fish markets, such as orange roughy, arctic queen, wahoo, and so forth.

Since I used to be a serious amateur fisherman, I'll tell you a little story about shark meat. Do you remember in the '70s when swordfish was virtually banned and became hard to get because of the stringent mercury concentration limits that were imposed? If you do, then you probably also recall that the price of swordfish skyrocketed overnight. Even today, swordfish enjoys an exalted status on any seafood menu, largely because of over-fishing and the imposition of mercury concentration limits for this species. I'll never understand why people pay so much for such a large, bland, flaky and near-tasteless type of flesh, but then there are many things that I don't understand.

Anyway, what I want to tell you is that back in the days when people in this country would have been repulsed by the very thought, many were eating shark meat that was illegally and surreptitiously labeled as swordfish. Just ask any old-time fisherman of the sea.

I remember being in England back in the early '70s and really developing a taste for a type of fish that they called plaice. Later, when I found out that plaice was nothing more than the repugnant skate, I almost threw up! Have you ever seen a skate? It doesn't look like something you'd want to eat. A lot of the fish that are highly sought after in classy eating establishments today used to be thrown back in disgust whenever anyone was unlucky enough to catch them. There are some fish that you wouldn't even hoist into your boat, let alone eat. You'd rather cut the line.

There is one called the sea eel that has encouraged many chicken-hearted fisherman to cut their lines, including this writer. It's one of the ugliest, most vicious-looking sea monsters you'd ever want to see — and, preferably, from a distance! Yet real fishermen know that this slimy green monster possesses some of the tastiest flesh in the sea.

Another example is the ling cod. I loathed this species. There was a time when they would only be used for cat food or chum. So one time when I took one home and tried to eat it, guess what: It tasted just like cat food! Now I've never eaten cat food, but I'm sure that if I did, it would taste just like ling cod. Call it a mental thing if you want to. Afterwards, I always regarded ling cod as some type of downgraded cod, which it is not. Cod is fine, but you put the word "ling" before it and you derive something that is highly undesirable.

So, returning to the question put before you: What's in a name? The answer is: Everything!

While I'm on the subject, let's consider the case of the lowly snail. Of course, we all know that they aren't called snails in expensive French restaurants. The haughty French waiter would be highly insulted if you asked if they had any fresh snails in the kitchen. He'd probably throw you out on your ear. It sounds much more appetizing to say, "I'll have the *escargots au buerre*," than "Gimme some of them snails!"

Of course, I will never be rich enough to eat escargots. There isn't enough money in Fort Knox. I wouldn't eat them if they renamed them filet mignon. It is said that a rose by any other name...still, is not a snail.

Now there are people who like legumes but detest peas.

Notice that restaurants prefer to advertise "calamari" rather than "squid," when, in fact, they are one and the same? Their reasoning is transparent. Who the heck wants to eat squid?

When I was growing up, my mother used to cook oxtails to such a level of culinary perfection that cows would march up to our doorstep and commit suicide. We're talking extraordinary on the scale of yummy.

Now I have this sister who used to love neck bones, which my mother also stewed to perfection. But oddly enough, she hated ox-tails. One day she bolted in from school as hungry as a soldier on bivouac, opened the pot from which the enchanting aroma derived, and asked Mom, "What is this that smells go good?"

Mom assured her that, of course, it was her favorite course, neck bones. Thirty minutes later, after my teen-age sister had wolfed down a respectable helping or two, my mother told her that she had just proven that oxtails couldn't really be all that bad. My sister proceeded to get sick right there on the spot, as well as exceedingly angry. Or maybe it was the anger that made her sick. Whatever — you get the point.

Okay, so just what IS in a name? Look at all the actors and singers who have changed their names to increase their marketability. People like Elton John, the late Redd Foxx, Englebert Humperdink, Marilyn Monroe, Lawrence Welk, Ann Landers, Prince, Stevie Wonder, Bob Dylan, John Denver, Michael Landon and so many others. If you know their original names, then it is clear to you why they changed.

I once thought of changing mine. I estimated that *Bernard Jackson* just doesn't sound like a famous name. Then I decided, "Awww, to heck with it. I don't give a hoot if I ever become famous or not, anyhow." I figured that I could best expend my energy learning how to be real, whatever my name, and leave the rest of those games to the world. In the final analysis that's the only thing that will count anyhow. How real are you?

Now when it comes to the realm of medicine, it's the same thing. Take the word *leprosy*, for instance. Over the centuries, there probably hasn't been a more negatively-tinged word in medical history. Is it any surprise that today's health professionals refer to this age-old scourge as Hansen's disease? I'm sure you will agree that the latter name is so much more acceptable and less stigmatized. Given a choice, no one would ever prefer to be called a leper. On this I'd wager. You could talk about Hansen's disease at the dinner table without raising an eyebrow, but it you substituted the word *leprosy* some people would lose their appetite.

The word "cancer" has a depressingly fatalistic ring to it. And then there's the twin scourges of gonorrhea and syphilis — two awfully tainted words. It sounds so much more benign to say that you have had the "clap," which is a colloquialism for gonorrhea.

It's easier to admit to having a "social disease" in polite society than to say that you have syphilis. Many of our most famous people throughout history, including some from the ranks of Old World royalty, allegedly died from complications of — shhh — "social diseases."

The health industry doesn't even use the terminology *venereal disease* anymore. VD has become such a negative label that they had to come us with something more psychologically neutral. Today, the accepted phraseology is *sexually transmissible disease*, or STD.

The moment you say *syphilis*, someone will immediately think *brain damage*. It's one of the most automatic word associations in existence. Try it sometime among a group of your closest friends, or, perhaps, when you're the M.C. for the company's year-end awards banquet.

Then there's the word *AIDS*. Now this is an amazingly benign name for something that society considers to be such a menace. For comparison, it certainly sounds better than the word *leprosy*. It is no wonder to me its proponents have encountered so much trouble getting Congress to give it the attention that it deserves. By no means am I trying to make light of AIDS, but perhaps if it had been given a name as connotatively-grave as leprosy, it would have been taken more seriously sooner.

Among all of the diseases of this so-called modern era, I don't think I have ever heard of one with such a negatively-tainted and charged nomenclature as herpes. Legionnaires disease was more toxic than HS2 or AIDS, yet it sounds like something you might want to don a banner in a patriotic parade for.

It's no accident that we have had AIDS telethons, but no herpes telethons. Who the hell wants to be affiliated with herpes? Not only that, but two facts have served to keep people from dealing with it publicly: (1) People aren't comfortable admitting that they have it, and (2) almost everybody has it, if not in an active state, at least in a latent state. In one form or another, virtually everyone in the United States has evidence of some form of herpesvirus in their blood.

In reviewing the literature, I found that many writers of magazine articles refer to HS2 as the "new leprosy" or the "virus of love." It has been interesting to observe how gingerly writers have skittered around the fringes of the subject over the past couple of decades. There's been a hush-hush tone surrounding this subject from the beginning.

When I first began this project, my approach was to cloak this subject in nice-sounding euphemisms, but then a change came over me. I bit the bullet and decided to use this opportunity to go ahead and heal my own fears. I made the decision to be strictly honest, which later became the official name of my spiritual publishing and teaching enterprise.

Names like the *new leprosy*, I can do without; and *love virus*, I personally deplore. They are much too cute. In the beginning I hadn't considered the possibility of being totally candid. This was a hurdle that I first had to surmount in my own mind — how I perceived the HS2 condition. Why was *I* so uncomfortable with the word *herpes*? How much power was I imputing to this illusory condition by having such a strong reaction to this word? After dealing with this consciously for some time, I finally got it all cleared up in my head. Then I realized that to subscribe to euphemisms such as *love virus* would be to evade the truth.

What we're after is a means and a mechanism through which true healing can take place. There is no transformative power in using words that avoid the issue. Euphemisms certainly do not convey the truth about HS2, nor do they signify the truth about love. Thus they are a bastardization and a sham. HS2 is not even remotely associated with love, so it cannot be defined as the result of love. Just think about it. LOVE IS NOT A VIRUS! If anything, HS2 is one of a plethora of circumstances that can result from the AB-SENCE of love, or the adulteration thereof.

It is unfortunate that the word love is used so loosely in modern society. Regardless, like all eternal verities, its nature is not altered one iota by our ignorance of it.

Now I am not one to play games with my mind or try to suppress, deny, or otherwise turn away from the hard cold reality of HS2 and make it seem trivial. To one who may have had HS2 for a few months, or perhaps a year, there are stages that he or she must pass through before any of this will make sense.

Back when I was going to attempt to rename the condition something cute like "virus of love" or "love bug," my girlfriend at the time, Elise, was straight-forward in sharing with me her opinion. She thought it was a lousy idea. Elise was one of those people who was always right on the money in correcting me whenever I wavered away from principle. Today, my wife does the same thing. Do you have a friend like that?

Elise always reminded me of the truth that I professed to already know. I remember her telling me point-blank after having read the first 20 pages of my budding manuscript: "Bernard, I don't like what you're saying. First of all, HS2 is not a result of love. Why make it sound like something else? Why not call it what it is?" I thought for a second before finally agreeing, "Okay Elise. I think I finally understand." That was in 1985. Elise's advice put a major kink in my plans. What I thought would be a one-year project turned out to take seven. Unbeknown to me at the time, there was so much more growing that I had to do before I could be strictly honest.

To be frank, I was hypersensitive in those days, but not too sensitive to realize that Elise was absolutely right. Indeed I did have a distorted concept of love. That was my whole problem in a capsule. She went on to tell me that if I was going to produce a book that was going to be useful at all, first I was going to have to become crystal clear in my own mind so as not to attempt to deceive anybody.

The project demanded that I dig deep down into my truth center and then recount that truth straightforwardly. Although I knew that she was right, it took a number of additional years before I could do what I had already agreed was the right thing to do. It takes time sometimes to embody a discomforting and harsh truth.

CHAPTER 7: EXHAUSTING HUMAN OPTIONS

MYTHS SHATTERED

Over the years I have encountered a number of myths about HS2 and myriad touted claims of cures and miracle drugs. Without exception, these cures have turned out to be just that — myths! Of the estimated 30 million people in the United States who have HS2, I doubt if any can honestly say that they've escaped being preoccupied with word-of-mouth cures at some point. The obsessive seeking of cures is a peculiar trait of a group that I refer to as the "privileged class."

By "privileged class" I mean those who are college-educated, professional people, Yuppies, and virtually anyone of means, which includes self-made successes. Somehow, this class of people got misled into believing that they could use their analytical, size-up-the-situation-and-take-charge powers to cure themselves of even this condition. Ask me how I know. Sheepishly, I must admit that I evolved from this line of thinking. In their jobs, at home, and in their professional organizations, the members of this class are so accustomed to taking control of intractable situations and working out solutions. After all, this is what made them the successful people that they are — their ability to reason and think logically. Conversely, this very thinking militates against spiritual healing.

Often, this class of person sees himself or herself as one who, for whatever reasons, has been infused with superior intellectual ability and big-picture vision that is far beyond average. I have worked with and studied on the college level with many people like this. I, too, must shamefully admit that I once thought along these lines. I wish I had a dime for everybody that I've met who regarded themselves as above average in intelligence. If ours were a country of royalty, the privileged class would undoubtedly think of themselves as just a tad below royalty in birth.

One could infer quite easily that, in a just universe, those who think of themselves as privileged might attract into their lives some special lessons. There is no way that any of us are going to get through life with such a convoluted attitude without having it challenged. There is a price for thinking this way. Rich or poor, so-called privileged or so-called under-privileged, life is simply an experience from whatever perspective we happen to be looking. Whatever lie we hold most dear will be exposed before we complete this journey. Otherwise, there really wouldn't be much meaning to it all, would there?

That which created heaven and Earth couldn't care less whether you and I are rich or poor. If we are still here, then there must be a reason for it, and it couldn't possibly be to teach a world full of "poor creatures" what *they* need to learn. This is the self-deceiving fallacy that so many self-professed "enlightened" people buy into — you know, the religious types, the missionaries, the New Thought practitioners, the gurus, and veterans of est and the Summit and Life Springers, *et cetera*. I can poke fun at these people because I've come from among their ranks. For good, I hope.

Seriously, I'm sure that God doesn't need me to teach the world what it ought to be doing, at least not as a primary or deliberate occupation. There's not a one of us who doesn't have enough personal stuff to work out every day in terms of our own lives and decisions, morals and ethics. Hence, if we devote ourselves to doing the best job that we can to straighten out our own lives, we will accomplish more teaching as a side effect than would have ever been possible intentionally. In other words, teaching is a side effect of LIVING a spiritually-consistent life, not its main purpose.

The belief that we belong to some kind of privileged class is nothing but vaunted pomposity and false pride. It's vacuous ego garbage and other traps of "privilege" that prevent us from seeing clearly enough to overcome the afflictions that crop up in our lives from time to time. In that sense, the so-called common man or woman is more able to spring back and carry on with life than the jaded intellectual or professional. If you are truly down-to-earth, you won't be preoccupied with feelings of shame, secrecy, and fear that your colleagues may one day find out that you have HS2. Yet I know for a fact that so many of the so-called enlightened practitioners and New Agers are carrying around so much guilt and embarrassment concerning HS2. So who's fooling whom?

I know we all do it at times, but what is it but pure bull when we allow ourselves to get caught up in the feeling that we aren't supposed to have certain conditions. Why not? The universe is totally impersonal. It neither protects nor harbors any privileged positions or privileged people. It's like no one ever thinks of a minister as having gonorrhea. Such a thing would be awfully embarrassing for a person of such status. Cancer — yes. Gonorrhea — no! Or the President of the United States throwing up at a state dinner, or perhaps, having diarrhea. Certain things are unthinkable, as unthinkable as it is for most people to imagine their parents making love.

President Carter once made a joke about catching Montezuma's Revenge during a presidential trip to Mexico, and he was roundly criticized for it. That same President was severely criticized while in office for admitting that he occasionally lusted in his mind. What has the world come to when a world leader is not allowed to lust in his or her mind? All of these examples indicate how screwed up we all are as we become too intellectually-significant and start taking ourselves and our roles in life so blasted seriously.

I'm convinced that so much of our neurosis and physical illnesses come from so much effort that we exert to keep the lid on personal and family problems that need to be brought out into the open. The big bad wolf isn't so big or bad, you know, not after we expose him to the light of day. We might get laughed at a little, but so what? If the so-called common man contracts gonorrhea, we don't think that much about it. Likewise, if he lusts in his mind, we tend to think nothing of it. Then why can't a minister or a president?

We entertain so many myths in our lives. For those with HS2 who desire to be healed, it is absolutely mandatory that these myths be identified, exposed for what they are and expunged. If we are going to approach God to help us, we need to clear our minds of all distortions and relative, partial truths. After all, a partial truth is not truth.

Here's my list of 10 of the most popular HS2-related myths which seems to have mentally hamstrung the HS2 population.

* Myth No. 1: Vitamin and/or mineral therapy can cure you.

* Myth No. 2: Natural herbs can cure you.

* Myth No. 3: Positive thinking, meditation, affirmations, or visualization can cure you.

* Myth No. 4: Being a good person, going to church, and praying can cure you.

* Myth No. 5: Avoiding stress can prevent outbreaks of HS2.

* Myth No. 6: Avoiding sugar can cure or prevent recurrences of HS2.

* Myth No. 7: A vegetarian diet can cure you.

* Myth No. 8: Avoiding alcoholic beverages can cure or control HS2.

* Myth No. 9. Avoiding sex (celibacy) can cure or prevent recurrences of HS2.

* Myth No. 10: Avoiding relationships can help to arrest or prevent recurrences of HS2.

Before we explore the relative truth or error of these 10 great myths, let me first say that there is a single antidote to all of the above: **THE PRACTICE OF TRUE SPIRITUAL LOVE.** There is no secret. The answer is simple in theory, but it's awfully difficult to practice. There are many subtleties that need to be identified and mastered. The reason that I've written this book is to try to put some teeth into what New Agers and metaphysicians often try to gloss over with nice-sounding platitudes. If the answer were so simple, there wouldn't be 30 million people with HS2 and over a million with HIV in the United States. After devoting years and hours and dollars trying every panacea on this list, the practice of continuous love and acceptance in our relationships with ALL of our fellow men and women is the only healing elixir that I have found, but few there be who are able to practice this.

There is no bitterness here. I am simply reporting on what I have found. Instead of putting so much energy into avoidance behaviors, it is paramount that we choose an attitude that will induce health, and that is the attitude and belief system of divine love. Don't be fooled by the seeming simplicity of this prescription. This is one of the most profound principles ever handed down to humankind. It could not be repeated often enough.

Now I'm no Bible thumper. Do you know what a *Bible* thumper is? That's a person who is so overzealous about saving your soul that he practically thumps you over the head with his *Bible*. He or she is one who see the Good Book as a weapon to be used like a blunt-edged sword.

Both medical authorities and many HS2 subjects assert that stress triggers outbreaks of HS2, and should therefore be avoided. Seldom, however, can these same authorities and subjects explain just how one is supposed to go about doing this. Many of these same people attribute like powers to nuts, chocolate, cheese, and alcohol, for instance. Personally, my lifestyle involves all of the above-listed no-no's, except for drinking, a habit that I have finally kicked for other reasons. Being the busy bee, high achiever that I am, I have always thrived on stress. Still do. Whereas I can do without chocolate and sugar-laden products on a good day, I must admit to being a freak for a good can of nuts and a hunk of cheese. One has to enjoy some pleasures, or else what good is it to be alive?

I remember risking my life as a boy to climb tall, swaying pecan trees back in my native Georgia. Sometimes I'd slither so high up that the branches would become tiny and begin popping and cracking under my feet. Then I'd be afraid to attempt the climb down. You see, I've always had a fear of heights. Ah — the things we do for pleasure!

Strangely enough, when I was practicing the extremes (no meat, no salt, no caffeinated tea, etc.), I was constantly assaulted by HS2 outbreaks. Despite the maintenance of a spiritual regimen that would have done St. Francis proud — prayer, worship, reading, meditation, counseling, healing sessions, etc. — I didn't even come close to being healed. Granted, there could have been many reasons for this, and I'm of the opinion that there were. Maybe I didn't allow enough time, maybe my teachers weren't that good, or maybe — just maybe — I wasn't the world's brightest student. Unless I'm way off base, I doubt if any of these reasons captures the essence of the problem, which was that I was simply trying too hard. The problem was that *I* was trying to do it myself, instead of totally surrendering and letting Spirit — or even better, the *Law* of Spirit — assist me.

Who wants to surrender when there is so much fun to be had by being naughty? Honestly...think about this for a moment. We cry foul and act pious, but many of us rather like being naughty. Today, I realize that part of my problem was that I enjoyed being naughty. In the world, being the life of the party is often synonymous with being naughty. I don't talk about it much today, but I spent about 12 years trying to be a comedian. Obviously, it didn't work for me, but I learned a lot about myself in the process, and I met a number of comedians backstage who are famous today. Ironic though it may seem, there is none so negative as the average comedian. It's not intentional but it comes with the territory. A comedian is a person who must spend hours on end standing in front of a mirror saturating his subconscious mind with what too often is some of the most negative, nonredeeming accounts of human behavior.

Try living that way for a few years and see if chronic depression and self doubt don't invade your mental atmosphere and color your heart black.

How could we learn to trust God if it were possible to attain healings by doing cookbook exercises in predictable ways? Unfortunately — or, perhaps, it's fortunate — God doesn't work that way. Yet most churches, as well as metaphysical and New Thought organizations, are still teaching this method. The various teachings may be overt or they may be suggestive, but the message is the same. Despite the fact that I had been trying for well over five years to do it the dutiful way, eventually I had to give up trying to be "good." Consequently, I re-adopted a number of my previous nutritional habits. Oh, I continued to proscribe alcohol usage and sexual misconduct, but otherwise, I opened up my diet to include everything within reason. It was then that I achieved the most prolonged state of happiness and general well being thus far.

To be sure, I still see God as the center of all creation, but what I have discarded are all of my previous superstitious beliefs concerning food. I believe now more than ever that it's not which foods I eat; it's how true I am to my higher self, which is the spiritual man. Knowing that the soul of man is anchored in God, it's how much at peace I am with my own life, regardless of how imperfect it may seem to be.

Previously, I stated that I don't believe that diet is all that important in healing. This does not mean that I have totally ignored the role diet plays in the evolution of consciousness. At times it may be of the utmost importance.

Do whatever is right for you, and by all means don't partake of any food substance that your doctor advises is bad for you. I am only sharing with you the thought processes that I have gone through to arrive at what works for me. Personally, I don't believe that the average person has to practice extremes in order to be healthy. If there's a God at all, the answer has to be found in a lifestyle of balance in conjunction with true alignment to the nature of God. Any decent deity has to allow you to progress from where you are to where you wish to be, and you can only do this through balance.

The goal cannot be accomplished by total abstinence and rejection of pleasures that you inwardly still crave. Think about it. **ACCEPTANCE AND GRADUALISM IS THE WAY.**

In my community, I maintain an impeccable image. Others see me as this super responsible guy. You know the type — Mr. Perfect Role Model for young people. I'm not bragging but this is another aspect of life that needs to be exposed. I want people to realize how even the best of us have to battle constantly with our own private demons. Unless we are brutally honest about these compulsions and addictions, we will get caught up in trying to make our lives fit the images that our friends and supporters have painted of us. As a result, we will end up being compromised while suffering silently in the closet, afraid that somebody will find us out. It's better not to be put on a pedestal in the first place.

Much has been written about the relationship between HS2 and stress. Surveys have revealed that many subjects feel that they have more outbreaks during times when they are under severe stress. Now it is well-known that there are two major kinds of stress and that all stress is not bad. One type of stress results from extremely negative circumstances; the other type results from unusual, positive or happy circumstances. In an attempt to get cured, the angry, manic state of mind in which many new HS2 subjects find themselves often leads to an obsessive, over-reactionary avoidance of all stress, regardless of type. As a result, they become boring people who stay home with the shades drawn whenever they're not at work, totally withdrawn from society and friends. This may sound extreme, but I can tell you that I have known real people who reacted to HS2 this way.

Life is indeed stranger than fiction. It is not my place to say that this is bad. On the contrary, I suppose that it could be the perfect prescription for certain people at particular stages of their self development. However — and there's always a however — anyone who thinks that that kind of 100 percent regulated behavior is going to solve his problem is setting himself (or herself) up for a surprise, or more aptly stated, a disappointment. The acquisition of HS2 does not exempt you from needing to take occasional risks. To gain any semblance of mastery in life means to take intelligent risks.

As it must forever be, the taking of risks can lead one into trouble or into freedom. And after awhile, you even begin to embrace the trouble.

In this paradoxical, continuously upward spiral of the consciously-lived life, I must inform whosoever will listen:

I HAVE FOUND NO EASY ANSWERS OR SINGULAR, ONE-DIMENSIONAL SOLUTIONS.

Mind you, my "failure" is not due to any lack of effort. This may be the world's first self-help book with no easy answers.

My metaphysical teachers and friends will pillory me for stating this, but as a devout student of truth, client or patient in need of healing, you can do everything "right" so far as your consciousness is able to discern and still not receive any evidence of healing. This is the unavoidable truth that nobody seems to want to admit. As a result there are lots of devotees walking around bearing loads of unnecessary guilt. One example that immediately comes to mind is Kim, whose story I will share in this chapter. She is typical of a group of would-be metaphysical devotees who are trapped in the tragic web of Catch-22. Those who feel guilty from not being able to induce self-healings are unbeknowingly feeding subjective thought patterns which are making them sicker than they were in the beginning. And the saddest part of the whole debacle is that they don't feel that they can tell anybody about it. They've bought into a philosophy where all of the fault for failing to be healed circles right back to their shoulders. This is a problem that is endemic to the occidental mind. We are much too caught up in results and effects and conditions as they appear to be, none of which means didley squat!

What these enlightened sufferers don't understand is that the only parts of the equation we're responsible for are the praying, the meditating and keeping our minds centered in spiritual reality. The other side of the equation — results — is not our domain. This is unfortunate or fortunate, depending on the individual's point of view. But this is the way it is, and it is what we must eventually accept.

The only job of true spiritual teachers, or agents for healing, is to exemplify the truth and uphold the light in our own lives.

KIM

I can think of a number of women and men presently who typify the attitude that I'm talking about. Let me give you one example of an experience that I had with a woman in one of the workshops that I produced and facilitated. I'll call her Kim. I asked everybody in the workshop to make a list of the issues that they wanted to work on during the four-week workshop and to organize their desires according to priority.

I had known Kim for some years. She was a beautiful woman in her 30's, the type whom it appeared could have any man that she desired. Over the years, Kim had often complained about how difficult it was to find a decent man. Many were the times that she assaulted my ears with her lamentations about the wimpy nature of most men who passed through her life. To my great surprise, after she made out her list and prioritized it, as I had instructed, I noticed that she listed a relationship with a man as the third and final priority.

I knew that Kim was involved in an intensely competitive, time-consuming, high stakes business enterprise. I also knew that Kim's primary purpose in life at the time was to get rich. It was no secret. She was utterly shameless in her pursuit of financial success and wealth beyond everything else on this Earth, and she was literally running herself into the ground trying to attain it. In fact, Kim had made me aware that she had a serious health problem, which was the other biggie that she enumerated on her priority list ahead of a good relationship. But number one, of course, was to get rich.

Exactly what this health problem was, I wasn't exactly sure, but it was characterized by a severe allergic reaction to just about every food product in existence. At least that's the story she told me. I recall at the time thinking, "Funny...she always seemed normal to me." You wouldn't have ever guessed that she was anything but perfectly healthy and remarkably stunning if you had known her. However, knowing her as I did, it was clear to me that this woman lived predominantly within the boundaries of her own head. In other words, she was relentlessly mental. She got involved in every way-out philosophy this side of the moon, as well as a few beyond. In brief, she wasn't spiritually balanced.

But let there be no mistake about it, Kim was a functional, sane, high achiever by the world's standards, but spiritually, she was merely flittering on the fringes and blowing pipe dreams, while hoping beyond hope to get lucky. She was not unlike many students of metaphysics and other New Age philosophies, sprouting arguments that were blatantly illogical and inconsistent, while cleverly evading any opportunity to be pinned down. Just as she refused to be challenged by anyone, she was content to float around uttering simplistic affirmations like some airy fairy zombie.

Deep down inside, I sensed that Kim was fighting with herself, whipping herself for her self-perceived failings and relating to life as if it were hundreds of times more difficult than it was. Privately, I wondered why, but figured, as with all things, in due time the answer would make itself known. One thing was for sure: What she had shared with me wasn't the whole story about her health.

Kim wore the persona of one who was highly evolved. She made sure that her spirituality, as well as most issues germane to her life, were beyond question. She must have reasoned either consciously or subconsciously that if she couldn't be questioned, she would never have to deal with being real. This belies the fact that she thought of herself as one who was completely open. I'll say this for Kim: She was one tough cookie. I mean, she didn't crumble easily. She hadn't survived in this jungle of a world by getting forced into checkmate too often. No, Kim was a winner through the eyes of that world whose opinion she valued so much, except for one problem: She was wasting away due to some kind of physical illness, undoubtedly fueled by an insidious mental maladjustment.

Isn't that always the story? We are so smart. We have this thing called life almost figured out, except for one little nettlesome flaw. So we spend all of our time trying to eliminate that flaw. There is always one little flaw that we either overlooked, or else it's something beyond our control that enters into the picture in the eleventh hour from way out in left field and blind-sides us. And humankind's greatest error is that they assign the blame to bad luck, bad timing, human sabotage or insufficient planning. In their insistence upon proving themselves self sufficient from God, they fail to realize that all human endeavors will and must eventually fail unless they are consistent with the pre-existent spiritual laws. At some point in our maturation, each one of us thinks that we wrote the book on mental perspicacity and human craftiness. Well we didn't.

Though this story is about Kim, I can think of many men and women whom I have met during the last decade who fit the same profile, flittering around like spiritual butterflies, touting big pipe dreams, ungrounded, unhappy, and as philosophically-evasive as a congressman. Enlightened spiritual movements attract these people in droves.

Gradually, I came to realize that there was one part of the world that Kim kept at a safe distance from her life: ALL MEN! To listen to her cant, one moment she loved men, the next moment she hated them. Eventually I began to wonder if, perhaps, the source of Kim's conflict and erratic behavior was HS2 or something similar. Something was going on with this woman. Clearly, there was a conflict lurking within and it was making her crazy. As the years have rolled by, I have encountered similar cases where identical patterns of vacillating logic, love and hate, on again/off again fixations, and sensible/illogical behavior were present, and where the problem was eventually revealed to be HS2.

I have a good friend now, a male, who exhibits this same driven, erratic behavior, especially in his relationships with women. It took me a long time but eventually I found out that he has HS2. To this day, it's not something that he is very open about or is able to handle. It's been decades (really!) since he's allowed himself to get emotionally close to a woman, and unfortunately, there's a good chance that he never will. The self-assumed shame of having an "incurable" sexual disorder will cause you to go bonkers if you try to hide it.

Now understand that I am neither judging nor condemning Kim.

I'm living in a glass house myself. Contrariwise, I have great empathy for people like Kim. They think that they wrote the book on sublimation, which is funny to me since I'm sure that I am the author of that book. From the early teens until about 30, I mastered in anger and minored in neuroses. Also, I was well on my way to earning a second master's in gamesmanship. My games were called "Snow the World," "Keep 'Em All Confused," "Let No One Into Your Life," and "Feign Superiority."

It would be safe to say that between the ages of 15 and 30, I didn't learn enough to fill a 30 second essay about my true identity. Due to ignorance I maintained a tight noose around my true feelings. Naturally, I was the most miserable person you'd ever want to meet. The image that I had of myself at 30 was about the same as the image that I had had of myself at 15, except that I possessed a few more ostensible accomplishments, which only rendered me a little more arrogant. For some stupid reason, I enjoyed playing out my game. So when people like Kim — who was just past 30 at the time — come to me reading a chapter from the book that I wrote, it's all I can do to act as if I'm hearing this story for the first time. Sure, the story is always interesting. Each one will have a different twist, but what the suffering raconteur doesn't know is: I already know the ending. That's the part that never changes. Why else do soap operas never end? Though I don't play games anymore, I certainly haven't lost the ability to recognize them.

The thing that made Kim's story so memorable was that she was so haughty and impressed by her self-professed purity. She waxed on and on about the things that she didn't do. You know the type: pure by default.

I am forever suspicious of those who deem themselves pure by default. Some would call this the sin of *omission*, and I would tend to agree, except that the word *sin* is so loaded that it can be misconstrued. What theologians call sins are, in effect, errors in thinking and judgment that students of Truth fall into at times. The error of assuming purity by omission is equivalent to a person trying to win a photographic contest by submitting only the negatives.

There was my friend Kim putting so much energy into convincing the world concerning things she had NOT done. I asked for volunteers from among those in the workshop to share with the group what their desires were so that we could all support each other in daily prayer. As always in my groups, I explained that it was totally voluntary on their part. I have always honored the philosophy that people have every right in the world to refuse to grow, without being judged by *me*. This is not to say that everybody who declined to participate in group prayer was necessarily refusing to grow. I also believe that people have the right to make whatever choices please them. One thing I do believe, along with the mystics of the ages, is that group prayer is a powerful and effective tool.

Personally, I have facilitated and witnessed a number of absolutely miraculous healings through group prayer — at least they seemed as much at the time. Though I say this, I am quite cautious about claiming miracles. The scientist in me still respects the skepticism that exists in the world at large concerning claims of spiritual healings, especially among intellectuals and rational-minded people. As ironic as it may sound, I think there is far too much emphasis placed on miracles in the spiritual community. First of all, spiritual healing is something that, by definition, you cannot prove. No one ever has and no one ever will prove a single spiritual principle.

When I called upon Kim, she agreed to recite her list of desires to the group. After reading her third and final one, I openly questioned her level of conviction.

"Kim, how important is it for you to develop a good relationship with a man?"

"Gee, I don't know," she whined. "The main thing right now is my health, and of course, I want my business to be successful. I've put so much into it now. Besides, I've gotta eat." Our previous conversations had led me to believe that money was more important than health, but she presented them to the group in the reverse order. Was she being sincere or merely vocalizing what was spiritually correct?

"Yeah, I understand that, Kim, but what surprises me is that you put 'relationship' on your list at all. So far, all you've been talking about is your health and your job. I've never heard you say before that you were ready to accept a man into your life, so I have to admit that I'm a wee bit surprised. Are you really saying that you're ready to make the commitment to a relationship?"

I asked her these questions to help her clarify exactly where she stood on this issue. Somehow, I had not received through the conviction in her voice or body language that she was serious about a relationship. It seemed as if she had sort of thrown it in as an afterthought, and I wasn't going to buy that. It was as if she was saying, "What the hell, since these people are going to be praying for me, I might as well throw in a wild card. I might luck out and get everything on my list." It wouldn't have been the first time that I'd encountered wild card prayers in working with spiritual aspirants before. If this was the case with Kim, I wasn't going to let her off the hook until she got in touch with what her true desires were.

It was Kim's turn to reply. "Well, look, let me be honest, I would really like to find somebody to do stuff with — I mean, it's lonely sometimes not having somebody to talk to at the end of a rough day, especially in the kind of business I'm in, but at the same time, he would have to be a special kind of man. He would have to understand the kind of tough and competitive business that I'm in, 'cause when the phone rings, I have to go. I get calls in the middle of the night and early in the morning — you know what I mean? See, I've got contacts who call me from all over the world. When they call I have to move on things right away because if I don't work, I don't get paid. And believe it or not, there aren't that many men who can understand that.

"And the other thing is, this kind of business doesn't leave much time for dating and stuff like that. That's why I didn't put finding a mate first on my list."

Kim was giving me the old smoke screen, what with all this ceaseless prattle about her job and her self importance. By golly, it was high time somebody got real honest with her. "KIM, WHY DON'T YOU JUST GET OFF IT! Gee whiz, kid, you aren't the only one who has an important job in this world. You're simply not being honest. You're not facing up to what the real issues are here. Either you want a relationship with a man or you don't, and what I'm hearing is that you aren't nearly ready for that — not yet. All of that talk about your job is just a lot of baloney — a smoke screen if I've ever seen one. If you really want something, you can't be wishy-washy with God. You certainly can't *fool* the Universe. [When capitalized, Universe refers to God, or the Infinite Mind of God.]

"You can tell the people in this workshop anything you want, but the Universe knows what's in your heart, and that's exactly what it's going to return to you. Where the Universe is concerned, you've got to put up a united front. I'm sorry, Kim, but you can't have it both ways. And it's perfectly all right, as far as I'm concerned. You don't have to be ready for a relationship right now. Look at me. I don't have one myself. But — I'm crystal clear on the fact that the reason I don't have one is because I, Bernard Jackson, am not ready for one right now. When I get ready, I'm going to simply ask for it, and I will absolutely expect to get it."

I don't remember exactly what her response was, but I know that it fell in the category of weak defenses. Kim knew that I was on to her, and on some level, I assume that she appreciated the honesty. At least then she didn't have to pretend anymore. Just for the record, I let her know that I didn't doubt the validity of what she said about men not understanding the exigencies of her kind of job. Kim knew where I was coming from in our workshop. No way was I going to let her or anybody else off the hook just because the odds seemed to be against them, or because they were able to conjure up so much palpable pain and emotion.

"Okay Kim, you still have not answered my question. I hope you're tough enough to stand up to this kind of questioning — "

"Oh yes, go right ahead. This is not a problem for me," she rapidly assured me — almost too rapidly, if you know what I mean.

I repeated my question. "Then what about commitment? Are you ready to make it? You know it's going to take commitment to be in a good relationship. You're going to have to make room for another person in your well-regulated life. Otherwise, you're just kidding yourself. When you tell God that you want something, you have to be willing to do whatever it takes to make your desire a reality. You have to have your entire heart and soul behind your desire, because it's not just your words that the Universe is listening to. As a matter of fact, your words don't mean much as all. It's the conviction of your heart that is going to make this thing happen, and right now I don't feel anything emanating from you that is convincing. Correct me if I'm wrong."

"Well, look," she chimed in, "I realize a relationship is not the highest priority in my life right now. That's why I didn't put it higher on my list. Still, I don't see why you can't have your career and a relationship too. I feel like, er, well, I'm gonna have it my way or not at all! Like I said, I've only got so much time..."

"Kim!" I interrupted her, "you're only evading the question and constantly repeating your well-worn refrain. I understand what you're saying. Yeah, you can do it your way, but don't fool yourself. Without making a resolve towards absolute commitment, you're not going to be able to have what you want. This is a cause and effect universe — you know that — and there is no way you can fool it. If you want what you say you want, you MUST conform. The Universe doesn't have to change for you.

"Oh sure, you'll eventually meet somebody. You'll get a man, no doubt, but he won't be the one you want. In this universe, we're always attracting something and repelling something else. The question is, what are you attracting? Are you attracting what you *say* you want?"

I couldn't say this in front of the other workshop participants, but I had spent a number of hours on the phone listening to Kim wail about one bad relationship after another. It never ceases to amaze me how different a person's public persona can be from the real person underneath. Of course, I'm not claiming that I, or anybody else, can ever know the real person underneath, but I do know that there is always a difference. We always hold something back. Some of us are so accomplished in wearing the mask of social approval that we ourselves don't even know who is underneath. It's been said that the worst form of deception takes place when people fool themselves.

Anyway, Kim was the cantankerous type. She was always embroiled in one dispute or another. It didn't seem to matter if the other party was male or female. In this sense, Kim was totally androgynous. She fought with everyone equally.

The thing about Kim was that she reminded me so much of myself. Hers was a tough, unyielding intellect. She was going to have what she wanted, and wasn't anybody going to stop her. She had one speed: fast! — and one direction: straight ahead! It was just too bad if you happened to be in the way of this juggernaut. Yet she embarked upon the study of a little metaphysics, coupled with a little religiosity. This mixture can be more deadly than TNT.

Every time I looked up, Kim was threatening to sue one of her business partners or associates for defamation of her character. In other words, every time she got wind that someone had passed an unkind word about her to another, she was ready to go to battle. I suppose we have really come up in this world when we can assume such self-importance as to think that someone can say something about us that will make any real difference. In her case, she claimed that what certain competitors said was detrimental to the extent that it could result in a loss of income to her. It's no wonder that we like to think of ourselves as "modern" people living in an advanced civilization. We had to contrive some way to justify our ability to creatively manufacture nonsense.

One time Kim went into this lengthy diatribe about this man whom she had been working with in a business situation and who presented himself to be so trustworthy, but turned out to be a flake. As I sat and listened, I immediately began to wonder why all of their dealings were done either in a restaurant or in her home. This is one of those "poor me" stories that only a friend would try to sell you, yet as you sit and listen you notice that things just don't seem to add up? Yet you know that you aren't supposed to point out the obvious to the "friend" who is bending your ear. At the same time, you don't want to be judgmental or presumptuous.

I wasn't going to jump to the conclusion that Kim was having an affair with her business associate, but at the same time, there was something pulling at the coattails of my mind. Something was trying to remind me: "Hey buddy, haven't you heard all of this before? Remember? Remember the friend whose husband was spending a lot of time away from the family on his private boat because he needed some time alone to 'sort out his feelings'? And because they were middle-aged, devout Catholics, she swore up and down that her husband couldn't possibly be having an affair? Remember how you told her that you had a feeling that indeed he was having an affair, and eventually it turned out that the devout, middle-aged Catholic father of three was indeed 'getting his head together' on his boat with a cute young thing some 25 years his junior? (Of course, the naïve little wife was devastated.) Even though you don't like the tone of some of your deeper inner feelings, don't ignore them Bernard. Sometimes, you're right, you know."

It was obvious to me that Kim was putting way too much negative energy into her relationship with that man, whom she now saw as the scum of the earth, for their relationship to be as purely business-related as she would have had me believe. When I asked her why didn't she just let him go and stop dealing with him, she replied that he was an important person in her business, with whom she needed to remain in good grace if she was going to succeed. A good story, but it's been played before.

Those who counsel know that people usually come to them with partial stories. They seldom are willing to tell the whole story for fear of indicting themselves and, perhaps, smearing their characters in the process. Their intent is usually to go no further than is necessary to smear the other person's character. Well, this isn't really a problem for the seasoned professional counselor. It would, however, constitute a problem for amateurs and the overly-sympathetic, and there are many who fall into this category. They are bleeding hearts, really. Counselors who are willing to buy into myriad fabrications that people offer concerning their lives will have lots of business, for the universe will serve them with an endless stream of clients. Regardless, these counselors will soon find themselves becoming as confused as their clients, and will, in turn, end up searching for someone to counsel themselves. I've seen this pattern occur with a number of my friends who are professional counselors — both spiritual and psychological.

There were a couple of other telltale events that occurred with

Kim that eventually helped me to assist her in resolving her conflict, one of which I'll recount. It involved an assignment that I gave her to do during the first three weeks of the workshop.

I'll never forget how shocked I was the first time I went to consult with my first spiritual counselor and he gave me an assignment that would require large chunks of my time twice a day. At the time I had a demanding job with lots of responsibilities, as well as a very busy life. I didn't believe that there was any way that I could squeeze in a single new activity, but I did. My counselor put it to me point blank. If I wanted to be healed, I was going to have to change my life. The reason my life wasn't working in the first place was because of the way *I* had structured it. It only made sense, logically, that if I wanted it to improve, I had to be willing to make some changes. Somehow that had never dawned on me before.

Isn't it often this way? We say that we want something new in our lives, but we don't want it badly enough to give up certain patterns that have grown familiar. I'm sure there are times when we all want to have our cake and eat it too.

The assignment that I gave to Kim was this: I told her to take an hour a day, three days a week, and leave home and go for a walk, leaving her notes, tapes, Walk-Mans™ and all other trappings of our "modern," technological society behind. I knew that this would be difficult for her to do. Sure enough, she protested even before I could finish giving her the assignment.

"Where am I gonna find time to go for a walk? You obviously don't understand what my schedule is like."

"For crying out loud, Kim," I countered. "Here you are racked by some kind of physical ailment that is threatening your life, but you don't want to change one thing to facilitate the process of your own healing. Are you willing to make a commitment to your life or not? The decision is entirely up to you."

Not to be deterred, she shot back, "Sure, I'm willing to do whatever it takes to get well, but you don't know all the things that I'm already doing."

"Maybe you're doing too much," I suggested.

"Well look, I have this special diet that I eat every day. It takes me a couple of hours to shop for all these really hard-to-find ingredients that I have to have, and then to cook them on top of that."

I would have fared better talking to a wall. Having gone off on another one of her defensive tangents, she wasn't even hearing me. Still, I tried to contact her. "I understand, Kim. I know it's not easy dealing with what you're dealing with. Believe me, we are all behind you in this workshop. We all want you to get well, and we are going to support you in every way that we can. All I'm saying is that what you're doing apparently is not working, at least so far as I can tell.

"I understand your concern about diet. On one level, I know that diet is very important, but on another level, it won't make any difference at all what you eat — within reason. Food is good. Food is not your enemy. But if you feel that the special diet that you're maintaining is helping you right now, then by all means, keep it. It's your life. I certainly don't know what's good for you. All I'm saying is that you are so intense and self-absorbed. It's imperative that you do something to break out of that vicious cycle. You need to literally stop and smell the roses. Do you have any flowers or plants in your house?"

She had calmed down a bit by that time. "No, but I used to have a couple of houseplants — what do you call the one with the green leaves that's shaped like this (she circumscribed a shape like a small oval in thin air)? You know, they're real common. Everybody has them because they're supposed to be easy to grow. Somebody gave me one of those, but it died. I just can't be bothered. That's why I don't have any children or pets; I just don't need the responsibility of taking care of anything right now."

What fascinated me about Kim was how closely her logic paralleled how I used to think when I was miserable. It was as if God had cloned me and changed me to the opposite sex and then sent me to participate in my own workshop. I was beginning to think that maybe He had. I even knew what was coming next. Her next ploy would be to justify her current attitude to the group. She'd probably tell them a tale about a noble service she'd rendered on behalf of a friend, an animal or plant.

"What you all ought to understand is that I came from a large family back East where I grew up with dogs and plants and everything. There was always a dog around our house, and I used to feed him and take him for walks and everything. I don't know why, but animals always seem to like me. We get along so well. When I make the money that I'm expecting to make in this new business, I can get the house that I want and get out of this apartment that I'm in, and then I can have plants and a dog too. That's the way I really want to live. After all, that's the kind of life that I'm used to."

"Okay Kim, I understand that, but all I'm suggesting is that you take some time off about three times a week and go for a stroll. Engage yourself in a walking meditation during which you attune yourself to everything around you. Listen to all the interesting sounds. Listen to nature. Listen to the birds. Listen to the flowers and see if you can hear them whispering. Maybe they're trying to talk to you."

Again she interrupted with a protest. "I just don't see what going for a walk is gonna do for me. I'm up to about six miles already in my jogging, whenever I have a chance to go to the track. I used to jog twice a week, although lately I haven't been feeling good enough to go. As you can see, I'm already out there exposed to nature."

"I understand that, Kim, but what you're talking about and what I'm talking about are two different things. When you're out on the track, you're engaged in a competitive thing. You're always telling me about the men that you compete with. That's good, too, but I want you to do something entirely different. I can't explain to you exactly how this exercise is going to work. If you want promises and guarantees concerning the outcome, I can't give you that. This is an exploratory, spiritual process that is going to put you in touch with ethereal forces that will reveal new information to you about your body, your job, and that perfect relationship that you desire. After you get clear, it will all begin to happen quite naturally."

Our dialogue moved in circles as she tried to convince me that she was already meditating more hours a day than everyone else she knew. In fact, she periodically engaged in marathon meditations, reminiscent of how college students stay up all night to cram for final exams. She just couldn't understand why she wasn't getting more benefits, considering all the work that she was doing.

Eventually, I let her be. I told her that it was totally up to her whether she chose to do the exercise or not. By the final week of the workshop, when I asked everyone to share accounts of their transformational experiences, I learned that Kim hadn't completed a single exercise or inconvenienced herself by taking a single walk. I was not surprised. Kim was the archetypal bottom line businesswoman. She couldn't foresee any benefit, so she didn't waste any of her resources.

There was something about Kim that bothered me, however. I could never quite get a bead on what it was that was driving Kim in what seemed like a helter-skelter, discombobulated life. In a sense, she was truly an enigma, and it was clear to me that she wanted it to remain that way. Nonetheless, it eventually all made sense. Eventually I found out that Kim had HS2. It came out many months after the workshop was over during one of our lengthy telephone sessions.

You have to use your imagination to understand how Kim must have felt. She had already accepted that the essence of her womanhood was ruined. On the first level, that is exactly what HS2 does to you; it destroys whatever sexual image you may have had of yourself. Thus Kim must have reasoned that since she could never be fulfilled, she might as well opt for the next best thing and be rich. Thus she was literally killing herself trying to compensate for the loss of her womanhood. I'm not saying that she really lost it, but only that she probably held that perception.

There was just too much commonality between Kim's history and mine for our meeting to have been merely accidental, and it's a testimony to my own naïveté that the possibility didn't occur to me earlier. There are no accidents in God's Universe. I had always believed that like attracts like. Now I really know it.

It has occurred to me, and I'm convinced that it's true, a lot of single people who are so afraid of getting married or risking a relationship have HS2. They are simply using their careers and all that madness about weird diets and spiritual purity and not wanting to be used or held back as excuses for not opening up. They are deathly afraid to face up to the truth about their lives. This is not to say that everyone should want to be in a committed relationship. They shouldn't and they won't. There's room enough in this world for all points of view and every conceivable lifestyle, but it is still true that most people both want and need a faithful companion. When people *en masse* begin turning against the grain of innate human desire, there must always be a cause behind it. Though it's the nature of us intellectuals to fabricate complex causes for everything, I believe that true causes are always simple.

MORE ON MYTHS

Jesus, the greatest semi-recorded spiritual healer, was no more concerned with what happened to a person *after* he spoke the word of truth for him or her. Even at his advanced state of enlightenment, he was not overly concerned with results.

Some may argue, yes, but he healed everyone he prayed for. Don't believe it! In the parable of the 10 lepers that he prayed for, only one remained healed — the one who came back to thank him. Now he didn't put a curse on the ungrateful nine or neutralize his prayer to punish them for their ungratefulness. It was not necessary. No — what the parable teaches is that their attitudes, or consciousness, was not sufficiently developed to sustain the healings that he had invoked. Such is life.

Now I can apply the same deduction to myself, but it leads me to a startling and uncomfortable revelation: **I DON'T HAVE THE CONSCIOUSNESS TO SUSTAIN A HEALING.** This is true! — painful, but true nevertheless. Some of my teachers would condemn me for uttering such a statement, but I say screw those narrow-minded pedagogues. By so doing, I am able to release a whole lot of guilt and go on with my life, laughing and smiling and having quite a bit of fun — at my admittedly lesser level of consciousness. This does not mean that I am complacent. Though I am satisfied, I am never complacent. It is necessary by universal edict that I, like everyone else, continue to develop spiritually and expand in consciousness, but I cannot force this process. This thing must unfold to each one of us according to God's own timetable, not according to what's written in some book. Our bodies don't care a thing about what's written in some book. Sufficient unto today is the goodness thereof. Thus I accept my life the way it is — no apologies.

Is it possible to gain something that you have not yet earned by the gradual development of your consciousness? If so, then why does it take a doctor four or more additional years of specialized practice to learn how to perform brain surgery? If the way some metaphysicians and New Agers think were correct, any medical student should be able to utter a few affirmations and then qualify as a brain surgeon. We students of Truth have to be careful not to get caught up in using the power of mind to manipulate effects. Students of New Thought/metaphysics do this all the time — bear witness to or demonstrate a single dramatic event and then soar off proclaiming themselves healers. But I've been around these spiritual circles long enough to observe the course that the lives of some of these sensationalists have taken. After all, time does reveal all. The reputed healings either shifted, did not last, or turned out to be incomplete. Their benefactors rarely seemed better off a few months later. How could they? It would be antithetical to principle if it were possible.

My role in this life is to practice the Presence of God every day as consistently as I can until the day arrives when my consciousness is truly changed. Then, and only then, so-called healing will be as natural as so-called disease is today. Now I don't know if that day will arrive in this life or in lives to come, and neither do I care. Honestly, if one really believes in the eternality of life, as I do, why would he ever shackle himself or herself with such a concern? This is where all the heaviness originates, the mental anguish and so forth. Rightly regarded, the occurrence of HS2 is as awesome and phenomenal as any instantaneous healing of cancer. It certainly amazes me.

There are moments when I'm able to glimpse this thing just right and it almost brings tears of joy to my eyes just to ponder how magnificent the mind must be that could create HS2. If you think

I'm crazy, that's understandable, but this is the truth. Each case of HS2 should exemplify to us how marvelously and perfectly the principles of life work. This is not to extol the virtues of being sick or diseased. What I'm alluding to is hard to explain, but I can grasp the potential for all possibilities as much in disease as in so-called miracle healings. The same mind that produces one can produce the other. What we have to do is figure out how to reverse the laws that we have been using and commence to create the consciousness that can produce the opposite. Admittedly, this is no small order, but all we need do at this juncture is get a grasp of this idea conceptually. It is the epitome of faith to be willing to work hard to embody an abstract idea without having definitive evidence of where it will lead you.

Things can only remain in place as long as there's a corresponding force sufficient to keep them there. In the domain of the individual, that force is consciousness. With all due respect to what the *Bible* says in one reference about transformation taking place in the twinkling of an eye, it takes years for the average one of us to change our consciousness. I'm a fairly intelligent and disciplined student of spiritual principle, and I can tell you that I haven't been able to make this thing work instantaneously where HS2 is concerned. Neither have most of my New Thought friends. In a few instances I have seen my prayers result in instantaneous healing, but I don't want to tout those cases as the norm.

The "twinkling of an eye" experiences are 10-point, "oh wow!" experiences but they don't usually last. They merely mark the point at which the long and arduous struggle to change one's consciousness begins to take place. Eat a piece of cheese cake and it tastes good. There are people who would die for a piece — do they not jeopardize their diets and health for it? — but the joy of eating it doesn't last. Unfortunately. And look what people put themselves through for the intense pleasure of sexual orgasm. Even congressmen and ministers who have everything to lose have been known to make fools of themselves for ill-advised romps in the hay, in spite of the fact that the pleasure that they risked so much for is ephemeral. In the ideal, the only thing lasting about a sexual encounter is the love that's fomented, the marriage that's initiated or nurtured and the child that's conceived as a result of the encounter.

If Earth is a school and if God placed you here for the long haul, what sense would it make to rush through the experience of being here? What kind of school would it be if you could instantaneously bypass all the classes and avoid enduring the time that it takes to learn meaningful lessons?

When you allow yourself to probe deeply enough to ponder the true meaning of time, you will realize that no time is sacred or special or even real in an ultimate sense. Time is real on the relative or human plane, but in Spirit there is no time or space. The more we align our thinking and being and feeling with the truth about Spirit, the more we shall realize that we are connected to all of our possibilities at any given time. When the realization finally sets in, it will take the urgency out of all our desires.

In metaphysics cancer is considered to be a perfect manifestation of repressed stress. Likewise, heart attacks and strokes are considered to be perfect solutions to over-reactionary, insensitive or unloving ways of dealing with stress. You witness a lot of these diseases in office environments. I've seen people manifest horrible automobile accidents, strokes, aneurysms, heart attacks, and triple bypass operations just to get some time off from work. I won't even mention alcohol and drug dependencies.

If you ask for time off because you can't cope, you might be laughed at or fired. Isn't this how we think? At the minimum your peers and management will begin to question whether you are professional or serious or tough enough to handle the assignment at hand. They'll get even with you at your annual review. Everybody knows this to be true. Or is it? However, if you tell them you're going to have a triple bypass operation, you'll receive lots of sympathy, and when you do go back, they'll understand when you tell them that you don't want to take on certain stressful, special assignments.

I've talked about this confidentially with a number of co-workers over the years. Many have agreed with me after honestly reviewing their own histories that most of their accidents and medical emergencies were totally unnecessary. These people were just over-stressed time bombs waiting to explode.

Industrial workers should also thank God for car pools. They are the only devices which have assisted many a burnt-out career worker in saving face. One of the standing jokes at work is how various of the old-timers use this convenient alibi for cutting out on time each day instead of habitually working late to impress the boss.

Many of us who are careerists, when forced to miss work for an extended period due to a medical emergency, undergo a veritable cornucopia of mixed emotions? On one hand, we hate to take the time off for fear that we will lose momentum in our careers. On the other hand, if we take the time off, we tend to feel relieved from the everyday business pressures. Then there's the darker side of our natures where I believe we often receive a rush of twisted pleasure from becoming the center of attention at work for a change. All of a sudden, and perhaps for the first time, we are being noticed. Who hasn't daydreamed at one time or another of being able to do exactly what he or she wanted to do *with* the company's blessings? I'd wager that we all have. It's just too bad that the average person has to wind up strapped to a hospital bed before he or she can enjoy this freedom.

We live in an age where most Americans are literate. Ours is an age where we are encouraged — indeed, forewarned — that we had better take control over our own lives. When it comes to our bodies and the whole milieu of health, homeostasis, preventive measures, exercise and medicine, our approach today is very sophisticated and interventionist. No longer are we expected to sit idly by while the doctor pricks and probes and works his or her magic upon our person from on high. Thus we feel that it is our right to intervene in our own wellness processes.

Being so literate, we go to the library and bone up on whatever it is that we have. Else, we borrow one of those "Everything You Ever Wanted To Know" books from a neighbor or co-worker down at the office and spend an evening becoming educated on whatever it is that ails us. While we are pursuing this approach to "Name that Symptom," chances are that we will just happen upon some list article in *Essence, Cosmopolitan* or *Readers' Digest* while idling in the supermarket check-out line. It will have a catchy title, such as "Seven Easy Steps To Determining If You Have...." If not that, surely we will happen upon a radio or television talk show or weekly news magazine feature proffering a panel of experts sprouting all kinds of wisdom from between the pages or each one's latest book on the disease of the hour.

Though all of this may sound great so far, it is riddled throughout by a common problem: There is only so much good news to go around. Let's face it. There just isn't enough good news of high entertainment value to sustain the daily broadcasting of news programs and publication of thousands of newspapers and magazines across this land. I see no reason why any newspaper should be published more than once a week.

Good news, like truth, is often bland and non-sensational, and it certainly doesn't sell! As a result, most of what you're going to hear or read is chock-full of horror stories and negative statistics, stories concerning how many people have whatever, and how it's going to become an epidemic within five years, etc. We have heard such horror stories about AIDS, and before that, about HS2. This is the way it is and this is the way it is going to be for as long as this is the material that sells books and magazines and news stories. After discovering all of this "knowledge," in most cases a person will be worse off than before. The human mind just isn't equipped to handle such a constant barrage of negative material without paying a dear price, especially when a person is in the early stages of experiencing disorder.

You know how we humans are when we think we're coming down with something. We would swear that we have every symptom listed in the medical encyclopedia. Then every time we stumble across an article warning of a new threat, there we go assuming a brand new worry all over again. It's easy to see why studies have shown that at least 80 percent of patient visits to physicians turn out to be mental or psychosomatic in nature. Let's face it: we're all nuts! When you are at home alone lying in bed and you suddenly experience a sharp pain in your chest, what is your first thought? Depending on your age and history, of course, chances are you are certain that you are having the long-feared heart attack. Well sure, it could be, but just think of all the false alarms you and I probably have had over our lifetimes.

I developed a series of neurologically-induced problems characterized by this kind of drama when I was just 20. How could something then construed to have been so serious seem so preposterous in retrospect? What justification is there for a normal, healthy, 20-year-old male to be obsessed with the fear of having a heart attack? How can we expect doctors to seriously consider our every complaint when it is clear that at least 80 percent of the time we are experiencing conditions that don't even exist? In many cases we may not be any better off than if we did not know nearly as much. As frightening as it may sound, we might be better off to simply live until we die. Maybe that's why the *Bible* asks, "What man by taking thought can add one cubit to his stature?"

The times that I have been most affected by HS2 have been when I've allowed my life to gradually get out of balance. It can be so subtle. I tend to work assiduously on a number of different projects day in and day out, dividing my time between my aerospace engineering job and my writing and publishing business. Thus I arise with the early morning sun and seldom rest or retire before midnight, even on weekends. Even then, I hate going to bed. So this is one of the areas in which I am prone to become unbalanced. Then I have to remind myself to retire an hour earlier each night, take a short vacation with my wife or, perhaps, just run down to the beach and fritter away some time during the weekend with no intention of being accountable.

Another major area that I have to watch is my diet. I tend to go on binges, especially when I'm working under that stress of a deadline over a long period of time, which occurs often. It might be a situation where I binge on junk food or vending machine food, especially if I'm working in my engineering office after hours. During such times, only junk food is available on the premises. Of course, with a little planning all of this could be overcome. Clearly, there is no excuse for not taking control over one's life. But...this is another part of my reality, and if I'm going to be honest, I need to admit how things really are, as opposed to how they *should* be.

The net result of all of this is that my system tends to get out of balance — not only in my body, but also in my mind. You know the old expression: You are what you eat. Whereas I refuse to take this to extremes, I can attest to the fact that when I recapture my control and pull myself back into balance, HS2 episodes subside and I become normal again in due time — usually. Lest I sound too smug, let me re-emphasize that there are no absolute formulas.

Despite what some New Age practitioners may tout, healing is not just an issue of diet. It's more than a physical issue. Even when my diet has been "perfect" — for example during the 14 months that I practiced vegetarianism and fasted and meditated — I still experienced flare-ups. It's a complicated issue. It can't be completely figured out mentally or reduced to a recipe, or else somebody would have written that book by now.

Another observation. I have many friends on the spiritual path who are vegetarians of one category or another. You know that there are many types of veggies, right? Some don't eat any eggs, some avoid milk and there's still this larger class who eat only fish and chicken because they don't consider these flesh products to be "meat." Well, I'll accept that argument the day I'm able to plant an egg and lettuce seeds and have chicken salad grow in my garden. I have news for these people: Fish is meat! And so is chicken. Today, I'm no longer a veggie, nor do I think it's necessary to be one. Though vegetarianism works marvelously for some people, I have known too many mystics who ate pig feet and barbecue chicken for the avoidance of meat to be a prerequisite for healing. Why else in Luke 8:55 would Jesus have ordered that meat be given to Jairus' daughter immediately after he snatched her from the jaws of death?

Anyhow, the most common feature among the overwhelming majority of the veggies that I have encountered over the years is self righteousness. You can feel it when you are in their presence. But here's the rub: I haven't known one yet who didn't binge on desserts and other sugar-laden sweets. Don't give me that brown sugar or honey substitution argument either, because there really isn't any difference. When you're out of balance, you're out of balance and you have to deal with it. However, you can never deal with a problem unless you first admit it. In most cases when someone is acting holier-than-thou, all you have to do is peer a wee bit under their rugs or peep through their back doors and you'll find that they are merely exchanging one obvious indulgence for another, more subtle one. Speaking for myself, every time I have gotten on my high horse, I have found this to be true in my life. Life is humbling and I am no longer going to be a hypocrite.

Up until about 1986 I was an alcoholic − not an obvious one, but a quiet, respectable one. I was the kind that would have become self righteously indignant had someone suggested that I was an alcoholic. Though I started on scotch, rum, vodka and mixed cocktails of every sort, I later forsook hard liquor completely for wine, which I thought was better. I convinced myself that there was no way that I could be an alcoholic at that point, although I was consuming large quantities of wine. How self righteous I was concerning my newfound passion. I fashioned myself to be a connoisseur, which is a far cry from being a common drunk, isn't it? I mean I was even a member of a prestigious enology club. Oh, to be honest I was quite a scholar on wines. I loved studying wines, visiting wineries and participating in tasting events, but guess what: At my job I went out for lunch three or four times each week and rather tidily siphoned away upwards of half a liter of wine every day. Though I categorized my case under the broad heading of "social drinker," the truth is that I was never satisfied until I felt that all too familiar buzz that only alcohol can produce. Still, I wasn't an alcoholic, mind you.

Although my fondness for the grape used to cause many non-HS2-related problems in my life, my drinking was one crutch that I could not seem to kick. For years I suffered from a condition that I later found out was called narcolepsy. I was known for falling asleep at every conceivable inopportune moment − at important meetings on the job, at parties, at movies, at night clubs, on dates, while driving. Of course, no one could convince me that anything was wrong with me. Sometimes in night clubs I would fall asleep while sitting up front directly in front of the band! Clearly, I had a problem.

At one time, at Marsha's behest, I even submitted to treatment by a psychiatrist for narcolepsy, but the medication didn't do me much good. Nothing helped until I finally got fed up with being tired and sleepy all the time. It was then that I faced the truth, bit the bullet and let go of all forms of alcohol — forever.

Now I realize that those who have been inducted into the Alcoholics Anonymous (AA) tradition will cry, "No, no, don't ever say 'forever.' " Their theory is that you are never cured of alcoholism. Well, that's their theory. I have my own. Whereas I have great respect for AA and their marvelous record, AA is not mysticism. They employ spiritual methods but stop far short of conforming to an inherently consistent spiritual philosophy. At best, AA is an intermediate step between total dysfunction and spiritual understanding. Once you attain true unity with Spirit through meditation, understanding and, eventually, transformation, you don't have to spend the rest of your life saying "I am an alcoholic"; you can declare with authority: "I am cured!" I know that I am cured of alcoholic desire. Unlike so many disciples of AA — and I bless them — my goal in life is not merely to get through another day or just function in the world, I want to truly know God. What I'm touting is above humanism, above psychology, beyond self-help benefits and even above self actualization. What I am talking about is absolute and complete transformation.

When I looked soberly at how alcohol made me feel and act, I thought, "How ridiculous for an intelligent man to act this way! The stuff isn't doing anything positive for me." All of a sudden it hit me: This isn't the way God wants us to use our free will. Miraculously, I have never experienced another single problem with narcolepsy since that moment. Of course, I also let go of Marsha, as well. That was a move which alleviated a major cause of stress. As a fringe benefit of giving up alcohol, I seemed to experience a significant drop in HS2 flare-ups. I don't want to make too much out of this factor, but that's the way it seemed at the time.

Another one of my dietary addictions is caffeinated teas. I've experienced quite a few negative effects from tanking up on caffeinated teas. Given all that I've read and heard about the negative effects of caffeine on HS2 activation, I don't know how much of my experience is real and how much is a result of suggestion. This is a continuous problems that all metaphysicians face. As a reaction to my reaction, I have learned to tolerate some of the non-caffeinated teas that are so popular today, but I must admit that I am not sold on that weak, *new agey*, ersatz stuff. I still enjoy the solid punch that you can only receive from a stiff shot of caffeine. It's amazing how many addictions there are, many of which we aren't even aware until we begin giving up old habits. Ever since I discovered hot tea, heaven to me has been the experience of sipping a cup of super Ceylon, Earl Grey or Irish blend to neutralize the briskness of an early morning chill. There's nothing that breaks in the morning more appropriately. And oh how I love those black pekoe/orange pekoe blends!

You may question, "Is caffeine really harmful? Is it necessary for a person with HS2 to give it up?" Well, I certainly haven't found it to be harmful to me, but it should come as no surprise that when I find myself drinking too much of it mindlessly, I can get pretty wired. I've read that a sufficient quantity of caffeine will do that to you. Again, balance seems to be the best policy. I don't know what's good for others and I don't know what's harmful. The problem with hard and fast dietary rules for persons in need of healing is this: If they hear that a certain substance is deleterious to their condition, a certain percentage are prone to apply linear thinking and deduce that if they eliminate all of the suspected agent, they will then be healed. If a lot is harmful, a little is better, so none must be best. Well, this sounds logical enough, but in this case I doubt if it's true.

I refuse to be fanatical (anymore). Life is too beautiful not to be fully enjoyed and lived. I deliberately shy away from giving specific lifestyle advice. What people put into their bodies is important, but no more important than their accumulated histories, and definitely no more important than what they allow to enter their minds.

The following question is one that I've had to ask myself many times. You may also want to ask it of yourself:

WOULD YOU AND COULD YOU GIVE UP ALL OF YOUR ADDICTIONS JUST TO IMPROVE YOUR HEALTH?

Some may think, "Certainly a person would give us anything to be rid of HS2," but such is not necessarily the case. Although it sounds good in theory, I doubt if most people would or could. Many times I have tried to give up lists of habits because I read somewhere that I would be healthier, but I found myself relapsing into old comfortable habits in due time. One thing I've discovered: Change is extremely difficult. I'm talking about real, lasting change.

We shouldn't be too hasty in getting rid of habits. The first step we need to take is that of respecting our habits. They are there for a reason. I've experimented with my cravings, addictions, fasting and discipline, and what I have found is that as soon as I stop indulging in one addiction, I tend to find myself replacing it with another one. The scam is that some addictions are public (for example, smoking), while others are not (for example, sex or masturbation). Eventually, we must ask ourselves: Who's fooling whom? This is why it is so cynical to be holier-than-thou. More than likely, the pious or religious person is the one with the most private addictions.

I was unable to master my addictions and break out of my on-again/off-again cycles until I first *embraced* my habits. This doesn't mean that I advocate making excuses for our habits. It is paradoxical that you have to first respect or embrace your habits before you can effectively get rid of them. In this sense, embracing is the opposite of condemning. It is not effective to condemn your habits – or yourself for having them. You have to *lovingly* let them go. In other words, I had to first train my mind to stop believing that certain foods were bad. [Note: This does not pertain to hard drugs or illegal drugs. Except for marijuana, I have no experience with illegal drugs. If you have problems with hard drugs, please consult with a chemical dependency professional.]

Today, I refuse to regard sweets or caffeinated teas as harmful or bad. So far as I have been able to discern, everything has its purpose in different people's lives at different times. For many years, these substances have served my needs and I have enjoyed them. I want to praise everything that God has created, so let me now bless them, rather than knock them. I'm not the same person today. Something is leading me toward a more disciplined lifestyle. Every aspect of my being is screaming out the message that I'm past due for a change.

During one three-year experiment, I completely avoided eating sweets. Ironically, I'm healthier now than I was then, and a whole lot less self righteous. During my self-imposed purity, I was so preachy and intolerant of others that it was sickening — even to me! It's a wonder I had any friends at all. Not to say that I'm not still obnoxious, but a deeper, more sincere spirituality has rendered me so mellow that it's even surprised me. I'm certainly tolerant of others when I see them treading in my old footsteps.

My approach to life today is one of balance and moderation. I don't celebrate Christmas or exchange gifts, but I certainly respect the joy such rituals bring in the lives of my friends. If I could indulge in these practices in good conscience, I would. But something within my mental makeup has changed irreversibly, and I can no longer engage in certain practices.

I want to eat sweets occasionally. I want to enjoy all kinds of teas from time to time, but without going overboard. The key is enjoy these substances without letting them control me. And the key to enjoying them is to first learn to respect them. Sex in a committed relationship is enjoyable, but without respect for your partner there will be no enjoyment. At least, not for long.

Discipline is a major ingredient in this process, but it's not the whole cake. I can do discipline. It's no longer a challenge to avoid whole categories of things. The problem is, I haven't discovered any way to avoid certain essentials, such as sugar, without becoming weird.

Does God want us to live ascetic, pleasureless lives? I should think not. We aren't glorifying the Father when we live this way — at least that's not my idea of God. To exude a cheerful, joyous spirit is also an appropriate way of demonstrating the glory of God. I have no desire to live each day as an ascetic with a self-sacrificing scowl on my face. To understand the true nature of God is to discover that there is no power in sugar or caffeine or any normal, legal food stuff when taken in balance, but that all power rests in Spirit. I guess what I'm saying is this:

IF YOU MUST HAVE HS2, YOU MAY AS WELL BE HAPPY.

My situation has changed dramatically in recent years. I have become so comfortable with myself as I am that HS2 just doesn't bother me much anymore. Since getting married to a most remarkable woman in 1988, I have been basking in the warm glow of unconditional acceptance. Of course, it was I who initiated the change by setting the right laws in motion way back in 1981, long before I ever met my wife. What more could one ask from life? I have finally validated what I had always accepted on faith: Unconditional love *is* the greatest healing agent in existence.

In summarizing my beliefs concerning all of the 10 great myths, I have come to realize the fatuity of adhering to false beliefs or folklore concerning the alleged power inherent in any practice, habit, list item or formula as a way of impoving or controlling my life. Therefore, I released all undue concern with taking vitamins, minerals or natural herbs, avoiding stress, sugar, meat, sex or relationships. I even released the thought that I could become a good person by going to church or praying, When I gave up smoking and drinking, it was not to gain relief from HS2. As I eventually learned, the motivating principle had to be purer than that.

Finally, I realized that there is no power in what is commonly referred to as positive thinking, nor is there any magic or miracle power in meditation, affirmations or visualization. The paradox is that many of these practices are helpful and necessary in the expansion of our consciousness and the fulfillment of our higher purpose for living, but the student who invokes them with the hope that they are going to magically heal him or her of HS2 within a certain time frame may be in for a major disappointment.

UCLA EXPERIMENTAL DRUG PROGRAM

Humanistic professionals, sociologists and medical researchers alike, despite all efforts to date, have not even begun to appreciate the impact of HS2 on the life of the individual. Sure, there have been studies, but they have been few and of narrow impact. None has come close to uncovering the deep, dark truth which underlies the surface niceties of some of the associated clinical questionnaires. I know. I have participated in a few studies of this sort myself. Even when talking to the doctors and other professionals who apparently are devoting their lives to helping those with HS2, I can tell you that there is still a large part of ourselves as patients that we hold back. Though these professional groups are among the most caring in dealing with the sensitivities of HS2 subjects, they are still severely lacking. Maybe it's them; maybe it's us. Still, the thing that dominates during programs like this is the shame, at least that was the case with me when I participated in a study of an experimental drug for treating HS2 at the prestigious University of California at Los Angeles (UCLA).

To my great surprise, even the staff associated with this program turned out to be ill-equipped to deal with my deeper emotional problems as an HS2 experimental patient. I mean, there was absolutely no sensitivity to be found among the entire staff. Mind you, back in those days during the early '80s, I was neither in touch with nor verbal about my deeper emotional problems as they related to HS2. All I knew was that I was angry, that life had cheated me and that the medical profession ought to be coming up with some answers soon. But the philanthropic staff of do-gooders at UCLA were so clinical and remote as they asked me the questions about my behavior, sex life, and frequency of outbreaks. They didn't have a clue concerning how to make me or others in my study group feel comfortable. The result of all this was that I tended toward prevarication when responding to some of their questions. I wasn't that spiritually-aware in those days, my main motivation being a desperate desire to be cured. I lied because I didn't want to look bad in comparison to the others in the study.

This may sound fatuous to someone who has never suffered the shame of having a socially unmentionable disease, but I wondered what would the program administrators think of me if I turned out to be the only one in the study group who didn't respond to the treatment. Or what if I was having more frequent outbreaks than the rest of the population? When I would provide the doctor with a trial number in response to his question concerning "frequency of outbreaks," he would inform me with characteristic monotonic clinical detachment that my response was about normal, less than, or greater than the norm. I don't think that he thought I was paying attention to every cue as I seemed to casually drop certain data on him. I strived to make every gesture seem casual. You know how it is: You can't let on that you are as desperate as you are. If I was going to participate in a program like this, I certainly wasn't going to let the doctor know how frightened I was of every sign or implication. While he was testing me, I was testing him. I was simply floating trial balloons by him to see how *he* would react.

Unbeknown to him, I was watching his very body English: every blink of his eye, frown, gasp, or involuntary tightening up of facial muscles as I sat there and responded to his questions. What you have to remember is that my life was obsessed by HS2 at the time. I thought that having HS2 was the worst thing in the world. My self esteem was zilch, relationships were horrible and everything seemed to be going to pot, and I blamed it all on HS2. I was convinced that if I could just rid myself of this blight I would be happy. It was with this attitude that I eagerly signed up for the experimental program at UCLA. When a patient is desperate, he is prone to cling to the slightest nuance as a sign of hope. If someone in a white coat says *maybe*, the patient interprets it as meaning *absolutely*!

It may be that doctors don't often think of the possibility that their patients may be reasonably intelligent (if this kind of behavior can be considered intelligent). I can't speak for others, but I was able to read my doctor's emotions like a book. My sole motivation for participating in the program was to find out what the doctor knew. I was still fairly naïve in those days. I harbored the belief that if I could just put my life in the hands of a doctor, everything would be all right. They were supposed to know things that were beyond the reaches of mere mortals like myself. Since I was in a blind study which consisted of a control group, I didn't know if I was even supposed to be getting better, or if, perhaps, others on the same medication as I were getting better results. Of course, I wanted to know these things, and I wanted to know them instantly. As I said, I was desperate! I had no intention of waiting until the end of the study (which seemed like an eternity at the time) to be cured. I figured, "Hey, they've got the drug and I'm gonna get it." I had no doubt but that it would work. Thus, during my little five-minute sessions with the doctor every week of so, I was searching for any sign of a hint in his face or in his body language concerning the efficacy of his concoction.

Then there was the office staff...his assistants. Confiding in the doctor was one thing, but I wasn't too comfortable having all of these people know my business. Although the doctor donned the traditional garb of objectivity — the mandatory, sterile white lab jacket — and, I trust, he had taken the Hippocratic Oath, what about the hospital's administrative staff? They weren't required to take the oath, and you know how people who work in offices are. What if somebody worked there who happened to know me? What if one of the staff knew somebody that I worked with? At that time such a revelation would have been devastating to the personality that I thought I was. I had no desire to be outed. There was no way that anybody was going to convince me that the office staff could be depended upon to maintain my confidence.

Let's face it. Many of these people get their kicks the same way that people in the world at large titillate themselves — by making fun of other people's misfortunes. Apparently, these are concerns that aren't often addressed in experimental medical research of this nature. Besides, how much could the doctors do anyway? Just because a person has an M.D. doesn't mean that he or she can control all of the variables necessary to protect my best interests. And if the truth be told, the doctor wasn't that great himself. Oh, I was thankful to be in the program. When you're desperate, you're desperate. Nevertheless, this particular doctor had this thick foreign accent which was all but unintelligible, and to boot, he was about as sensitive as a shoe.

So I realized right away that it was up to me to protect my image. I have three sisters who work in hospitals as nurses or technical specialists. They are all skeptical of hospitals based on their awareness of what sometimes goes on behind the scene. Plus a number of my friends have gone through medical school and some of the stories they've told me would make a sailor wince. There are real human beings behind those sterile facades in hospitals — unfortunately. They are no worse than anybody else, which everyone knows. What everyone may not know is that neither are they any better than anybody else.

Yes, it was up to me to protect my image. If I was just emerging from a particularly difficult bout of infections, I just wasn't equipped to bring myself to admit that to the doctor. After all, what did he really care? He did nothing to destroy the notion in my mind that I was just another statistic in his blind research study. I was convinced that he didn't care about me as a person. Besides the accent and complete absence of personal charisma, he did nothing at all to help break down the wall between us.

He didn't even look up from his note pad to make eye contact with me when he asked questions of the most personal nature. In the hands of a doctor who was personable and who cared about his patients, my impressions from this study could have been totally different. After all, that's all healing really is — caring. First and foremost, healing takes place when the patient is made to feel genuinely cared for, or even loved. There's nothing else that a human being can do as a professional, because in Truth, God is the only healer. Even when the surgeon puts you under the knife, he or she must depend on God to take over and make you better. After he sews you up, his or her part is finished, whereas God's role has just begun. No doctor can tell you what will happen to you after that point. Like the least of us, all he or she can do after that point is trust and hope.

I knew that this research doctor wasn't particularly tuned into me as a person because he put me through the horrors of a placebo-based protocol, i.e., a new drug study where half the patients get the real thing and half receive a placebo. You can bet that the overwhelming concern of any intelligent patient in such a study is the fear that he may not be receiving the real drug, and thereby, is wasting his valuable time. This is a totally selfish attitude, I admit, but then the unaware person tends to be motivated primarily by selfish ends. There is no worse feeling than to agree to be a human guinea pig and not know whether you are taking harmless sugar pills or the real McCoy, especially when you think that the latter *might* make you better.

The flip side of the coin is that the experimental drug could make you worse. Actually, this is what I believe happened to me. My records indicated that the incidence, region, and severity of outbreaks dramatically increased under the medication that I was given. I was so embarrassed by this. I even felt empathy for the doctor to the point that I didn't want to disappoint him by telling him that his "wonder drug" was making me worse. That's not what he wanted to hear, professional objectivity notwithstanding. Remember: I was trained as a scientist, too. Scientific objectivity isn't all that it's cracked up to be. This may not be rational, but it is the truth about how I felt. Let me repeat that I was not a man who was spiritually-committed or aware at that time. I was still very much in the world — selfish, hedonistic and most definitely lost.

Of course, I realize today that my reactions to the experimental protocol were all mental. The "medicine" probably wasn't making me worse and it probably wasn't making me any better. Being as depressed, fearful and all around mentally confused as I was, there was no way that I was going to have a normal or neutral reaction to the placebo or medication. I didn't know it then, but the mind is just that powerful. What I brought to the progam was a highly confused mental atmosphere.

There is another subtlety to the experience of participating in a medical case study. By the time a person, such as I was, applies and is accepted to participate in such a program, he is ecstatic beyond belief. At that instant, I thought I had died and gone to heaven. When one is suffering, it doesn't take much to pump new hope into his or her life. Most of us live on promises and prayers, anyway.

Considering that all of the experts had repeatedly pronounced my condition as incurable, and here I had finally hooked up with a doctor who at least believed in the *possibility* of a cure, I knew right away that he was my kind of medical man. What's difficult as a patient is to remain objective, sensible and level-headed. As I mentioned before, if a doctor says "maybe," we tend to translate that to mean "absolutely." Reasonable or naught, it's hard not to.

Initially, when one is reeling from the shock of being forced to deal with the unmentionable, he or she will tend to defy all that is rational and put 100 percent faith in the doctor and his program. At such times, we are at maximum vulnerability and we wish so desperately to believe that it will work. Such unfounded hope provides the perfect setup for a calamitous fall. I must be Humpty Dumpty because in my life I have experienced a number of great falls, which have often led me to wonder just how many one person can take.

It is often said that a little bit of knowledge can be a dangerous thing. We humans are so comical, and in some ways so predictable, are we not? I knew very well what the literature said about the norms for HS2 flare-ups. My case seemed to be much worse, i.e., more active, than the norm, which created lots of anxiety within my mind — anxiety that I did not need.

Why is it that we are always comparing ourselves to somebody else's norm? I don't suppose that I'm the only person who's ever done this. We do this in hopes that we will discover that we are at least as good as, and preferably better than, the average person in the same boat as we. That would give us a little more hope and make us feel a little bit better. One thing is certain: We never wish to discover that we are the three sigma outlier on the negative side of the Gaussian curve (meaning much worse than average). But if one believes in norms, he must also believe in outliers, i.e., individual cases that are much better than or much worse than the norm. Today, I'm sure that the anxiety associated with my own vaunted knowledge was the greatest contributor to the higher level of outbreaks that I experienced. In my case the cure may have been part of the problem.

My anxiety was also heightened by having to leave work and

take significant blocks of time off to participate in this program. It's all so backwards. The amount of money we pay doctors in this society, you would think that they would schedule their hours for our convenience! But I had to take off frequently during the work day, which I managed without ever telling my co-workers and bosses the truth about where I was going. So I was stealthy. Lying has always been a problem for me, even in my unawakened state, but there was no way I was going to tell people on my job about this situation. I would have rather committed suicide.

Every time I arrived at UCLA, I was forever worried that I would run into someone that I knew. What if I ran into a close friend or a co-worker who was in the same program? Don't think that such an experience would have been a relief. The way I thought back then, I might have just fainted or suffered cardiac arrest. And what if I ran into someone as I was waiting in the venereal disease (this was before the term *sexually transmissible disease* became popular) section of the facility who didn't have HS2, and while he or she was talking to me, the receptionist came out and announced, "THIS SECTION IS FOR HERPES PATIENTS ONLY!"? Even if you're an exalted guru of assertiveness training, you still quake at the thought of these notions. I wouldn't have been able to tiptoe away or pretend that I was in the wrong area, because the receptionist was also the administrator for this special research program, and she knew me by sight. And the entire medical team was just that casual about calling your name or making announcements such as this. I guess none of them had HS2. Either that, or I was just too sensitive.

Despite all the jokes that have been made about hospital insensitivity, I guess it's just the nature of the beast. They've seen it all, so it must be hard for them to comprehend how a person could be so sensitive about having his business blasted from loud speakers throughout their hallowed halls.

Just recently, I converted out of a group practice medical plan that was conveniently-located and comfortable for me because of an inexcusably bad habit on the part of my primary care physician. After seeing a patient, he would go outside and stand next to his secretary's desk, within earshot of waiting patients, nurses and bustling medical center activity and dictate his medical case history into a tape recorder. Every time I bore witness to that scene, it made me cringe.

At UCLA not only did I fear the waiting room, but I also feared the laboratory. There was a laboratory at UCLA where we had to go regularly to have blood drawn and cultures sampled from lesions, but the discomforting thing about it was that this lab was not a dedicated HS2 lab. Neither was it co-located within the wing set up for the experimental HS2 study in the hospital. No, it was on another floor, in an entirely different wing of the hospital. Now the UCLA hospital complex is a mammoth, bewildering labyrinth of floors, corridors, elevators and basements. You could be murdered in one of its niches and not be discovered for days (as someone was recently). It's the kind of place that would intimidate Sherlock Holmes.

What must also be understood is that those of us in this program were marked people. We were labeled and tagged. When we went wandering around the halls, they knew who we were, and those in the know certainly didn't want to rub elbows with us. In this day of AIDS hysteria, the scene I'm describing may be difficult to imagine, especially since AIDS was not an American issue at that time. Regardless, we felt like lepers walking through the hallways side by side with "normal" patients.

If you've ever had to walk through the open corridors of a hospital with a bottle of fresh, warm pee in your hand, you know about one-tenth of the magnitude of the embarrassment that I felt. If you've ever been left in a hospital room stripped naked while various members of the hospital staff casually darted in and out of the vicinity to take care of routine hospital business, then you are beginning to get close. I realize, however, that these perceptions and complaints were my problem.

Here I am, like so many others in our privileged society, looking the proverbial gift horse in the mouth. Don't get me wrong, I was thankful for what the medical staff at UCLA did for me, and I often verbalized this to the individuals involved. For every staff member who shunned us and shunted us aside, there were dedicated laboratory technicians and administrators who did everything within their power and tight schedules to make us feel comfortable. It made an indelible impression on me to discover that such people actually exist. It also helped me to realize with unquestionable finality that I don't have the special stuff that is required to work in the medical profession. I forever tip my hat to the people who do. Thank you, UCLA, for at least trying.

What I've just described are some of the personal issues that I was dealing with while trying to find a way to be healed. Little did I suspect back then that one's mental state has a tremendous bearing on one's receptivity to healing. In fact, today I know that the state of mind that kept me prisoner in a totally degrading relationship for three long years was the very reason why I was ill in the first place. These factors cannot be treated as separate issues.

Though I believe that medicine alone can cure physical effects in many cases, studies such as the one in which I participated clearly point to the lack of consideration conventional medicine gives to the intangible mental and spiritual factors. Even if the subject were included in the medical school curriculum, it would be difficult for them to do it justice. To seriously treat such a subject, their teachers would have to be trained in spiritual and metaphysical principles. By design, physical science shall forever separate itself from in-depth investigation of the mental and spiritual aspects of healing, the true treatment of which could easily take the dedicated student a length of time equal to that of his regular medical curriculum.

Should a seriously disturbed, guilt-driven person, such as I was, enroll in a particular protocol run by a medical doctor who is neither sufficiently aware or properly trained to deal with the spiritual and mental factors, the chance of being healed of the causal condition is virtually nil. Sure, I may have had a bug in my bloodstream, but I also had a gaping hole in my spirit! Even if the medicine had worked, at best I would have had a temporary physical cure. How can an individual sustain good health when his or her spirit is sick? This clearly is not possible. Even if the physicians had been able to cure the bug, I would not have been healed because the underlying mental state would have remained the same. Thus in due time, I would have re-manifested a similar or worse condition.

There's another significant factor on which I wish to comment while I'm on the subject of doctors and researchers and how they deal with HS2. I have read articles about a number of doctors and nurses that have HS2 themselves. Possibly, some of those who were working in the UCLA program, or else someone dear to them, had it. Individuals seldom end up dedicating their lives to causes like this for no reason at all. It would have been comforting if some of them had dared to share their personal experiences with us. But that entails risk. It's always the reaching out and making personal contact that heals, but no, that scenario wasn't to be. It's so much easier to play the no-risk game and perpetuate the myth of objectivity.

The same argument would apply later when I consulted with spiritual healing practitioners. Some of them, as well, must have had HS2, or at least a similar experience with STD's. This just points out how deeply rooted the stigma is. I can't imagine a better way for professionals to establish rapport with a scared, anxious patient than to share their own personal experiences.

It is interesting to me that the people who were in the treatment program were never brought together to talk to each other. Although I can imagine how forbidden it must be from a researcher's perspective, it would at least be emotionally comforting to the participants. Having been trained as an engineer, I certainly understand how such a methodology violates the rules of scientific objectivity needed to pass the scrutiny of the ultra-critical medical community, and perhaps, the FDA as well. Be that as it may, I can still imagine a great, intangible benefit accruing from such a methodology. We can become slaves to our own rules, and we often do. The so called objective scientific method is geared toward eliminating all non-material factors from research efforts. *Wouldn't it be ironic if one day they discover that what they have been eliminating is the essential healing factor?*

By and large, people just weren't sharing personal accounts of having HS2 a decade ago. We were walking around in a vacuum, each feeling like an isolated leper. Each must have thought that he or she was the only one going through the continuum of self-flagellation and self-doubt. Based on everything I had read about HS2, I felt that we were all hopelessly doomed, so what would be the use of talking to anyone about it? Secretly, I was hoping against hope that someone would touch me, confide in me and convince me that "it ain't so."

Eventually, I dropped out of the UCLA program. As I mentioned, the program was run blind, which means that some of the participants were given placebos. That was another reason why I dropped out. As a scientically-trained professional, I understand the necessity of the placebo in a controlled drug effectiveness study. Still the practical and the selfish side of me dictated that if I was going to take off from work and drive that far every week, there was no way that I was going to settle for a placebo.

There are metaphysical lessons in my UCLA trials. It's amazing how all of life forces us to ultimately deal with what is real, even though the deeper message sometimes eludes us. Without necessarily understanding the underlying metaphysics involved, doctors accept without question the power of the almighty placebo. This is an interesting revelation to explore. By including this factor in their studies, they are in effect acknowledging that they believe that a certain percentage of people can get well simply by *believing* that they will get well. They have accepted that just the soothing effect of being cared for by a medical authority is enough to make some people well. When you think about it, this placebo concept is quite a potent drug. An odd thing happened to me during my quest for the magic cure. In spite of promising medical research, I eventually decided:

I WANTED MORE OF THAT BELIEF WHICH CONTAINED THE POWER TO HEAL SOME OF THOSE WHO WERE ON PLACEBOS.

This is why I often wished that the medical cure for HS2 would not come too soon. As masochistic as this may seem, I preferred to hold out for that cure which would be lasting.

It is unfortunate that I grew up so sexually-repressed without ever becoming comfortable with my body. I'm sure that my attitude was the single biggest factor that I needed to heal, rather than the

HS2 condition itself. I had to conjure up a mind-changing regimen which could enable me to get over the embarrassment and guilt and become comfortable with my sexuality before I could be healed. I realized that through a lifetime of limited thinking and mental misalignment, I had gotten myself in a "mell of a hess" and that it was going to be up to me to get myself out of it — with God's help, of course.

At the time of the UCLA experiment, I simply could not accept the fact that I had HS2. For me HS2 represented the worst thing that a person could have. As one of my future girlfriends, Elise, would later point out, I had never accepted that it was all right to have HS2. What she was saying was profound: I was at war with myself. Before I could realize a happy future, I had to learn to accept the present — as is. I can't say how the great UCLA experiment ended, since I didn't stick around until the end of the program. But I have a fairly good idea.

CHAPTER 8: EXPLORING HIGHER OPTIONS

EDUCATED FOOLS

I do not consider myself to be religious, neither am I what you would call a goody-goody or holier-than-thou kind of guy. True, I consider myself to be spiritually-oriented and reasonably knowledgeable about existential issues and eternal verities: the nature of God, Life, Love, Truth and Consciousness, the meaning of existence and individual purpose. These are the subjects that matter to me. Although I am devoting the rest of my life to the quest for greater understanding in this area, I realize that I still don't know enough to feel smug. The point I'm making is that, whereas men and women who care about cars will tend to learn all there is to know about cars, those who are naturally interested in spiritual philosophy will devote most of their discretionary hours to this singular pursuit. We all know people who care only about money. Nothing written on the subject of investments and changes in income tax laws is likely to escape their attention. But few there be in life, relatively speaking, who know very much about their relationship to the big picture. What most people know about God at 30 is little more than they knew on the subject at the age of 10.

That's the way it works. What we care about, we illuminate with our attention. I don't know why, but ever since I was a child, I have cared predominantly for things spiritual, metaphysical and philosophical. This has held true in spite of all my wandering and diversions. As an adolescent, I recall sitting around musing about the irreducible nature of matter and wondering if my senses were sufficiently keen to detect its finer essence. I didn't have anyone to talk with about these things, but that didn't stop me from thinking about them. It wasn't until I was about 30 that I was inclined to pursue these burning issues in a systematic, satisfying way. Despite it all, make no mistake about it; I had as much prodigal in me as any other lad. Maybe more.

Whatever I've learned, I've learned because I've read and read, and read and studied, and studied and studied, practically without ceasing. And I continue to carry on the same regimen to this day. You might say I am on an eternal quest. Even while I'm on my job, quite often I find myself meditating, reading or writing about God and Truth and my relationship to the Big Picture. Naturally, I tend to gravitate toward those who share a similar passion.

Despite all of this, I am definitely not religious. If anything, I am trans-religious. What I espouse is far beyond religion, though spiritually consistent with the original aim of all religion. What I am talking about isn't taught in church.

My life is dedicated to **LEARNING** and **KNOWING.** The two are not synonymous. You've probably heard the cliche that there are two types of fools: plain fools and educated fools. The only difference is the amount of time each class of fool has wasted to arrive at where he or she is today. I know a lot about the educated version of fool because that's basically what I am. Educated fools accumulate an impressive storehouse of facts and commit them to memory, but they still don't KNOW very much. Like many contemporary intellectuals, I've got credentials thick enough; but you won't believe the countless nights during my post-collegiate 20's that I found myself sitting right smack in the middle of my living room floor utterly dejected, emotionally hemorrhaging, riddled by so much depression and pain. I would have gladly traded every intellectual accomplishment that I possessed for one day of true wisdom.

During those years while I was still living in the Boston/Cambridge area, it was common for me to come home from my engineering job and collapse in tears in the middle of my living room floor, screaming out requests to God only knows whom: **"HEY UP THERE! IS THIS ALL THERE IS? PLEASE DON'T LIE TO ME! HEY! — TELL ME THE TRUTH — I CAN TAKE IT. IS THERE MORE? I CAN TAKE IT, I TELL YOU! SURELY THERE'S MORE, ISN'T THERE?**

"THERE HAS TO BE MORE!"

The folks back home — parents, siblings, friends, teachers, mentors and counselors — thought I had done exceedingly well. They thought I had made it (whatever that means). I thought it ironic how miserable I was. The average one of them may not have accomplished as much in the ways of the world, but I envied their happiness. In my mind I was a failure. They had something that I had lost, something I feared I could never regain. Somehow, everything I had learned just didn't seem like enough. I had played by the rules and yet I still was miserable. Do you know what I mean? Have you ever been there?

Then there are people like my father who never had the opportunity to be educated in a formal, academic sense, but still seems to know more than one would ever guess. In spite of his long-term battle with alcoholism, he possesses a natural wisdom that is impressive by any standard. Psychologists would have a field day studying the incredible enigma that is my ol' man. His life, and the lives of so many of our wise, old, "ignorant" ancestors have led me to believe that, perhaps, we've gotten it all wrong and that the concept of modernity and advancement is nothing but a big misconception.

There is quite a sizeable gap between what I have learned (facts) and what I know (wisdom). I like to refer to this as the **"EMBODIMENT GAP."** During my aforementioned prodigal 20's, I learned many facts, but one fact that I did not learn was that the accumulation of facts does not constitute wisdom. With all of us, save for a handful of mystics, there is a significant Embodiment Gap in our lives. One of the keys to living life successfully is learning how to close this gap. To live successfully is to learn how to build bridges across this gap.

Ancient Biblical writers used to say that a certain man *knew* a woman, meaning that he was intimate with her sexually. That's sort of what I mean by embodiment, to know the soul of an issue. To embody a concept, you must go way beyond mere learning, or the ability to memorize and regurgitate facts, and become so *intimate* with the principles of Truth in which you say you believe until every pore of your body breathes it, every cell of your being accepts it, and all of your actions reflect that new concept.

As for me, with each passing year I find that the gap is shrinking. This pleases me. More and more, the way that I behave naturally, without thinking about it, is beginning to approximate the way that I profess to believe. I have already learned to pattern most of my conscious thinking along the highest plane of my ideological paradigm. Like many, I would like to believe that I could see dramatic change taking place from day-to-day, but such isn't the case. I'm just not that enlightened. Historically, I have proven to be a slow learner, which would surprise many who know me, because on the surface it seems as if I have done well. Some of my friends think that I have all the faith in the world. I guess it could have been worse. My shortcomings could have been made more dramatic.

Admittedly, I haven't died. That is, I haven't had to lose my physical life to learn my lessons — at least, not quite. Nevertheless, I've been banged up fairly badly. The Prodigal Son (in the fifteenth chapter of Luke) was a model of obedience compared to me. For most of my life, people have considered me to be obstinate, angry, uncooperative, iconoclastic, arrogant, smug, nonconformist, individualistic, stubborn and mean — and, as the old joke goes, these are just the compliments! The thing about it all is that everything that I've been called, I deserved (deliberate past tense). I haven't exactly relinquished all of my chutzpah, but I have softened considerably around the edges.

So no, no, no, I am not one of those goody-goody holier-than-thou types — not by a long shot. I am not always proud of my human actions. Ignorance may have gotten me into some horrible situations in the past, but I'd rather be damned than let it control what I can be tomorrow. Humanly, I may not have yet attained the perfect ideal, but I am working diligently to close that Embodiment Gap. So I must request, as is taught in many truth teachings: *Please don't be too hard on me, for God hasn't finished with me yet.*

It's an interesting phenomenon how people can be quickly turned off by positive, uplifting books written by celebrities and promoted on talk show circuits, because they figure that such people are different than "normal" folk like themselves. Such people are often believed to have special advantages, or I suppose, even special dispensations from God. Ha, ha! That's the biggest joke in town. In fact, the exact opposite is true. These people have gone through some of the most degrading and despicable horrors and human misery to learn what they have learned. Their lessons didn't come cheaply.

I wish I had a nickel for every psychologist who has cracked up, or every minister who, in a moment of weakness, has yielded to the temptation of the flesh. I'd be rich for sure. Who do we think these people are?

I remember when I was a teen-ager and stumbled upon some male teachers who had gotten together one day after school to watch a stag film. This predated VCR's and X-rated video rentals. Smut was hard to come by in those days. I couldn't believe it — my role models! Yet another nail was pounded into the coffin of my innocence that day. Up to that time, I had put all teachers on a pedestal, high above the level at which my life was being lived. It had never occurred to me that they were people just like me.

Those things used to bother me. Oh how much fun being a kid can be. Learning about life can be such a rude awakening.

Ministers are such convenient scapegoats. I've heard many folks say, "The reason I don't go to church is that ministers are so corrupt. They aren't any better than anybody else. All they want is your money." Even I used to think that. That's why for the first 15 years of my post-high school life I avoided churches as if they were the plague. As soon as I was old enough to defy my mama's wishes, I got out of the church. Oh, to be sure, I felt plenty guilty. You see, I was brought up in the church — the orthodox, Southern Baptist, fire and brimstone, God-fearing church. If you were brought up under a similar brand of forced faith, I bet you, too, felt guilty for every Sunday that you finagled your way out of church. I think one of the things that I enjoyed most about going to college was that it was one of the few legitimate excuses that I could give to parents and other adult pillars of the community for not regularly attending church. And look what I chose: MIT! That was about as far as you could stray from God without becoming a communist.

Lest I be misunderstood, let me say a good word about churches and money. I have learned that it really does not make any difference what the church or the ministers do with the money that we give. For those who do not yet understand the law of universal supply and circulation, as I didn't understand it back in those days, you are probably blocking yourself from happiness, prosperity, and other blessings just as I did.

This is not a lightweight subject. There are immutable principles which govern life just as surely as the law of gravity governs your fate if you jump off a 10-story building, regardless of whether you intended to jump. Even if you decide to change your mind in mid-air, the law of gravity will not care. It is the same with the law of giving. Today, I actively seek places to circulate my money (you can't really give anything away, anyhow) for the simple reason that I know that my giving blesses ME. What the minister or those in charitable organizations do with the money once I give it is none of my business. Of course, I wouldn't want them to squander or misappropriate it, but even if they do, my blessings will not cease. I will be blessed by my actions and they will be blessed — or not blessed — by theirs. The Law of God which serves us is perfect. It serves each of us individually. If your minister jumps off a 10-story building, gravity will affect the quality of *his* or *her* future, not yours.

Now, I am always one for practicality and common sense, two elements that are sorely missing from the metaphysical/New Age movement. I am not suggesting that we should knowingly support corrupt causes or operations. Why should we? I certainly would not. All I'm getting at here is that it's important to realize that the higher laws of life are both inherently consistent and totally impersonal. Each one will be blessed according to his or her own nature. You may recall Jesus saying that the sins of the father are not visited upon the child, or Joseph telling his brothers in the Old Testament that they might have intended evil against him, but God meant it for good. In spite of their evil plot against him, Joseph was blessed.

In choosing a college, I had two strong criteria. The second one I've never admitted to anybody, not even my mother. The first was that I wanted to get the heck out of Georgia. No kidding! I wanted to be farther away than you could drive in a weekend. That excluded Georgia Tech, which, otherwise, would have been a natural choice for me.

The second and more important criterion was that I wasn't going to go to any college that was either affiliated with a church or that required its students to take even one course in religion. As far as I was concerned, that excluded the entire South. Conversely — or *perversely* — it included just about anywhere in New England or California! My mother was dead set against my trekking clear across country to Berkeley, so I compromised and settled for MIT. Many were the times that I regretted the choice.

Let me interject something here. Earlier I stated that I have always been interested in spiritual and existential pursuits, even as an adolescent. It should come as no surprise that I strived to get away from religious doctrines at the age of 18. This was just part of the process of breaking out of the fold so that I could begin to investigate Truth freely and independently. Even now, I feel that that part of my process was the best decision I've ever made.

I was not happy at MIT. I haven't always thought that my choice of schools was the best. Sure, I busted my butt, graduated with a respectable cum and all of that. Considering that I was not overly fond of failure, after being accepted, graduating with a good grade point average seemed to be the easiest way to get the heck out. Once I got out, you might say that I went overboard: I moved to California of all places. Surely you know that California is considered to be some kind of haven for weirdos, fruits, freaks and nuts (okay, California *and* New York).

A popular joke is told concerning a certain sign on the border as you leave California. It reads: You are now leaving California. You may resume normal behavior.

My experiences at MIT were weird and bizarre. It was like living in the twilight zone. If I have another MacLainian-type incarnation wherein education is as important as it is in today's world, I'm going to chose some great fun school where students go to football games and basketball games and drink beer and get drunk. What I didn't know upon entering MIT was that therein resides some of the most sacrilegious humanoids that God, evolution or machine has ever created (manufactured?). I needed a breather from the orthodox, stifling religious vice grips of my childhood, but never had I known people who were irreverent, fearless or just plain loony enough to openly crack jokes about God. Man! Even if I didn't believe in God, I couldn't see myself taking chances like that. I spent four years looking overhead for lightning bolts. My aim was not to stand too close to their intended targets. Oh well...

What I've been trying to do by sharing personal details of my life is shed light on how I got into the mindset that eventually attracted negative experiences, including HS2, to me. Despite the woe-is-me tales that we spin, things don't just happen to us. The stage is usually set long before we find ourselves all tied up in a logjam.

This irrepressible desire for Truth led me to spend the first 32 years of my life getting into all kinds of jams. Even the act of fleeing the church as a teen-ager was a definite move to discover some kind of truth which transcends religion. When I go back today and read some of the papers that I wrote in college for my various humanities classes, to my great amazement I find that I was almost always writing about this quest to know God. It's weird how I don't remember writing those papers. Clearly, I was asleep. But though I was unconscious, something was conscious within me. Those experiences were a forgotten part of my life until I was about 36. Today I'm sure that I was subconsciously trying to offset some of the agnostic intellectualism that was so prevalent among the majority of my smug, self-sufficient, "I-don't-need-God," super brainy, colleagues.

Even after I contracted HS2, if you think I changed my life in any significant way, forget it! Not this eductated fool. I didn't have that much sense, or perhaps, I should say *maturity*. Common sense would have suggested that a change was in order, but I was such a stubborn fellow in those days. As you may know, if you've ever been a smoker or drinker or druggie, habits are hard to break. Oftentimes, the evidence of pain and self destruction is not enough to make you undergo the agony of change. **We often prefer old vices to unknown virtues.**

THE SPIRITUAL QUEST

I have read many of the books and listened open-mindedly to most of the outlandish New Age claims. Not only that, but I have joined the movements, taken the workshops, and listened to the lectures. In short, I have experimented with living an endless sequence of alternative lifestyles. What I have witnessed indicates that so-called New Age fads come and go. We've had our Ramthas, Shirley MacLaines, rebirthing, channeling, crystals, harmonic convergences, Sidonas, energy vortexes and treading on hot coals. The latest fad that has found my "enlightened" friends shelling out big bucks is the native American Indian sweat lodge experience. I know students of metaphysics who have sworn by all these processes, some of them with HS2, some with AIDS, and some who won't say. Despite it all, I haven't seen a single one healed yet. The ones who had HS2 still have it, and some of those who had AIDS are now dead. Some of them have adopted a lower profile, while others have dropped out and joined more esoteric spiritual orders, characterized by the donning of funny garbs, way out rituals and the whole nine yards. As I've said, challenges like HS2 can make you weird if you aren't careful.

Regardless of whether I'm healed or not on the physical level, what I know is that I am a spiritual being beyond all else. Nothing can change that. I know beyond a shadow of doubt that God is Absolute First Cause. Yet I am not even close to being a born again, charismatic or pentecostal. No guilt nor apologies either, for God is not going to strike me down. If anything, He is going to lift me up and bless me even more for thinking for myself and refusing to get caught up in all of this foolishness.

This may be difficult for some to accept, because in this society we tend to expect people to fall into neat little categories. If someone is a scientist or engineer, and loves it, it's hard to think of him or her as professing a strong faith in God. And if someone reads the *Bible* and tries to live according to its word (ignoring for the moment the obvious inconsistencies and contradictions), we tend to think of him or her as being religious or belonging to a particular congregation. Well, I have no denomination or category other than free-thinking spiritual being and child of God. Consider this: I belong to the same religion as God. Though I was raised a conventional Baptist in the deep South, my present concept of God and religion would not meet with the approval of my former religious body.

Today, there are investigators from the scientific community who have made a career by researching and exposing spiritual healing frauds, but I am not among them. They tend to be skeptics of long standing who are caught up in the traditional science versus religion dichotomy that has characterized man since the dawning of the Scientific Age. In that framework, scientists tend to be either atheists or agnostics who believe doggedly in evolution, while believers in God promote only Creationism. The only common denominator between these two camps seems to be weapons. Put weapons in their hands and either side is willing to fight to the bitter end for what it believes.

My philosophy does not satisfy either of these paradigms. I am a technologist who sees good in science and enjoys working as an engineer, manufacturing products that are sometimes practical, sometimes exotic, and sometimes profligate with no redeeming human value. I enjoy the people whom I meet in my technological world, along with their errantly precise, left-brained personalities, ignorant conservatism and predictably humdrum lifestyles. Of course, there are exceptions, but, regardless, I find it all rather fascinating to observe — as a mirror and as a revealer of my own soul. Everything that we experience is about ourselves, because we are the observer and the interpreter of our universe. I mean this, not in a selfish way, but in a painful, soul-searching way.

My whole thesis is about how one person can apply *pragmatic* spiritual healing principles in dealing with HS2. Unlike so many publications in this genre, I am not making a single phenomenal or miraculous claim. There have been no cascades of light, instant illumination, distinct voices or hunches telling me to turn left when I wanted to turn right. When I have wanted to turn right, I have simply turned right and that was that. No mini-cams had to be set up and no news conferences called. No apologies, no after-thoughts and no guilt. It's all been fairly simple. I'm sorry to have to report this, but there have been no hunches other than my own human greed telling me which numbers to play in the lottery or which slot machine in Las Vegas holds my fortune in waiting. Of course, at this juncture in my spiritual evolution, I have completely sworn off games of chance, other than an occasional dollar bet in a pool at work. My good will continue to come to me, and it will have nothing whatsoever to do with luck. Of this I'm sure — let the rabbit keep its paw.

It is my responsibility as a spiritual teacher to resist misleading anyone. Thus I must report that I don't feel compelled to buy the *Bible*-as-literal-word-of-God theory in any way, shape or fashion. As I repeatedly drill students in my classes and workshops, everyone has the right to believe whatever he or she wants to believe. I grant other people that right because I claim that right for myself. Without this freedom none of us would have a chance of finding God. I do not bear any guilt about past sins, wanton pleasures or desires. Despite my ex-girlfriend Marsha's psychological assessment of me, I am not a religious zealot, fanatic, or sociopath who, after having failed in more conventional approaches, is now attempting to lose myself in faith. I don't have a problem with making it in the world — even *this* world, one that sometimes seems so evil, inhumane and unfair. *Au Contraire*, I see this world as incomparably beautiful and challenging and fun. I'm so glad God placed me here. Their limitations notwithstanding, capitalism and competition are as good a game as any other that will ever be on Earth — and as bad. I love everything without being bullish on anything. In short, I believe myself to be a mentally healthy person. If I am correct, then it is axiomatic that steadily improving physical health will continue to follow, as it most certainly has since I surrendered to this attitude. Of course, there may be occasional setbacks, but I doubt if they will affect the big picture.

Though I believe in God more than ever, I am repulsed by the abuses and manipulation that are being foisted on the desperate "sheep" by churches and spiritual organizations, whether orthodox, New Age, New Thought or whatever. I have searched far and wide and I have found no pure religious organizations.

Though I consider myself to be a serious metaphysician — an absolute *spiritual* metaphysician, which is an important distinction — I shall not attempt to deceive you. I have received no special favors from God, which in a way is good news. Why? Because in my discovery of God and acceptance of his natural goodness, I have become totally satisfied. I can perceive of nothing that is missing. This is what I want to share with others. You, too, can attain total peace and contentment, even if there are no light shows or miraculous demonstrations. But if you're uninterested, that's your prerogative, too, and I respect you for exercising your God-given free will.

It doesn't matter if you don't see me as being enlightened. It won't change what I really am, or diminish the effusive joy that I presently feel. Whether I say that I'm healed or not healed won't change whether I really am in my soul, and there's no one who can peer into my soul. Likewise, whether I say that I'm enlightened or not won't change the truth, so I won't bother. It is sufficient that my soul knows the truth, I know the truth and God knows the truth.

When you are sure that your life is in God's hands — I mean, really sure — you will suddenly lose all interest in effects, whether those effects are considered to be pleasant to human consciousness or unpleasant to human consciousness. What I'm hinting at is difficult, and perhaps, impossible, to explain. One of the great mystics admonished us over and over: Judge not by appearances. If you find it necessary to have appearances set up around you in a certain manner before you can be happy, you will never be happy.

Can you imagine not being healed when you are perfectly at peace and effervescing with joy? I believe that everyone wants to be rooted in joy, but may not know the way. Like Dorothy in the *Wizard of Oz*, they have lost their way and do not know how to get back home. Admittedly, it's not a trivial undertaking to find that perfect center of joy in this society. I have no cookbook recipes. There are many circumstances which befall us in this life, but I believe that we place far too much emphasis on our problems. Something happens, prompting us to react defensively and to over-analyze the situation. We gather advice from friends, and we conclude that it means this or that. If we can't get rid of it or resolve it in one way, such as through conventional medicine, we indulge ourselves in some other discipline, such as spiritual or mental healing. We clean up our lives and attempt to take control over our minds, applying principles of thinking and living that promise to restore us to our natural state of perfection. Then we feel good about ourselves because we have finally gotten back in alignment with nature, or God, or the universe.

But we're still entertaining a concept of healing. Some condition is still kicking our figurative butts, which we cannot dislodge from our minds. Now we're really confused! We have done everything that is known to humankind, and we have adjusted every element of our lifestyle that could possibly be out of sync. The only thing left to question is the very foundation around which we have constructed our lives. Are we to conclude with agnostics, scientists, and heathens that man is but a random being in a universe governed by chance with no control over his destiny? Or that we reached into the cosmic hat and it was just our luck to draw the shortest straw? Are we to prove false the mystical teaching that ours is a spiritual universe of Law and Order, governed by the immutable principle of cause and effect, and that we are spiritual entities who are in touch with and governed by an infinite, omniscient, and omnipresent Power? If our original premise, along with that of the mystics of the ages, is correct, we should be able to change any condition though the practices that we have been employing. But as it is, when we look at our lives we're forced to conclude that we have not been able to do that. As a result, we find our minds tied up in a knot, and now we're more confused than ever!

The scenario that I just painted describes the stalemate in which so many metaphysicians, New Agers and other self-styled spiritual healers have found themselves. I have been there, and I know that so many of my friends, ministers, and teachers have been there, yet I've never heard an open, honest discussion on this subject. Under the guise of "enlightenment," each one seems to be privately bearing the pain and everyone is afraid to question the obvious. One minister has a nervous breakdown; another one dies from cancer, while a well known metaphysical healer succumbs to AIDS.

Privately, they summon me in a continuous stream for answers to these issues, because they cannot discuss them openly in their own organizations and classrooms. Let's just deal with pure spiritual logic for a moment. To my simple way of thinking, it's axiomatic that something is missing in the healing formula that is being applied, is it not? Either (1) the fundamental premises are wrong; (2) the fundamental premises are right but they're being misinterpreted; or (3) something of major importance must be missing from some of these premises. There is no way around this logic.

Throughout the remainder of this chapter, I will undertake to prove that the fundamental premises of spiritual healing are correct. The sad fact is that they are being grossly misinterpreted, not just by lay persons, but also by ministers, New Agers and metaphysicians as well. It could be that people haven't yet learned enough or labored diligently enough for the evidence to appear. From experience, I would have to reject this. I have seen so many students running from course-to-course, organization-to-organization and philosophy-to-philosophy in search of Truth. Some have flown all over the United States, and even the world, to sit at the feet of various gurus and fad healers that are forever springing up. With many of these people, the lack of money is no obstacle. I have encountered people who have tried to tap into every conceivable fad and convert it into a religion. The only thing that I have found in common among all of these seekers is that most of them have lost their bearings, and nearly their minds, without even knowing it. In my humble opinion, I'm telling you that I haven't met one of this ilk who was even close to finding contentment. The problem is that people are trying so hard. In many cases, too hard.

The pattern is always the same. They take on some highfalutin title, adorn themselves in some kind of weird garb, learn a new language that is replete with obscure, foreign words that English-speaking tongues aren't equipped to pronounce, and while hypnotically convincing you that they "love you," somehow manage to reduce you to feeling inferior. The unspoken theory seems to be this: The more inferior they make you feel, the more money you will be willing to pay to have them build you up again. Think about it. It works just this way. This is essentially the way all religious organizations and fringe spiritual groups work. The larger the gap between them and you, the more you will be likely to pay to close that gap.

I am aware that to some this may sound like an unusually harsh, and possibly even unfounded, attack, but I am not kidding. This is exactly what is going on in the name of spiritual healing. And what's going on in the churches is absolutely unforgivable. If Jesus came back today, I guarantee you he'd kick 99 percent of all existing Christian, New Thought and metaphysical ministers clean out of the church. Not only that, but I guarantee you that most of those who are teaching Jesus-as-the-only-way doctrines would not even recognize him. They would attack him as being from the devil. If fact, they would crucify him all over again.

Now there are the fundamentalists who are quick to say, "You fools, of course something is missing. You have to accept Jesus Christ as your personal Lord and Savior." Well, that's a big guilt pill that you can swallow at your own risk. These United States are saturated with obedient, orthodox Christians, and yet they are the epitome of long-suffering. They have the same problems that the New Age aspirants have, plus guilt and the feeling of doctrinal worthlessness. While pointing the finger at those who won't be saved, this group awaits its results "by and by." While I believe in most of the recorded teachings of Jesus and probably adhere to them more scrupulously than most born agains, it's obvious that this isn't the answer on the individual level that so many have been seeking.

So what is the answer? What's missing? As you would expect, it has to be so simple that most people would miss it. Nothing that is rooted in the eternal is ever complex or arcane in this world. The Truth is always simple, but its very simplicity makes it appear to be impractical. If it were complex, we'd figure it out. We're good at unraveling puzzles, but place something simple before our eyes and we're buffaloed. Our "normal" system of life is so replete with static and confusion that simple things are almost impossible to see. The problem is that we are looking in the wrong places for Truth.

Our purpose for existing is, primarily, to achieve a state of true understanding about God, about ourselves, and about the relationship that unites us. And the true relationship is not the one that is taught in Christian churches. This must not be an intellectual under-standing, but an inner, soul-level understanding that goes far beyond words and effects. Like I said, this thing is so utterly simple that it's hard for our jaded, modernized minds to grasp.

It's the attainment of a state of happiness, peace, and objectless joy that literally goes beyond all reason. It's the embodiment of the love-of-God principle, based on nothing that makes any sense to the mores of this world. When we arrive at that point, we won't even be able to talk about conditions, effects, diseases, cures, healings and so forth. Our only question will be: How can I be or service to my fellow man? We will also begin to ask: What is there to heal?

No matter how strenuously I try, I cannot imagine being deserted by God, not even for one second. I cannot even imagine being separated from God. It is impossible to hold this point of view and think of yourself as not being healed, or being in need of anything, even a healing.

Patrick Henry was known to have said that he had only one life to give for his country. Well, in that same vein I have only one life to *commit* — not to my country, but to God — so I'm going to commit it for Truth and God and principle, no matter the conse-quences. If this means that I die tomorrow, so be it. If this means that the doctors and all of society condemn me as a fool and declare my teachings wrong, so be it. If this means that I never become a legend or amass a fortune, or receive my just due on Earth, so be it. Sink or swim, I have chosen to cast my lot with God. Spirit is real. Just look around you. Babies are being born, flowers are blooming, birds are flying, the wind is blowing, fish are hatching... These are all such astounding miracles. There is no way to remain depressed or hopeless when we ponder these things.

Here is what's been missing. Many people are still looking outside themselves at conditions. Many are still worrying and fretting about what others think, and what they're going to tell others by way of explanation. They are still worrying about insignificant elements such as time. "How long is it going to take?" they cry out. Who are they asking, and who could possibly know? Most of the time, God has no idea of what they're talking about, because they aren't speaking the language of the Infinite Knower. Time, fear and conditions have no relationship to the language of true spiritual knowing. I know that this is not easy, but it's awfully simple — at least in concept. It is ultra-simple, because its attainment does not involve any of the common factors of merit in which we place so much value: a certain amount of money, a certain IQ, travel or a degree. Heretofore, we have been willing to travel anywhere, pay almost any amount of money, and force our way to the front of the line to grovel at the feet of the anointed prophet who could provide us with the final answer. But what we're going to find out now, just like the great prophets and mystics have all promised, is that we already possess the key to unlocking the great secret, but do not know it.

This is simple and yet it is not simple. It is human nature, I surmise, that we have been influenced to search everywhere else for the elixir of truth before we can relax in the assurance that it's ever available right here at home.

The things we argue, worry and fret over are trivial and insignificant once we develop a true relationship with God. When individuals do not have a true concept of God, they judge themselves as needing to be healed *from* some condition. In their angst, they may also become distraught with others. A relationship with the true God frees you from all of this and renders the subject of physical healing moot.

Now don't get me wrong. I understand how important the body and the perfect functioning of its organs are to normal humans. I am not about to belittle that connection, or to take the common metaphysical cop-out by declaring that none of the things that are important to you are real. The body *is* important, else you can be sure that you wouldn't have one. And people are justified in worrying about their various expressions of disease; they just want to know the objective truth about the effectiveness of various forms of spiritual healing, and that is perfectly reasonable.

Obviously, I do not advocate worrying, but I respect the need of worriers to worry. They are justified in their worrying. It is absolutely necessary to be unconditionally loving, but to do so is to unconditionally accept people right where they are, which includes worriers. I'm only here to allow the light of truth to radiate through me, not to attempt to prevent people from choosing from among an endless host of more Earthly alternatives. Humbling though it is to admit, God has not appointed me to be their savior. If Spirit wants them saved, It will certainly take care of that. What Spirit has appointed me to do is to stand here firmly, holding my ground, while being willing to radiate the light of Truth, to reflect its goodness, and to sense its goodness in others. That's the most that I can ever hope to do. I may not achieve worldly fame, but to do these simple things is to be a hero.

I am convinced that we weren't put here to "save" people. One bird doesn't tell another bird how to fly. He simply leads on the wing and lets God determine which ones will follow suit — and which ones won't. What could be simpler? Yet we humans have no faith in acting this way. We have to interfere in everything and impose the trademark of our personalities upon the process.

Skepticism is healthy, especially in light of our recent history. If I did not understand these things from a personal viewpoint, I could not write anything that would be of benefit to the average person. And I should add, it is the average person in whom I am interested. As it is, I have labored long and hard through a veritable mine field of physical diseases during my present life cycle. If anyone has a right to plea for pity, it is I. In other words, I've paid my dues with the coin of the proverbial realm. I know what it means to suffer, to doubt your religion, and to question whether there really is a God. For the first three-fourths of my life, I didn't see any evidence at all that the Universe was either fair or loving. And given that the Universe and God are one and the same, you can well believe that I once called into question the fairness of God.

CLASSES IN METAPHYSICS

There exists a phenomenon within spiritual healing circles which has often baffled me. No one warned me. In fact, everyone seems to be oblivious to it, but I am always able to detect it whenever I am in those circles. It hangs in the air like the ubiquitous inversion layer of smaze over Los Angeles. In metaphysical or New Thought congregations and classrooms, and in the private offices of spiritual healers, I have found that, with few exceptions, these teachers become markedly uncomfortable if one of their students or clients fails to become healed. This is particularly true if their charges admit it openly. I've observed this strange reaction in classrooms where sick students have raised questions about their own disease processes, especially after they've done everything that the ministers and healing practitioners have told them to do. Oh, I forgot. I shouldn't say *disease*. As New Thought students, we were drilled to say *dis-ease* instead (two syllables, meaning the absence of ease) and refer to all problems euphemistically as "challenges." Furthermore, it would be unthinkable for students to refer to themselves as being "sick" — God forbid.

In an absolute sense, these teachings appear to be consistent with Truth, but in a pragmatic sense, they represent pure, unadulterated distortions. Between the two extremes lies lots of pain and confusion. There is no way under the sun that such denial can help people become whole, perfect or complete. It certainly cannot help them to become healed. What it is is hypocrisy and the antithesis of unconditional love. If a person comes to me thinking that he or she is sick, I guarantee you that he or she really is sick. That's all there is to it. Metaphysical principle states: As a man thinks, so is he. If I am the light of Truth, it is incumbent upon me to stand steady and let that light shine on him until he declares himself healed on his own volition. I don't have to spoon-feed him the "right" point of view about his own condition. To do so proves that I don't truly believe that the principle works. Neither should I try to cajole him or convert him by chicanery. By no means do I have the right to cram my words about his (or her) condition down his throat. There's an old expression which says: A man convinced against his will is of the same opinion still.

I can't think of how many times I have been corrected or reprimanded in New Thought classes because I have used the "wrong" language to describe a situation. In the absence of real spiritual healing — which there is scant evidence of in the world today — we become overly picky, and even picayune, about semantics. You can't use words like *sin*, or *evil*. You're taught that there is no devil, or sickness; disease is not real; the world is an illusion; and so forth. As far as I can tell, these methods of teaching can only lead to withdrawal and uptightness — everything but spontaneity and openness, which are the keys to real spiritual healing. What happens eventually is that embarrassed students cease to ask questions after getting "the treatment" publicly once or twice. I almost quit my formal studies back in 1982 after I got "the treatment" from one such bull-headed instructor on more than a few occasions. How many are willing to subject themselves to public ridicule and embarrassment and continue to march on in their search for Truth?

I remember a confrontation I had with this vociferous, overpowering metaphysical teacher during one of my beginning courses. He posed a trick question to the class, as too many so-called spiritual teachers do, and as usual, I took the bait. We were discussing Ralph Waldo Emerson's essay on "Self Reliance," and expounding in general about Emersonian nonconformity. Then the teacher asked, "Is it possible to be a nonconformist?"

My response was, "Of course, it is." Then I went on to tell the class how I considered myself to be a nonconformist, because throughout my college years and professional career I have often marched in the vanguard that challenged outdated conventions and the status quo. What did I ever say that for? Before I even finished making my point, the instructor had jumped up into my face with his well-rehearsed argument. He couldn't wait for me to take the bait. Before I could slither away, there he was at the board drawing symbols and logic paths to prove that conformity and nonconformity were no different, and how each is part of the same system, and those who think otherwise are nothing more than fools. I felt so humiliated. The great professor had beaten me into a pulp. He had made himself right and me wrong. From that day forward, were we to ever face that question on one of his tests, we'd sure as heck know what the right answer was: his answer! He made sure of that — the big bully! He had bludgeoned his version of truth into me and my classmates, and I had the bruises to show it. Other than that, we hadn't learned very much at all. That ol' prof is still teaching, but to my knowledge, with all his pomposity, knowledge, and flawless arguments, he has yet to heal even a single flea.

Today I can see that based on the rules of logic under which the professor constructed his argument, I was never a nonconformist. He made his point. Since we live in a spiritual unity, there is no way to remove ourselves from any system of which we are a part. The universe is holistic. The more you try to resist or oppose, on some level you become locked in the same rhythm and vibration of that which you are trying to oppose. From the absolute framework of spiritual dynamics, there can be no nonconformist. I understand this today after many years of study. However, at that time there was no way that I could grasp the point that he was ramming down my throat.

Be that as it may, on the relative or material plane I was a nonconformist. By playing a game of semantics, the ol' prof made a very common metaphysical mistake. He failed to elucidate the difference between the absolute way of viewing things and the relative. Most people live and think in a relative framework, and it's the height of insensitivity and callousness to disrespect their point of view. Their world is as real to them — and maybe even more so — than the absolute world is real to metaphysicians. By the way, the professor was not perfect himself, by any means. It always struck me as a bit ironic that he could hardly wait for the scheduled class break to rush outside to puff on a cigarette.

The time has passed for making students wrong, even in spiritual and religious teachings. For the life of me, I cannot comprehend how anyone can ask a bad question. The only bad question I can imagine is the one not asked. As an airplane buff, I can tell you that a large percentage of airplane crashes would have been prevented if the copilot had asked a few more questions. But for years it has been a standing tradition that no one challenges the word of a plane's captain. Ever since I was a child, I have been too inquisitive for the authority figures in my life. People said that I would outgrow it, but now that I've passed 40 I guess it's safe to conclude that I never will. I certainly hope not. People are never wrong for believing as they believe. We are all evolving in a manner that is totally consistent with the pattern of our souls in the eyes of God. And because you and I can't understand it, that doesn't make it bad.

In the classroom, when the authorities who happen to be highly-reputed healers tell you that (1) you are not sick, and that you should never make such a claim about yourself again, and (2) that your condition is but a mere experience which you would be able to heal if you were doing your mental and spiritual work correctly, all of the protest is scuttled out of you.

It's an unfair debate. They have all the power and you have none. If you argue the simplest of points, you will be put down in the most pompous, arrogant manner. Not only will the teacher almost invariably lose patience with you, but your fellow classmates can be depended upon to show their disdain as they publicly align with the authority figure. You see, they ARE conformists! You will be left out there all alone. I experienced and witnessed this situation many times while I was studying to become a licensed practitioner of Religious Science.* My investigations have convinced me that it is no different in any of the other organized New Thought/metaphysical healing disciplines.

I have always been a nagging interrogator, a veritable thorn in the side for teachers, professors, ministers and other authority figures.

---

* New Thought is a religious teaching embraced by Religious Science, Unity and Divine Science, as well as hundreds of metaphysical splinter groups. It teaches the unity of all life, that thought is creative, and that the mind of man/woman is the mind of God.

Metaphysics, when used in this book, simply means "beyond the physical realm." In other words, it refers to the spiritual and mental realms. Mysticism, on the other hand, deals only with the spiritual realm.

Many have judged my demeanor obnoxious, and my intentions disruptive, but nothing could be further from the truth. I believe in challenging and being challenged, for there is no better way that I know of to really learn, and I'm always trying to learn something new or clarify what I already know. Not only that, but I don't consider argumentation and disagreement to be negative devices.

So many people seem to believe that if someone publicly disagrees with them, it means that they aren't well-liked by that person or that they have been disrespected. For instance, you seldom see a husband and wife take opposing views in public, unless they're engaged in battle. I'm more prone to think that if a good friend *doesn't* ever disagree with me, and verbally so, then *that* is disrespectful. Even my wife and I are willing to verbalize our individual points of view in public, regardless of the other's position. We don't check with each other before we speak our minds. This has led more than a few people to think that we were fighting, when we were not. So far, we have always been able to laugh about the whole thing afterwards. As strange as it may sound, we are more committed to Truth than we are to each other − and, so far as I'm concerned, that's the way it should be. But here's the paradox: As a consequence of putting Truth first, we are also committed to each other.

Another reason that I've often fallen in disfavor as a result of questioning authority figures is that I am quite slow in my comprehension. I have the reputation of being a gadfly. That, plus the fact that teachers tend to regard me as being bright, have often led them to the wrong conclusions. I am pathetically slow in my understanding of new concepts. Teachers think that I'm bright because the few things that I do know, I know very well. I'm crystal clear about what I do know, and I'll stand up and defend it to the bitter end. Even so, I often turn out to be wrong. And that's all right, too. But most often, I am classified as a kook and put out to pasture long before we exhaust all of the avenues of possibility.

As I mentioned, I have trouble comprehending the obvious facts, particularly those that seem so trivial to everyone else. While all of my fellow classmates seem to be nodding their heads in agreement with the impatient instructor, I am usually hopelessly befuddled. I would often wonder how they could understand so quickly when I couldn't. Yet I'm supposed to have a fairly decent IQ. Furthermore, I would always wonder what does this say about me? Am I retarded or something? It was like that as a child. More times than I care to recall, I prompted my parents to shout, "Shut up and stop asking questions!"

Others used to retort, "How come you want to know so much? How come, huh?"

Even then, I vowed, "One day I'm going to grow up and find the answers to some of my private questions about life." Meanwhile, I learned to button up and restrict my weirder thoughts to the confines of my own mind.

By the time I discovered Religious Science (not to be confused with Scientology), I was 30 years old. At that age it was quite difficult when teachers reacted contemptuously towards me as a result of my importunate nature. It was never my purpose to be obnoxious or show up the teacher or prevent him (or her) from covering his sacred course agenda. It was just that at that juncture in life, I had absolutely no desire to pay money to sit up in yet another classroom as someone's stool pigeon. I played that role for the last, sickening time when I was in college. When I ventured to enroll in another class at age 30, no longer was I content to be a passive observer. I'm sorry if 30 is not old enough to have your own opinions. When is anyone ever old enough in this society?

When I first embarked upon New Thought, I was ecstatic. "Wow! You mean there are other people who question life the same way that I do? And they teach courses in the philosophy of life, the spiritual principles of living, and the relationship between man, God, and the cosmos? Wow, I can't believe my good fortune." I was so excited. Finally, I could begin to openly discuss all of those weird questions that I had been storing up for so many years. I could begin to explore some of my unconventional, iconoclastic notions that had dominated my thinking for so long. I entered these studies with such a spirit of expectancy. Unfortunately, my elation didn't last long. One of my greatest spiritual teachers, the late mystic, Dr. Homer R. Johnson, used to say, "Wherever you find a human being, there you will find human consciousness." How right he was.

In no time I discovered that, along with their bodies, my teachers also lugged all of their unresolved stuff into the classroom, despite what the tenets of their philosophy espoused. New Thought philosophy was touted to be open at the top; well it isn't. Its trained ecclesiastical leaders profess to practice unconditional love, but, with few exceptions, they don't. Some years later, I was surprised to hear from a number of my classmates that they used to consider me to be a royal pain in the butt during classes. When I asked why, they responded that it was because of the havoc I caused in the classroom by asking all of those questions. The basis for finally confiding this great secret to me was that they wanted me to know that they finally understood that questions were constructive. The test of time had proven to them that I was a dedicated truth-seeker, even if I wasn't loyal to their particular organizations.

The bane of education is the course syllabus. So many times I recall bubbling over with excitement and anticipation upon reading the outline of a new course during my college years or during formal spiritual training. At last I was going to have a chance to explore the boundaries of thought in some chosen area. But there is always that stupid syllabus. No matter how excellent the teacher, he or she is always saddled with the responsibility of covering everything on the agenda for that particular week, regardless of the needs of the students. All of the spontaneity is taken out of the dynamics of the classroom by the imposition of that all too-sacred agenda. Who makes up these stupid rules in the first place? Just as soon as the discussion is properly kindled and begins to get really juicy, the teacher invariably announces, "Well, let's wrap it up. We have to curtail this discussion for now so that we can cover the other topics on the agenda for this week. If you desire, we can continue this discussion after class." Forget it. The moment is gone. No matter how well-intentioned the teacher or students, the moment can never be recreated.

Later, after graduating as a licensed practitioner of New Thought, I was shocked to discover that so much emphasis was placed on control. The New Thought charter was supposed to be different, loftier and more open. It was supposed to be more encouraging to the spirit than suppressive. In actuality, some teachers were loving and yielding, while others who hailed from more militaristic backgrounds were pleased to bring that hackneyed old form into the classroom. Regardless, everyone was forced to adhere to the sacred agenda much like a race car driver staying in his assigned lane while circling the oval loop at the Indy 500. He's going awfully fast but he's missing all of the scenery along the way.

Continuing my diatribe against fixed agenda, let me repeat my belief that spiritual enlightenment cannot be attained by following a menu. The instructions in the textbook may have worked very well for Ernest Holmes, Charles Fillmore, or Mary Baker Eddy, but they may not work the same way for you or me. In my opinion it is a mistake to try to teach courses in New Thought, metaphysical or advanced spiritual Laws in the same manner as college courses are taught. There is a vast difference between the intellectual and the spiritual, and the respective methods in which these two faculties in humans are developed. There is no way that one can be trained to be like Jesus and to develop Christlike consciousness while rushing through a fixed, rigid syllabus.

FINDING THAT PERFECT MATE

For me, the journey to awakening was a harrowing experience. To be sure, it was fun, but also bewildering and harrowing. I feel like a man who has walked through a forest of fire and been dragged through the metaphysical graveyard in search of a single straw of hope. In looking backward and examining my motives, I've come to the realization that I was laboring under the false belief that I could never live a normal life unless I was healed of HS2.

For many years I was desperately lonely, but being the archetypal man that I was, I wasn't about to admit it. Instead I felt compelled to rationalize my weird behavior. It was tearing me apart inside that I could not attract a regular, committed girlfriend — at least, not the kind that I desired — and get married and have a regular, intimate relationship with the possibility of kids, just like "normal" people. I just didn't see how I could have that, because there were these prolonged, all to frequent periods when I was festering with virulent sores, and depressed to nearly despondent levels. I wondered why in heaven's name would any decent woman tolerate me under such conditions.

HS2 represents a dysfunction and any dysfunction will force you toward acting out distorted or inverted behavior. On the other hand, it is the nature of the human mind to constantly strive to counter-balance any dysfunction or abnormality. When you encounter an otherwise normal person who consistently acts weird or anomalous and attempts to cover himself or herself with smoke screens such as, "I'm just different, that's all," "You have to understand that I'm not that sociable; I like being alone," "I don't feel anything for you; I have no sexual desires" — look out! The normal flow of life just doesn't work like that. Only through radical self-examination and open inquiry into the higher eschelons of Truth can we neutralize this distorting tendency which is always striving to rationalize our dysfunctions.

The most painful aspect of my entire debacle was that friends and co-workers were always bugging me about normalizing my be-havior. "Why aren't you married yet?" they'd persistently inquire. "What went wrong between you and Elise?" another would ask. "Why don't you ask Ella out?"

Well, Ella was a fine woman and a good friend. She was this charming, well-bred, high-achieving super sophisticate whom I just knew would be repulsed to no end if she had even the slightest hint concerning my little secret. We were great friends and I knew that she liked me a lot, but risking the ultimate blow with a woman like that was something else again. At the time I held the belief that a woman such as she deserved only the best out of life, and by no stretch of the imagination did I think that I was the best. What I thought was: "Ella expects only the best out of life and, I'm sure, the best is exactly what she's going to get. Just look at her. She even dresses for the part. Everything about her exudes style, class and expensive, impeccable taste — from her earrings to her perfume to her cultivated New England accent. It's as if her very aura broadcasts the warning, 'Don't even play with me, little boy, unless you're corporate executive material, refined and fully equipped to play in this arena.' " Yet there was nothing mercenary or callous about Ella. There's another class of calculating woman just a shade shy of a hustler, but Ella was not that kind of woman. In fact, she hailed from a class so naturally refined that I even agreed that she should have somebody better than I. There was simply something regal about Ella.

I didn't want to muss up Ella's life — not that a person can't live a normal life with HS2. Obviously, my whole thesis is that we can, but we have to be sure to select the right person. Again, it is not just an issue of blind faith, but I always advocate logic and practicality. With any contagious disease there are risks, and HS2 is a contagious disease. No one with HS2 should enter into a relationship without making a candid appraisal of the risk. No matter how spiritual, positive or faith-filled one is — assuming one isn't a mystic — there is still this very real risk.

Of course, there is also this new issue of asymptomatic transmission. The possibility exists that HS2 can be transmitted (1) even by people who don't know that they have HS2, and (2) in cases where the safest, risk-free sexual behavior is practiced. As I mentioned in Chapter 5, I haven't seen any evidence of this form of transmission in my various relationships over the years, but it is important to realize that there is no such thing as risk-free sexual activity.

There is this tendency for truth students to play the ostrich and stick their heads in the sand, pretending that God is going to protect them and their mates from all harm, but this is not the case. Often, their metaphysical teachers must share the blame for this, because the absoluteness of the principles being taught tends to encourage students to act with a certain boldness that is well beyond their level of consciousness. One of our problems as human beings is that we all tend to think that we are more enlightened than we are. There are biological and material laws that have to be obeyed, and the Truth student must never be so irresponsible as to subject another person to unreasonable risk. The problem for the aspiring spiritual student is that there is no room in metaphysics for doctrines of gradualism, such as I teach. The tone in which I am writing is widely considered to be negative by the enlightened set.

No matter how badly I may have craved having a relationship with Ella, I could never promise her that she wouldn't be infected. Not really. If you are sufficiently disciplined, mentally and physically, and if you are willing to do all the right things, then chances are great that your mate won't be compromised. But — and this is a major *but* — it is not you, but your mate who must decide to take that risk. Any other move, and you've just created an enemy for life. In this chess game that we call life, that's your mate's move. Where entering into a relationship with someone with HS2 is concerned, our job is to allow our mates to make an informed choice. As a single man, I wouldn't dare make that move for my mate, or even attempt to influence it. If you have to argue someone into accepting you with HS2, I can assure you that it's not going to work.

There are different kinds of people in the world. Some can handle adversity very well; others can't deal with it at all. It's not a matter of criticizing them for how they are, or trying to change them. The only issue is opening your eyes and being aware and being gracious enough to say "no thanks, I pass" when you know something is not exactly for you. In this case, almost is not good enough. You have to hold out until you find someone who accepts you *exactly* the way you are.

I had the greatest respect for Ella. I loved being around her and she loved being in my company, but it wouldn't have taken a Rhodes scholar to see that Ella wasn't the type to graciously accept any type of adversity or personal setback. She didn't have time for imperfections. She is an achiever of the highest ilk, one who's going to reach extraordinary heights in this world. You know the type. I'm sure there are some Ellas, both male and female, in your life. They are idealistic, insulated, soft types. When things go wrong, they tend toward denial and nervous breakdowns. All their lives they've been groomed for success — I mean in a regal, painless, yellow-brick-road sort of way. As an intelligent man, I just couldn't walk into that kind of woman's life knowing that I wasn't bearing the kind of news that was consistent with her program. That kind of woman can sulk silently for a long time, mostly in a state of insufferable catatonia while categorically denying this unplanned infringement of reality. Then when reality finally begins to set in, Ms. Super Sophisticate/Super Achiever is capable of turning on a man and suing him for all he's worth. The charge: not fulfilling her dreams — or better yet, not fulfilling her *mother's* dreams for her! — and not playing the exact role that she signed him up to play. This may sound negative, but by the time I met Ella I had already been around that block a couple of times. I knew the neighborhood.

This message is especially for my metaphysical and New Age friends. Even those on the spiritual path cannot afford to be naïve. There is a pragmatic and rather harsh side to this life that we are obliged to live through the medium of the flesh. Those who do not obey its laws will be scorched and burned.

There is another complicating factor that makes it difficult for men to deal with women like Ella, a factor that operates in such an insidious way that men rarely recognize its presence until it's too late. The very qualities of women like Ella are those qualities that most men will die for. It's women like Ella whom they want to conquer and possess. She's an achiever; she's sophisticated; she's everything that will help him elevate his status in society. Clearly, the kind of man that I'm addressing is one who hasn't invested much in his own spiritual, psychological and mental growth so that he wouldn't be coming from need and materialistic/superficial values in a situation such as this. Unfortunately, there are lots of highly successful, intelligent and educated men who fall in this category. They have invested no time in getting to know themselves, and in most cases, given a choice, they will opt for the most superficial values in a mate. Once this type of man "wins" the charms of the woman, she becomes nothing more than window-dressing for his ego, and should they enter into commitment, they rarely become happy campers.

Though some of my stories must obviously be told from a male perspective, we shouldn't get hung up on the gender issue in our search for truth. There is no question but that, for every female

Ella, there is a male "Ella," or perhaps, Elias, who also can't handle adversity — or, perhaps, I should say, who is *unwilling* to handle adversity. Everybody knows of men who won't commit and men who run away from responsibility, family, their children, the mortgage, and any other unpleasantness that strikes their families. In my eyes, there is no favored gender. All stories, if they speak of spiritual truths, must have an androgynous, universal appeal.

After the Ella situation, at least then I realized that what I really longed for were the same "normal" human values that I and my intellectual colleagues had mocked for many years. It sounds hokey for an iconoclast like me to utter the words, but I wanted love and acceptance, normal human relationships, commitment and family. I wanted to belong. But I didn't know how to break rank from the smug set that comprised my cherished circle of friends. When you're in your 20's, how do you stand up in the midst of a group of haughty, over-educated, self-righteously indignant, condescending friends and admit, "I've been wrong all along! I'm sorry but this way of thinking is not working for me. I'm miserable! I want to be like those people that we've been poking fun at — you know, Americana and apple pie — at least in part. Though I'm still a free-thinker, I want those good ol' family values that we have pooh-poohed and disdained for so long. I want to partake of those faithful, one man-to-one woman virtues that the middle class believes in." How do you ever explain this to your friends? It's hard enough to even admit it to yourself.

This is what I wanted, although it took me 10 years to admit it to myself. It didn't help me one iota all of those years that I prayed and fasted and meditated and paid healers to try to heal me, and ate vegetarian, and tithed, and volunteered in the church, and took natural herbs, and acted spiritual. The Law was simply waiting for me to exhaust myself in the field of metaphysical gamesmanship and return home to a set of simple truths and values. There is no mystery to life. It's simple in concept, but accepting it can be a bitter pill to swallow.

This is not to imply that everyone should want the same things that I wanted. Everyone must search their own souls and try to be as honest as they can.

While searching out there in the far country for substitute values, I missed heaven. This should be our premise:

GOD HAS NEVER MADE A SINGLE MISTAKE. SO IF I HAVE CONTRACTED THE EXPERIENCE OF HS2, LET ME GET IN TOUCH WITH WHAT HAVING THIS CONDITION IS ALL ABOUT, INSTEAD OF WASTING ENERGY BY FIGHTING IT.

As I began to do that, I discovered that nowhere is it written that I can't have those values that I really want − a satisfying, committed relationship, family, a normal sexual relationship, etc. − even though I have HS2. Where did I get that bogus information in the first place? It turned out that I had *assumed* this on my own. Of course, I had been influenced greatly by media-magnified herpes mania, articles, lawsuits and comments published in the newspapers, thoughtless comedians' jokes, water fountain wisecracks and other groundless lore, but I committed the error of believing in all of this baloney when Spirit hadn't revealed anything of the sort to me.

This is reminiscent of a mind set associated with many Catholics. At one time the Pope ruled that Catholics couldn't eat meat on Fridays, or else they'd end up in purgatory or somewhere equally warm. Later, the papal office reversed itself and decreed that it was okay for Catholics to eat meat on Fridays. What was the truth all along? Did God change his mind? Did God rewrite his criteria for getting into heaven? Absolutely not! As always, certain appointed spiritual interpreters came up with this nonsense. In some cases, assumed "truths" can confine us to such regimented modes of thinking that they block us from our healings.

After a couple of years of diligent meditation and practice, gradual but positive changes began to take place in my life. As I neared completion of my formal metaphysical training, it became clear to me that I had come a long way since Sophia and Marsha. After a couple of long, dry years, socially speaking, I began to meet an entirely different genre of woman. As if I had passed through a transforming barrier, all of a sudden there weren't any more Marshas in my life. I could only deduce that this new, more responsible, ordered philosophy of life must be working.

I am reminded of Angelica, a beautiful young lady whom I dated a few years ago. Our relationship marked an important milestone in my life in that she was the first spiritually-aware woman with whom I had a significant relationship after I embarked upon the spiritual path. Elise would come later. Finally, the triumvirate would be completed upon meeting my wife.

Angelica, a nonpracticing Catholic, was the living embodiment of grace and beauty and class. At the time, I wanted her in my life in the worst way. Meeting her was living proof that my karma was changing for the better. I was about 33 when I met her, and it was difficult at that time for me to stay in the moment. I was so enthralled by what was happening to me that I tended to press for every little thing to be perfect between us. The way of Truth is to stay in the moment and let life reveal itself one step at a time. I suppose I knew this intellectually, but I had never been in a spiritually-centered relationship before. So basically, I didn't know how to act. In the vernacular of the street, I didn't know how to lay low and be cool. After all, a relationship is going to be whatever it's going to be. Sure, it's important to put some effort into it, but one also has to know when to back off and let a relationship reveal itself. What complicated matters was that this was one relationship that I didn't want to blow.

From an HS2 perspective, it would have been much easier for me if, after I had given it my best shot, Angelica had not fallen for me; but as divine grace would have it, she did. She liked me a lot. The problem that forced me to face was that I couldn't just play around with her. After the Marsha experience, I had promised the Creator that if It would lift me up out of the gutter and change my life, I would never take advantage of women again. Now I had to honor my word by being brutally honest with Angelica, even if it meant that I might lose her.

The year was 1983. Now mind you, up to that point I had never had a sincere or decent relationship. My highest ideal of a romantic relationship had always involved the prosaic principle of mutual usage. I couldn't imagine a relationship with a woman that did not entail lying and cheating and suffering and heart-break. Though I had been working diligently to overcome the old pattern, it is difficult to accept it when the time finally arrives. I was comfortable in my misery. But that was before meeting Angelica.

It's awfully difficult to open your closet and expose all of your skeletons to someone that you really love. In all of my years of living, I have never found a right time to spring bad news on anyone. Here's someone who is totally enamored with me, who thinks I'm brilliant, honest, upright, special — how in the world do you tell a woman like this that you have HS2? It's not the kind of thing that's easy to face.

It would be so much easier to meet people who are horrible, and whom you don't love and never could. Then you could simply use each other and nobody would complain. It would be easier to meet someone who has become hardened and bitter and has been stripped of every vestige of innocence — the kind of person who expects every line to have a hook, the kind who has graduated from the school of hard knocks and has heard every line twice. Those kind of people can cope. You don't mind laying bad news on them, because they expect it. They never allow themselves to be too happy, so it's impossible for them to ever be too sad.

But Angelica was a genteel woman. She was so trusting that it instinctively made me want to protect her from shock, worldly realities and things unpleasant. Thus it was the hardest thing in the world to risk the whole enchilada by telling her that I had HS2. I toiled over this issue for days. I didn't want the relationship to progress too far before I leveled with her. It was only fair. Guided by my strong libido and weak mind, I had hurt too many before. If I was to advance in life, I couldn't bear to hurt anyone else. It was only right that she have the opportunity to pull out before becoming emotionally invested.

Since there never seems to be a right time to deliver unpleasant news, I decided that the best way was to write her a detailed confession letter and let her read it privately, away from my influence, so that she wouldn't have to maintain composure for my sake or feel pressured into continuing romantic involvement with me. Of course, during the moments of waiting, I felt like dung. You can't imagine how badly I wanted to be accepted by this lady, but I decided that I had to risk losing her rather than deceive her and have her become angry with me later. It was one of those "damned if you do, damned if you don't" situations. If you tell them up front, you risk disappointing them wholesalely. If you delay and tell them later, you risk making them angry. Either way, you become another dog, validating their prevailing suspicion that there are no decent men (or women, if you're a man). Today I realize that it's immaterial which way they react. Therefore, my current modus operandi would be to do whatever I think is right and let the chips fall where they must.

With trembling hands I somehow completed the letter. When she came over to visit, I made my disclosure the first order of business. Once you decide to act, it's important not to let the atmosphere be broken by pleasant banter and other more agreeable diversions. I still don't know how I did it, but with all the courage I could muster I handed the letter to her and left her alone so that she could be free with her emotions. In the meantime, I was sweating.

After she finished reading the letter, she came into the next room where I nervously waited and embraced me in a way that spoke louder than words. Before a word was spoken, I was sure that I knew everything that I needed to know. Not only did she want to continue the relationship, but she couldn't even understand how I could have ever imagined that something as trivial as HS2 would be allowed to come between us.

It turned out that the whole nightmarish debacle — the fear of rejection complex — existed only in my head. My dear Angelica saw life differently than I — or than I had even been able to imagine. I knew then that I was on the right track with this new approach to living. I took a risk and faced the ultimate dragon, and was rewarded — for the first time, I might add — with the immense joy of total acceptance. It's rare to receive unconditional love, but once you do, you immediately realize its awesome power. It can change your life.

Due to the impact that my letter had upon her consciousness, my friend informed me that there was something that had been eating her up, as well. Unbeknownst to me, due to my preoccupation with my own troubles, she, too, had been harboring this looming, dark secret which she had never had the nerve to share with anyone. I looked at her and I'm telling you that this woman was shaking like she had the D.T.'s. She couldn't keep her composure or command her own voice to speak. Next thing I know, she was crying uncontrollably, as I tried to comfort her and tell her that it was all right...whatever it was.

Can you imagine how difficult it was for me to remain patient during what seemed like an eternity, while my mind raced through all of the possible things that could possibly be wrong with this dear soul whom I loved? Just moments earlier I was worried because I was totally focused on how bad my condition was. In the very next instant, here I was totally preoccupied with what could possibly be wrong with *her*. Is life strange or what? Maybe she had something worse than I. AIDS wasn't a big thing back in '83, so that possibility never crossed my mind. Would I be able to handle it? What a paradox and a tragedy it would be if I ended up rejecting her because I couldn't handle her revelation after she had come through in such a grandiose way by accepting mine. Is life really this cruel? Cannot experiences exist which bring pure joy with no strings attached?

Some people say that God tests us. I summarily reject all such beliefs. Granted, it *seems* as if God tests us at times. By my reckoning, it has to be impossible for God to test us, for God is pure, absolute and unconditional love. Regardless, life is definitely structured such that it confronts us with enough hurdles or "tests," if you will, hierarchically-queued, to ensure that we are serious when we say that we want to grow. In metaphysics this is referred to as the *Law* of God, or the Law of Cause and Effect. Sometimes, it is also referred to as karma. The in-depth treatment of these issues is beyond the scope of this book. But the practical implication of this law is this: Don't pray for God to help you grow unless you're sure that you want to grow. Growth hurts!

So far I'm thinking that this woman must have done something or been subjected to something incredibly horrifying. Maybe she was raped. I dated one woman back in Chicago who had been raped, and in the 13 intervening years that I knew her since the rape, her life went progressively to pot.

Maybe my friend had accidentally killed someone with her car, perhaps a child. I once worked with an attractive young lady back in Cambridge who had fatally injured a child in this way, and she was darn near a basket case. So I figured it had to be something like this.

Finally, I got my friend to tell me what had happened to her. Her great "sin" was that she had undergone an abortion. As already alluded to, she had been raised a Catholic. One of the lessons that I learned when I lived with Sophia during the prodigal phase of my life is that there are no ex-Catholics.

Abortion — phew! I was so relieved. Not to trivialize the impact that abortion has on someone who had been brought up staunchly Catholic, I was relieved because at least *I* could deal with that. At least one of us needed to be able to accept whatever the problem was going to turn out to be.

Abortion was not one of my weak points. I had plenty of arguments to help her learn to accept and love herself despite what she had gone through. And, I could be unconditionally loving right on, which came as a total surprise to her. For the first time in her life, she had risked to invite somebody into her confidence and had been met with total acceptance. She was healed in that very moment, just as I had been healed by her acceptance of me. Mutually, we had just experienced our first real life lesson in unconditional love. Of course, each of us still had ample work to do. We had to continue to push ourselves to complete the personal healing work that was necessary during the subsequent months.

The verbalizing of acceptance marks only the beginning, and in truth no one is ever *totally* unconditional in his or her love. It's one of those phrases that's easy to say but difficult to practice. Total acceptance is an absolute standard and a lofty goal. One great thinker said, "A man's reach must be further than his grasp, or else what's a heaven for?"

I shared this story because it helps us see how everybody is going around protecting their own "worst possible" scenarios. It should be clear from this story that if there are those who want to continue believing that they are injured, there is no way that I can convince them that they aren't. On the other hand, the moment they decide that they're ready to give it up, they don't have to be injured anymore. My friend Angelica gave it up.

My other friend, the one in Chicago who had been raped, was never able to give it up. Last time I talked with her, she was continuing to subject herself to a succession of abusive, degrading relationships with men — usually married men. In all cases, they were men who weren't really available.

Lest someone be tempted to indulge in pop psychology here, let me cut him or her off at the pass. If the whole story were revealed here, it would be clear to those who might be tempted to draw simple conclusions that the fallout associated with this rape was only one of this woman's major life issues. Rape is bad enough. It's a horrible thing. I personally pained for what this woman must have gone through, but I can tell you that this woman thrived on the edge of disaster. She attracted, courted and created disaster in every aspect of her life.

As it were, I knew this woman's family quite well. I had worked under her father's tutelage as a summer engineering intern at a research facility for a major oil company in Chicago. What was clear to me was that she was trying desperately to strike back at her successful, perfectionist father who has always been somewhat disappointed with her performance in life. Her father was a Ph.D. and doted on his oldest son, who was my friend's picture perfect older brother and an M.D. Without spiritual intervention, my poor friend didn't have a chance. And she wasn't interested in things spiritual at all, at least not at that time.

The main point that I want to highlight here is that there was only one factor that was common to healing the great anxiety harbored by Angelica and by me, and it was neither understanding nor communication. It was this: **UNCONDITIONAL LOVE AND ACCEPTANCE.** This is the thing that the whole world is searching for today. I was hesitant to tell my romantic interest about my condition because I was afraid she would not accept me as I was, and she was hesitant to tell me about hers for the same reason. Once revealed, we both thought the other person's concerns to be overblown to the point of ridiculousness. Her concern was trivial to me and my concern was trivial to her. The happiness that ensued was beyond explanation, because we had each found somebody who loved us enough to look past our so-called defects and accept us unconditionally. Wouldn't it be nice to live in a world where you never had to worry about rejection? You and I must create microcosms of that world for ourselves and for our friends.

This is it, world. If you want to be healers, start learning how to accept everybody unconditionally right now. That's right, *everybody!* Work out a way in your own consciousness to accept everyone that you come into contact with, regardless of how obnoxious certain ones may appear to be or what you think they may have done to you. And be not mistaken; some of these people will be extremely obnoxious! Nonetheless, in Truth no one has done anything against any of us. No one has tricked us or duped us. We are getting back exactly what we have sent out, and it only *appears* as though someone has done us wrong.

Now I know this seems pie-in-the-sky and theoretical, but I'm telling you that this principle is practical. You just have to try it and prove it for yourself. Until then, there is just no way to realize the truth of this universal principle. If you will chance to totally accept someone who is obnoxious to you, or who has apparently duped you — without being a doormat, of course — you will be in for the surprise of your life. "Prove me now herewith, said the Lord of hosts..." (Malachi 3:10)

A strange thing happened during the days that followed. I became preoccupied with trying to keep Angelica in my life. It's like the preoccupation with accidents and death immediately after getting married. Some of you will know what I'm talking about. It's like that adjustment period right after purchasing a new car when you're hoping that nobody scratches or steals it. Whenever you find something good, it's natural to want to hold onto it. Once you've found that perfect one, you can't imagine ever finding someone a second time to love you just as perfectly. Is it reasonable to expect to hit the million dollar lottery twice? Little did I know that I was making another error in thinking so far as spiritual Laws are concerned, and thus setting the stage for another hard lesson: the loss of Angelica.

God would not have us hold onto anything out of fear, for to do so is tantamount to believing that perfect Spirit cannot provide for our needs in the future. If It did it one time, It certainly can do it again. But this is one of those indisputable truths that's easier to voice than to practice. I've often wondered: Why do my lessons have to be so hard? Just for one day, I want to have it easy.

After a few months, Angelica lost interest in me, severed the ties that bound us and moved on. The turnabout was as instantaneous as when she fell in love with me. She was young (mid-20's) and wide-eyed with lots of mountains to scale in her life. She would go on to enroll in graduate school and get involved in political movements to help liberate the small Caribbean country of her birth. In terms of our relationship, it had tremendous promise but the timing simply was not right. It would be awhile before I would recover from the loss of what could have been.

Exactly two years after meeting Angelica, the second important, spiritually-significant relationship was attracted into my life. Her name was Elise. After reaching rock bottom following rejection by Angelica, I was through licking my wounds and wallowing in self pity. A fresh shot of self esteem was slowly beginning to bud, and I was determined to get on with the process of living.

By this time I realized that I was so confused about relationships that nothing short of drastic action was going to help me clear my mind. I needed to forget about women for awhile, clean house and make a desperate, all-out attempt to get back to self. No longer was I aware of who or what my true self was. Who was thinking these thoughts through me? What was driving me? Why was I so consistently attracted to women who couldn't possibly do me any good? It was time to rediscover the true self of my being, the one that would be able to see clearly if my mind hadn't been enslaved by a lifetime of worldly experiences.

Finally, I said to myself: "Let's face it, Bernard. Your social life isn't working. Drastic action is called for." The only thing that

I could think to do was to take some time off from dating and all romantic involvement until I could recapture control over my own mind. Without realizing it, I had, in effect, come to the decision to be celibate. Yes, celibate! I decided to shoot for a year. Perhaps, by then, I would be rid of a gnawing feeling of persistent sexual need. Perhaps, in a year I could become uncluttered, clear and innocent again — like a child. Once upon a golden time, I did not know the feeling of missing anything and I was able to look upon attractive women innocently and neutrally. I was determined to get back there.

Many of the problems that I have been addressing are related to a single, prevalent human state: sensual desire. If sensual desire is too deeply-rooted, it blocks one ability to behold pure thoughts. A pure thought, by my own definition, is a thought that is not dependent upon anything external to you, as individual. To the degree that we can have pure thoughts, we can begin to slowly unravel the mystery of life and formulate clear answers that will reveal to us what is best for our lives. In other words, we will be able to interpret the will of God. Whatever temptation there may be before us at this time, a pure thought will reveal spontaneously whether it is in our best interest to pass or indulge.

Consider this. If there is a deeply-rooted subconscious desire that is associated with the human ego or human will, that desire will color everything concerning any decision to be made. No longer will the thought be pure. It will be tainted. It's sort of like trying to clean yourself off while standing in a puddle of mud. You can expend a lot of energy and feel real proud of yourself for the amount of work you've done, but your goal will never be accomplished until you find a pure vantage point from which to work. In other words, you've got to get out of the mud.

I had a strong feeling that if I could approach life as an observer, and not a participant, for a year or so, I might then be ready for a clean, clear and unfettered relationship. I needed time out. My mind had become corroded. Too many years of *Playboy* magazine and X-rated movies had taken their toll. I had bought into the liberal, humanistic lie which teaches that these devises do not lead to degeneracy. Well, one man's testimony does not constitute a scientific study, but I can testify that they degraded me. The effect was immediate and palpable. Every time I indulged in prurient entertainment, I became more and more restless and more obsessed with the physical aspects of sex. Certain impulses became deeply embedded in my subconscious mind and it was hard to dislodge them. Sex became increasingly more detached from personalities, relationships, growth or love. Instead, sex became an oppressive, weighty end in itself, consuming vast proportions of my unconscious thought. It was like a separate beast lurking within me, incapable of being satisfied. To regain my mental health, I had to vacuum clean my mind and start afresh. Only then would I be ready to accept the implications and responsibilities that go with meaningful involvement.

Granted, none of this is easy to accept. I expect many liberal-minded people to categorically reject my conclusions. In fact, I'm sorry to have to be the messenger. I never expected to arrive at these conclusions, or to be the one to have to announce them. I never liked people who go around condemning other people's way of life. To this day, it's still strange hearing myself speak this way. As difficult as it may be to believe, I'm not coming from a judgmental position. Unlike the Bible-thumpers, I still believe in free will and freedom of choice. I'm not preaching that everyone ought to stop indulging in these behaviors because they lead to degeneracy. I realize that everyone isn't interested in change any more than I wanted to change while I was operating in a more worldly way. It was my choice, and I was enjoying it at the time...I thought.

People have to learn at their own pace. That's the way God designed it, and that's the way it ought to be. My message is to help guide those through who are tired of suffering from the effects of HS2 and have firmly resolved that they are ready to change.

It's hard to see clearly while you're still caught up in the game. Pure, uncluttered thoughts cannot navigate through a foggy mind. It would be like trying to thread a needle through a Brillo pad. There just aren't any clear channels to get a pure thought through. I wanted to be able to approach relationships from a new place in consciousness, one free of certain habitual, deeply subconscious, primitive male impulses. I yearned to be in the driver's seat for once in my life, as opposed to my libido.

Those of us who are serious about change must continually struggle to regain control over our minds. My self-imposed "purification" process was designed to weed out the countercurrents of negative thought from my mental field, effectively building a new, attractive field around me that would function like a huge electromagnet. And afterwards, if my understanding of spiritual Laws was correct, I would no longer have to look for love, sex or what have you, but I would be able to attract whatever and whoever was right for me according to my own mental equivalent. With sex no longer the dominant issue, for the first time I would be able to see the true woman.

IF YOU WANT TO REGAIN THE ABILITY TO TASTE SUGAR, SOMETIMES YOU HAVE TO STOP EATING SWEETS ALTOGETHER.

The question was put earlier: How does one stop seeking outwardly for love so that the law of attraction can come into play? Well, this is how I did it. Taking some extended time off was effective for me, and I believe it can work wonders for others just as well. But we mustn't fool ourselves. Many times when we say that we are denying ourselves, whether it's food, sex or whatever, we are still stashing away hidden pleasures in the closet. We may be sneaking desserts when nobody's looking; i.e., we may be keeping a lover on the side. You know how we are. We may be saying that we aren't seeing anybody, while still maintaining an old standby who has a tendency to call at the last minute on those lonely Saturday nights when self pity and hormones conspire to overtake the will. If you are still playing that kind of game, nothing is going to change in your life. You mustn't attempt to fool yourself.

The process that is being outlined here is designed to change your very MIND. You CANNOT fool your mind! Don't get caught up in trying to fool people. If you slip, you slip. Go ahead and admit it; then get back on the wagon and try it again. Never say die. Just keep trying and trying, and praying and meditating and being patient, and finally the day will arrive when you will be able to look self pity and hormones both in the face on Saturday night and assert, "NO, I WILL NOT SUBMIT TO YOU ANYMORE!" From that day forward, you will have broken their power over you and you will know your true strength. Your subconscious mind will have finally gotten the message that YOU (the true self) are in control.

This method may sound far out, but it is totally consistent with universal spiritual principles. Now, by no means am I advocating seclusion or weird behavior, because, if you want to become normalized, I am a firm believer in staying grounded with your feet planted firmly on the ground, while interacting as normally as possible with people of all ilks and working hard at some kind of job. Except in rare cases, we should never detach ourselves from the world around us. We were placed here, and it's important that we learn to function here. It's important that we not try to escape. We just need to remain grounded while we growing, that's all.

It's so easy — and tempting — to develop a disdain for people and withdraw from them, especially as you develop a higher spiritual understanding. But this is not the answer. Furthermore, it is not healthy for students of Truth to surround themselves only with others who think the same as they think, or subscribe to the same spiritual philosophy, yet this is a standard form of behavior among aspirants in every religious or metaphysical order that I have investigated. Obviously, there may be times when people need to withdraw from certain influences, but as a consistent practice it can only lead to self righteousness and delusion.

Jesus appeared to be a fairly earthy, grounded dude. In violation of the religious standards of his day, he consorted with Samaritans, harlots, lowlifes and regular working class people, as well as the high and mighty. That's one of the things I like about this historic personality. Also, similar to the process that I underwent to cleanse my mind, Jesus understood the importance of purifying his mind on a regular basis. (Of course, I modeled my life after his, and not vice versa.) By devoting lots of time for meditation and prayer in places called "the wilderness," or "the mountaintop," he developed an attractive aura around himself that affected many who came into his presence. History reveals that he often fasted during his seclusion. I, too, found it necessary to fast during my year of abstinence — not so much from food as from sex. The object of a fast does not have to be food.

Omniscient Law of the creative Spirit attracts certain people into our lives at certain times for specific instructional purposes according to our readiness and receptivity. After my year of "fasting," It brought Elise into mine. She was a sensitive and loving woman, and she professed to be spiritually-committed. In her I found an unusual combination of mores.

Although Elise was a highly moral person, she was devoid of the slightest tinge of sexual repression and guilt such as had haunted me all my life. She had two young kids, a girl and a boy, and again, she was a tremendous role model in the way that she handled her sexuality. I couldn't help but wonder how different my adult life would have been if I had started out with such a healthy respect, understanding and openness about sexuality.

The reason I qualified her as the first "moral" person that I'd met who possessed this particular balance is because she was spiritually-aware, spiritually-oriented and spiritually-committed, *and* sexually healthy, a combination which, prior to then, I had not witnessed in a woman. I don't mean that she was kinky or way out. She just didn't have any neuroses about how her body looked. She was just very natural and open. Before her, I had known many physically attractive women who, once I got to know them, were amazingly insecure about their bodies (for example, my ex-girlfriends Marsha and Sophia). My earlier experiences had suggested that sexually-liberated people were hedonistic, while "spiritual" people were self-abnegating and puritanical, in the classical, Victorian, guilt-laden sense. In Elise I realized how stereotypical and false my beliefs had been.

By the way, Elise did not have HS2. Neither does my wife, D Renee. I suppose somebody will want to know these things. People are always looking for evidence and precedents in their attempts to develop greater faith, which is all right with me.

Regardless, in 1985 when I met Elise my whole world was still colored by the specter of HS2. There were all of those happy people out there, and then there was me. Forgive me if this doesn't sound enlightened, but that's the way I saw the world.

At the time I was about 95 percent certain that I had met my true soul mate. I thought that I wanted to be with Elise forever. Unfortunately, forever turned out to last for about six months. Or I should say, *fortunately*. Although the flames of our hope burned out faster than fireplace kindling, I still remember that relationship as a wonderful, loving experience, as well as an important transition point in my life. Like Angelica, Elise represented a relatively new experience for me: parting with a positive memory of an ex-girlfriend. So even though the relationship turned out to be a bust, it left me with something that I had never known before — confidence and hope. I knew right then that this new, attractive presence that I had been developing was indeed working. The verdict was in; spiritual Laws were real.

Elise was wonderful. She was tantalizingly close to what I thought I wanted. Instead of feeling disappointed, I began to think that if I could attract her, I could attract someone who was even more perfect for me. From this experience I developed a brand new respect for the stupendous power of our thoughts and words.

What I manifested in Elise was not the ultimate, highest or best relationship for me, but it was perfect enough to teach me what I needed to learn at the time. Why did we part? There were a number of small events that, lumped together, caused us to drift farther and farther apart. Taken separately, they are not important. Looking back, the central issue for me was Elise's craving for materialism. She was quite unhappy with her lot in life and, like so many others who are attracted to New Thought teachings, she expended a lot of her mental energy trying to figure out how to get rich. Her father had been a physician, but he had died while she was in adolescence, leaving her, her mother, and a couple of other siblings with little security. As a result, Elise couldn't get over the feeling that she had been cheated. She had been born to be a queen, with servants and all the works, but there she was a working class professional and a single parent struggling from paycheck to paycheck. This reality just didn't jibe with her image of herself as an enlightened spiritual being, and though I loved her I wasn't very sympathetic.

So Elise's materialism was one of our issues. Still, that wasn't enough to make me quit. Another incident occurred which caused her to undergo one of her numerous financial crises. But unlike the good, reliable boyfriend that I was supposed to be, I decided not to play the white knight by stepping in and bailing her out. I loved her, but I had firmly resolved that if that relationship was going to work, it was important that it be built on a foundation more solid than financial or material dependency. From that exact moment, Elise withdrew all of her love and affection for me and turned a deaf ear to all of my future attempts to establish communication.

I was extremely hurt. It seemed to me that Elise was using a perfectly surmountable issue to end a promising relationship. During the weeks that followed, I never stopped calling her or pleading with her to engage me in communication on a higher level. What were the underlying issues? — that's what I wanted to know. She wouldn't say, so we drifted apart and went our separate ways.

A few months later, the telephone rang. It was Elise. We spoke, but the tone was more befitting of strangers than close friends. The most important information that was imparted was Elise's confession to me that the real reason for her withdrawal from the relationship had everything to do with HS2. In the vacuum created by the lack of honest communication on her part, the fear that she would become infected had taken on gargantuan proportions in her mind and over-powered her.

Phew! I was relieved. At last closure had been established in one of the most perplexing episodes of my life at that juncture. I didn't blame Elise then, nor do I blame her now for making that particular decision. As I said before, I believe in free will and I commend people for exercising theirs, so long as they are willing to own up to it. It's too bad that Elise did not feel confident enough to communicate her true feelings to me in real time. The outcome would have been the same, because there was no way that I would have argued against a woman's intuitive feeling. There is one thing on which I have always been clear:

I DON'T WANT ANY RELATIONSHIP THAT IS HELD TOGETHER BY PITY OR ANY OTHER FORM OF EMOTIONAL OBLIGATION.

Where important principles and values are concerned, I ardently believe that compromise in relationships is completely unnecessary. I have had many arguments with people about this. Whether coupled or single, I am absolutely convinced that I am supposed to be happy in this life. If one person doesn't want me because of HS2, it doesn't mean that I am unlovable. In fact, it doesn't mean anything at all about me. This is where my faith in a Universal Loving Spirit comes in, a Spirit that is personal. So long as I'm being honest, loving, genuine and sincere, I can bless people like Elise and send them on their merry way, knowing that I will attract someone else who is even more perfect for me.

To be perfectly honest — as it is my pleasure and my burden to be — I must admit that I was not celibate for the entire year while I was undergoing mental cleansing prior to meeting Elise. You might say that I "fell" once, right smack in the middle of the year. Perhaps, this aside isn't germane to the main principle that I am presenting, but it is the truth. You need to know about the human side that is always involved in this process. You see, I am not doing this for you; I'm doing it for me. Sometimes, spiritual self-help books tend to make everything seem so easy. Well, it's not. It may be simple but it's not easy. The process is seldom, if ever, monotonically progressive. There are days when you are able to gallop ahead, but sometimes you have to trot two steps backward for every one forward.

Yes, I fell once. When you really understand principle, it's not even an issue of regret. This is life — real life. There are those who would like to hear me say that I regret it, for people's sake. But regret is useless. Regret is a backwards-looking function, whereas I am a forward-thinking person. Although I once may have been blind, I am certainly not blind anymore, and believe you me, that's all that matters.

On the average, you're going to do what you have to do when you have to do it. That's fine. It may as well be, because no one has yet figured out how to regulate human behavior. No prison official or human behavior expert has yet figured out how to stop male prisoners from having sex in prison cells — with each other. What is the moral of this extraneous point? It is this: Go ahead and play your hand. Short of committing crimes, do whatever it is that you have to do — BUT! — after you have done it and found yourself tired of living that life, cast it out of your mind forever. Then lay your cards on the table and get on with your life.

It's a noble idea to go on a diet, in this case a sexual diet. Nevertheless, any time we get so caught up in the ritual of denial and self-discipline to the exclusion of balance, we will not learn very much from the experience. Life is a process of constant re-appraisal, rechoosing and balancing. It is not a situation where we determine *a priori,* once and for all how we're going to be in every conceivable situation. Sometimes we fall off the horse. The value of actually living such an experience is that we get to learn how it feels to fall off the horse. Then we get to look at ourselves anew and rethink our futures. We don't get to be quite as unadulterated and self-righteous as the guy who made a one time declaration and never fell off the horse, but then who needs to be *that* right?

I broke the rules, every last one of them. I was the original rebel. Not a soul was going to tell me what I had to do or what I couldn't do. I was going to show them that, for once, someone had come along who was truly different. I was going to show them that I could indeed break society's sacred rules AND get away with it. As I look back, I can say that I did enjoy every indulgence in which I engaged...at the time. But this I can also say, unflinchingly: Sooner or later, I paid dearly for every indulgence. I can't think of a single self-indulgent action that I have taken in life that hasn't caused me grief and pain later. And in most cases, it wasn't that much later.

Am I saying that one should never break the rules? No! There are times when you just have to break the rules. This is the nature of human growth, evolution and learning. As I approached the end of my *almost* celibate year, I went through a couple of months when life was so difficult that I began questioning everything that I had ever believed in, including life itself. The good news is that I came out of it with the same kind of conviction that I had before, only stronger. I knew then that, yes, I wanted to live, and how!

The truth was that I hadn't even lived yet, not really. The only reason I was going through all of that weird business (such as celibacy) was so that I could spend the rest of my life living peacefully, joyfully, affirmatively and spiritually consistent. Thus it would have been counterproductive and wasteful to bow out after all of that effort. Of course, everything I'm saying now is intellectual and rational, none of which seemed to matter at all at the time that I was having serious doubts.

After my relationship with Elise folded in 1986, I found that I had advanced to a different plateau along the road to spiritual maturity. Strangely enough, there was no need to go out and meet new friends for the purpose of restoring my sense of self worth. I continued to feel lovable, peaceful, self-confident and contented in spite of the breakup. At last I had reached a state where my opinion of myself was independent of some woman's opinion of me. I was okay and that's all there was to it. There simply was no need for me to enter into another degrading cycle of playing the game.

As weekends approached I no longer felt anxious to make the rounds, or to keep up with where the parties were and which night spots were hot. Though the idea of celibacy never came to mind at this new level of awareness, I found myself staying home and working passionately on new plans and projects during most weekends. I had dreams to fulfill. Though I wasn't meeting any new dating prospects, that was perfectly all right. It's awesome when it happens, but after all of those years of meditating and praying and trying to surrender to God, peace finally came.

I hadn't known that it was possible to maintain such a state of contentment over such an extended period without having what I had always wanted − a committed relationship with a devoted mate to call my own. Despite having been dumped by the two most spiritually-enlightened women that I had ever attracted into my life up to that time − Elise and Angelica − I was neither depressed nor angry. Nor did I feel bereft of purpose.

After breaking up with Elise, I turned and peered into the mirror and realized that I was still a bachelor, 36, and with no progeny. I remember thinking: "Maybe it isn't supposed to happen for me. So now, what do I do with the rest of my life? I think it's time to draft plan number two." Though everyone knows that men don't have a biological clock, per se, this man figured it was still getting to be pretty late. For the previous 10 years, I had been deliberately trying to settle down with one woman, and if I could have found the right one, I would have married her. It never occurred to me that there was no *right* woman for me at that time, because I wasn't *right* myself.

Nineteen hundred and seventy-six marked the year when I had given up the old gaming life in Boston, met Sophia and set out for a complete rebirth in Los Angeles. During the intervening 10 years, life hadn't unfolded quite as I had expected, but then life seldom does. Little did I know that I would be dragged through a succession of horribly painful and disappointing relationships over all of those years. Glancing backward, I could clearly see how confused I'd been and all the mistakes I'd made. Obviously, there was a lot more to mastering this thing called life than I had ever imagined. If a reasonably intelligent, upright young man, such as I was, could miscalculate his social capabilities by such a wide margin, what did that suggest about his future? Maybe it would be 10 more years before he would really see the light. What a depressing notion!

Instead of pursuing a new relationship after Elise, I borrowed $10,000, took a leave-of-absence from my engineering job and founded a small grassroots magazine based on a simple but little-known philosophy called New Thought. I named this magazine THE UPSTAIRS JOURNAL. Since I had little capital with which to launch this venture, my staff consisted of volunteers recruited from among my students, clients and friends. They were people who had attended previous workshops, classes and seminars of mine over the years. Little did I know it at the time, but one of those volunteers would later become my wife. If somebody had predicted such a thing, I would have laughed in his or her face.

I first met Donna Renee Brooks (known as "D") in 1984, two

years before I met Elise. She was 10 years my junior. In stark contrast to every woman that I had dated before, it was definitely not love at first sight. In fact, unlike it was with Angelica and Elise, I did not pursue her as a romantic interest. At the time I was still trying to make a go of being a successful standup comedian in the most competitive entertainment mecca in the world, Los Angeles. To improve my stage presence and enhance my performance skills, I signed up for an inexpensive acting workshop at a little theatre in my community. So did D. As either fate or Divine Providence would have it, D and I both chose the same scene to study from the classic play, *A Raisin in the Sun*, so our drama coach had no choice but to assign us to do a scene together.

It wasn't something that D was looking forward to. She considered herself to be a serious actress, having earned a college degree in drama a few years earlier before moving to L.A. to take on Hollywood. She knew a hack acting student when she saw one. As a wannabe comedian, I was looked upon by her as basically a clown who couldn't bring anything to her program in terms of enhancing her acting career. Within 60 seconds of talking with her to arrange the first out-of-class rehearsal for our scene, I accurately homed in on her entire attitude about me.

"Miss D," as I playfully refer to her, had already mapped out a firm picture in her mind of what her perfect mate would look like. I didn't even come close to qualifying, and she didn't pull any punches in letting me know. She was a classy, yet tough and haughty, San Francisco chick who neither minced words nor worried about some poor bloke's feelings, particularly not this bloke. For what it was worth, I admired her for that. Cute, she certainly was, but then they're all cute in L.A., so that was nothing new. At best I figured she could be what the guys refer to as "a project," meaning that a relationship could be worked out given enough time. But as for myself, I reckoned that there wasn't that much time in the world. She'd just have to be some other guy's project.

It's wonderful when you can do business with a person of the opposite sex without having to worry about her feelings or trying to impress her. "Does she like me? I wonder what she thinks of me?"

are the kinds of questions that often occupy our minds while we pretend to be concentrating on the business at hand. With Miss D neither one of us had anything to lose — or to gain — so we just settled down to being ourselves.

It wasn't long before we began to trade discussions about individual interests. I found out that she was an avid reader, a rather deep thinker (which surprised me) and a rather unhappy person behind that brusque facade. She found out that, besides being an engineer (which did not impress her) and a wannabe commedian, I was also a teacher and practitioner of some kind of arcane metaphysical philosophy. But she was private and independent and skeptical. It would be many months, or even years, before she would trust my motives. I thought that my motives were pure, but she wondered if, perhaps, my program wasn't just a way-out, clever scheme by yet another smooth-talking brother trying to weasel his way into another woman's boudoir.

She was impressed that I had read Kurt Vonnegut's popular book from the antiwar era, *Slaughterhouse Five*. It wasn't so much that she was impressed with *moi* as she was about finding a literary friend — male or female — in Los Angeles. After all, it's no accident that Harvard and Yale are not located in L.A. After having grooved in the ubiquitous intellectual circles in the Boston area for years, I, too, was impressed that I had met someone who held an appreciation for the wonderful world of ideas. Although I didn't satisfy her sartorial or aesthetic requirements — I'm no Mr. G.Q. — we ended up sitting in a restaurant discussing *Slaughterhouse Five* over Chinese food during the stretch of an entire afternoon.

Because I seemed to have a consistent, workable, and even pragmatic philosophy of life, D began to show interest in various aspects of my personal growth program. This included a list of recommended books on spiritual transformation, classes and workshops. In due time she completed a number of my workshops, as well as a couple of formal, accredited classes at a local New Thought training institute where I was on staff. Not only that, but she began to employ me as a professional personal counselor for the continuing problems that she encountered in the areas of career and relationships. Clearly, our relationship was platonic. I emphasize the "professional" aspect of our relationship because, unlike the average "friend" who has approached me for professional spiritual assistance, she always insisted on paying my going rate for services. Nonetheless, in spite of appearances, she did not matriculate through this regimen without continuously challenging and fighting against everything that I said. In later years I would discover that she had wanted to believe with all her heart, but she just didn't want to be suckered.

During the next couple of years we traded stories about the women that I dated and the men that she dated. I took my dates to see her perform in community theatre and she dragged hers along to my parties. We laughed and cried about the most intimate details of our respective pasts, liberated by the unquestionable assumption that we would never date each other. If she had had a hint that we might date someday, she wouldn't have told me half of what she did. As my wife, she has told me as much. We shared so many secrets with each other, because our friendship was pure with no strings attached.

As I withdrew from the frenzied pace during the year and a half post-Elise, besides leaving my job, I severed my affiliation with the New Thought church where I was a member and surrendered my hard-earned license as one of their professional practitioners. Afterwards, the only people with whom I communicated on a personal level were my volunteers and freelance contributors to THE UPSTAIRS JOURNAL. I did not drop out in anger. I was simply a man on a mission. Together, my volunteers and I organized and presented several public seminars on subjects of practical metaphysical interest. Busy cranking out magazines and preparing materials for lectures and seminars, I did not set aside time for dating. There would be no more girlfriends or dates until October of 1987, when I would propose to my future wife.

Unbeknown to me at the time, D had also decided to withdraw from the dating scene over roughly the same 18-month period. As close friends with common spiritual interests, we were devoting our attention and time to the development of our consciousness and the pursuit of higher understanding over a definite interval of time. Yet there were no formal rules to conform to or be restricted by. We were free to date if we so desired. Finally, after more than a year of working together so intensely, it began to dawn on me that D and I had moved closer and closer together in temperament and ideology. At first it was frightening. What did this mean? At the time I had no idea that she wasn't seeing anyone. Conversely, I assumed that she was. After all, she was very attractive and young. It would have only made sense. Though we shared a lot, I had always known that she maintained two different sets of male friends — those who were still into playing the game, and those who were interested in spiritual values.

To be fair I must credit two other special women for playing a pivotal role in my preparation and cleansing during this period of intense focus. It is true that every teacher needs a teacher, which is something that I certainly appreciate. For my continued growth and development, I retained two outstanding practitioners of Religious Science, Ms. Bessie Pickett and Rev. Juanita Dunn. Ms. Pickett was in her 80's at the time and Rev. Juanita, though younger, was still a couple of decades my senior. Both were old enough to have been places in consciousness where I still wanted to go. Both were no-nonsense, strictly spiritual types with outstanding track records in their work, yet each was a quiet, simple soul who shied away from public adulation and fanfare. Thus I was thankful for having the opportunity to take my troubles to their doorsteps and lay them on their mantles. Likewise, I was exceedingly glad to pay their nominal fees for working with me, praying for me and keeping me in the healing light. These magnificent women knew that I was interested in attracting my true soul mate, so they continued to treat for me during this entire episode. [In New Thought, the verb form "to treat" means to pray scientifically.]

The day was October 27, 1987. I'll never forget it. D came by that evening to help me assemble the latest edition of our publication. As I mentioned, we were not dating, nor had we been fooling around or flirting with each other during the preceding years. But all of a sudden, something changed. It's as if a light came on and infused me with the knowledge: "Listen up buster, this is your wife!" Somehow I knew that the light was the truth. By golly, could it be that my soul mate had been there all along! – closer than my very breath, nearer than hands and feet? I waited until we had finished working for the evening and she had sat down to collect herself before hitting the freeway. If I was going to act, I had to do it then or else the moment would be lost. So nervously, with eyelids a-fluttering and a humongous frog in my throat, with no introduction or build-up, I swallowed hard and blurted out the naked question: "D, will you marry me?"

It was surreal. After 38 years, this was the first time that I had every uttered those four magic words, and I tell you it's strange hearing yourself say them.

She knew all along that her answer was going to be yes, but she still put off the decision for a month to allow time for all of her newly-perturbed emotions to settle down. To my utter amazement, my proposal had not caught her by surprise. I would later learn that as she sat outside in her car prior to ringing my doorbell on that particular autumn day, the same light that had consumed me also descended upon her. I don't know if our experiences were synchronous, but by the time she heard me pop the big Q she already knew what was coming.

Six months later we were married and we've been happy ever since. "But," someone is probably wondering, "what about HS2? Did D know that you had HS2 *before* she accepted your proposal?" Well, yes. As I already mentioned, during the many months of our close, platonic, working friendship we had shared the most intimate of secrets. Of course, that didn't make it an automatic decision. There is always risk when you divulge information of a personal nature. You see, I realized that D had always looked up to me and regarded me as a perennially positive person. She saw me as one who had it all figured out. Despite the risk, at some point I realized that she was sincere and loving enough for me to tell her about even the imperfect, darker manifestations in my life. There are friends in our lives, and then there are *friends*. We will boast about our joy and accomplishments and finer points with virtually any breed of friend, but it's only with those special, one-of-a-kind friends that we chance to share that darker side of our souls.

Even after laying it on the table for D, it was difficult for her to think of me as a sick or unhealed person. She was only able to think of me as a child of God, spiritual in essence and committed to the ways of Truth. Of course, at that point in her life — when I told her that I had HS2 — she didn't have to ponder the implications in any personal sense, because, after all, she was never going to date me.

During the month between proposal and acceptance, I'm sure that she worked through many concerns and arguments about my having HS2. However, I never apologized for having HS2. What was, was. I could make no promise beyond what was then being offered on the table.

Of course, during our six-month engagement we had serious discussions about HS2. Although she told me that it was no problem, I insisted that we force ourselves to discuss as many of the associated issues as we could think of. I did not want to sugar-coat this thing with spiritual platitudes. Instead, I preferred to deal with its ugliest implications and call it for what it was. If she was reticent to express her true feelings, I turned up the pressure until every last thought was brought out into the open.

Being deft in my argumentative and persuasive skills, I could have played a psychological game on D's mind and made her feel guilty, unfaithful or unspiritual for harboring doubts about someone with HS2, but I wouldn't dare. This is that pragmatic side of metaphysics that I believe in so adamantly. We mustn't shrink from dealing directly with worldly conditions and negative aspects of life just because we believe in an enlightened principle. It's all part of the course curriculum in this thing called life. We don't want to get caught up in cutting off parts of ourselves and labeling it "bad," while labeling others parts "good." With my chosen wife-to-be, everything had to be discussed — not just once, but over and over and over again until we were both satisfied that there were no more unresolved concerns.

In contrast to what many people believe, it is critically important that we committed students of Truth not put dampers on our disclosures, although fears may surface, tears may flow and the mind may attempt to shut down. We must learn to approach these processes like heavyweight fighters groping for transcendent powers to descend upon them and lift their tired, heavy arms to help them make it through the final grueling rounds. As they say in sports, "It ain't over 'til it's over"; thus we must learn to remain firmly planted in the center of the ring until the proverbial stout lady sings.

But still, the process should never be forced. We must respect the fact that everyone is not capable of processing at the same level of intensity. After having known D and subjected her to intensive spiritual processes over the previous three and a half years, I knew that she could handle the heat. In fact, she held me to the same tough standard. I used to kid her all the time about having "too much lip," because she was known for saying exactly what was on her mind. In the early days of our relationship, very little of what was on her mind was flattering. But, in due time, this kind of mutual intensity was one of the features that attracted us to each other. She knew that I would not let her take the easy way out.

At one point during our processing, it seemed that we might not be able to make it to the altar. As a result of becoming engaged, it seemed as if a pall of urgency had descended upon us. We seemed to be on a treadmill heading inexorably towards matrimony and couldn't get off. What started out as a decision of choice suddenly seemed to be on automatic pilot. Realizing that, I felt that we needed to get back to that place of choice and relieve ourselves of every vestige of external pressure. In other words, we needed to back up and get back in touch with the fact that we still didn't have to get married if we didn't want to, and that we still had free choice. I reminded her that right up until the day of the wedding, should there be any doubt we could still change our minds. Conditions weren't in control of us; we were in control of conditions.

I was not afraid of marriage. The actions that I took had nothing to do with fear. Speaking for my half of the responsibility, I just had to take whatever time was necessary to make sure that I was thinking clearly and that I wasn't just infatuated or desperate or otherwise caught up in an emotional whirlwind. After all, it was the *process* of unfolding in Truth, and not the marriage, that was of the greatest importance. Since my day of awakening, I have said to Spirit: Thy will be done. If the process had revealed to us that we shouldn't get married, then that would have been the highest and most noble move to make. If we ignored the process, or otherwise circumvented issues due to laziness or unwillingness to face pain, then we would marry based on an incomplete understanding of our deeper, sub-conscious feelings. In that case the resulting marriage could only turn out to be disastrous. Thus it clearly is the process that's most important, and not the marriage.

To complete our process we held many sessions and audio-taped every word that was said. As committed students of Truth, we needed to explore our true feelings, fears, and desires and ask ourselves if what we were embarking upon was consistent with our true life mis-sions. If the answer came back negative, then there would be no marriage. We realized at that point that we loved each other more than we had ever loved anyone else, but so what? Loving each other was not enough. It was all about loving God and Truth and the ways of Spirit and doing only those things that were consistent with its purpose for creating us.

Up to this point it may seem that D's life was pristine and un-fettered by anything as weighty as HS2. If that were the case, we would be entering into marriage unequally yoked and it would not work. I would be bargaining from a groveling, insecure position, sort of like begging this "perfect" woman to sacrifice her life to bring happiness to this poor little imperfect man. But that wasn't the truth and it certainly wasn't where I was coming from. One of the things that I did for D was to make her aware of the opportunity that she had through this marriage to work out some of her eternal soul problems.

How did I know that D had some unresolved soul issues to work out? Because we all do. Why else would we be living on Earth? There's no question in my mind but that we all come here with some excess baggage to heal and release. You might picture this baggage as a pair of police handcuffs, which has your wrists firmly clasped together behind your back. The only way to remove the handcuffs is to find the key. So you spend the better portion of your days on

Earth searching for the key. During the course of a lifetime, you will probably try many keys, but most of them won't fit. The mechanisms just don't quite mesh. It's the same way with your emotional baggage. You can't get rid of it until you find the right key, but when you do you're going to be so relieved. Then you're going to SOAR!

Different people are carrying different burdens in their bags. Some are carrying around the burden of incest; others can't break free from the shackles of poverty; still others are housing afflictions like HS2. On the surface, everyone's bag looks just about the same. They come crying, "Help me — I'm lonely. I can't find a mate." "I'm a victim." "I've been abused and discriminated against." "Life is not fair." "Nobody understands me." There's nothing unique about the outer skin which circumscribes and contains the garbage. It's the inner cargo that defines the individual's mission and quest.

D's burdens had been two-fold. Number one was a feeling of failure in finding a man with vision and intellectual interests to truly love her, a man who would care for, understand and accept her as she was. Plus she wanted all of this in a faithful, committed relationship. It was part of her soul's quest that she had been searching for it all her life — idealizing, romanticizing and fantasizing in her mind — but up to that point it had been painfully elusive. In place of fond memories was the residue of pompous, self-centered suitors and a long stream of burnt out romances that almost were. Who doesn't have memories of lost romances that almost were?

The other biggie in D's life was her acting career. She had moved to Los Angeles a few years before and rationed herself five years to make it in the dog-eat-dog world of Hollywood, but that hadn't happened. The net result was that she was facing some facts about her life that summed up to disappointment. She was distraught and tired of it all by the time we met, but she didn't know where to turn or what to do. Besides these two challenges, she also had some physical challenges, which, compared to mine, seemed to be trivial. One was a skin problem; the other, which was actually caused by the medication she took to cure the former, was a hair loss problem. She didn't consider either to be minor. In fact, she became as depressed over her physical challenges as I had been during my worst bouts of HS2 infection. It's so astounding — and at times, even comical — yet it's all so relative. You can't convince anyone that his or her problems aren't the worst that's ever been known to humankind.

It turned out that both D and I were able to conquer some of our lifelong issues by committing ourselves to each other in marriage. Once the situation was positioned in the proper light, it was easy to see that we were indeed equally yoked. I should note, however, that never during our discussions did I try to persuade her one way or the other. To the day that I shuffle off this mortal coil, I will remain a fervent believer in free will. This is the highest of the *concrete* spiritual laws (to love God, Spirit and Truth is the highest of the *abstract* spiritual laws). Regardless of the losses or pain that I may incur, I don't want anything that does not gravitate to me by right of its own free will. I know that I can never *possess* a wife or keep one attached to me a day longer than she desires to stay. Further-more, in my puristic way of reasoning, if a woman is confused and begins to vacillate back and forth concerning which way to go, then so far as I am concerned the decision has already been made. She must go. I know by her actions that she is not for me.

If you think about it, vacillation is indicative of confusion and indecision. There should be absolutely no compromise in the decision to select a life partner. No agreements should ever be final-ized until all parties are absolutely sure and committed.

It's been more than four years now since our marriage, and we are happier than ever with each other. I still have HS2 (though I rarely have symptoms anymore) and she still doesn't. There have been lots of adjustments, but the unconditional love, respect, trust and support continue to pour forth like a mighty waterfall. In my wildest dreams I never expected it to flow this smoothly. There have been spats and arguments, but none heated or out of control, no dogfights, no separations, no harsh or regrettable words spoken or accusations made. Indeed it has been more like a dream than reality. But neither of us can take credit. Instead, we recognize that all credit goes to God and the Universal Laws of Spirit that I have been addressing. We are simply allowing ourselves to live in the kingdom of heaven on Earth moment by moment, day by day.

The result of this entire saga is that I have proven for myself this principle:

HS2 WAS NOT THE DOMINANT PROBLEM IN MY LIFE IN THE FIRST PLACE. IT NEVER POSSESSED THE POWER TO PREVENT ME FROM LIVING A HAPPY, PRODUCTIVE AND FULFILLED LIFE.

There's nothing out there blocking us. We can have what we want so long as it is consistent with the Divine Plan. But first we have to be able to imagine ourselves having it. Then we have to be willing to work, and even sweat, for it. Then we have to bless it along with all of the people who may appear to be standing in our way. Then we have to be honest about what kind of garbage we're bringing to the table. Then we have to let go of our preconceptions, misconceptions and biases and be open to all possibilities. Finally, we have to recognize it when it shows up and simply accept it.

Like Job, when I turned away from my physical condition toward reaffirming my faith in Spirit and Truth, I was immediately blessed and set free. Everything that I really wanted, I now have. I have the perfect wife for me and ours is the most committed, loving relationship. She loves me as I am and I love her. Neither of us has the attitude that HS2 is something in our relationship that needs to be healed. I know that I'm not a healer; God is the healer. I will take care of my life and let God take care of the healings. D and I choose to spend our time thanking God for our respective families, for bringing perfect mates into our lives in the form of each other, for our creative abilities and creative avenues for expression, for our lovely home that we are privileged to own, and for money enough to pay our bills, purchase an array of appetizing foods to eat and travel occasionally. We thank God for the privilege of being alive, for peace and harmony in all of our relationships, for quietude, for a cadre of open, giving and supportive friends, wonderful in-laws, for the nice cars that we own, and for a continuous stream of nagging little obstacles that we are obliged to face every day. Everything that's worth anything, God has already given to us. So why would we choose to focus disproportionately on HS2, when it is in no way reducing the quality of our lives or the state of our joy?

This doesn't mean that I don't wish to be totally healed some day of every vestige of this malady. I wouldn't dare utter such a lie. I can wish anything that I want, but I believe in calling things as I see them. Yes, I have HS2; yes, it is a malady, and, yes, I would like to be completely healed. This may make some metaphysicians and New Thoughters cringe, but who cares? This is my life! Perhaps, I would also like a $42,000 Lexus and $5000 a month more income, but you won't find me praying for these things either. As a human being living on this Earth, I find that I can't help having desire for certain things, but as an intelligent, self-choosing child of God, I have discovered that I can spend the bulk of my time giving thanks for the good that has already come my way and appreciating the bountiful gifts that are already mine.

None of this is designed to appease or induce God to act on any secret motives that I may yet harbor. I am clear concerning the fact that if my body goes to its grave with HS2, it will be all right with me. Not only that, but if I should live on this plane for only one more week, that would surely be sufficient. This is no bid for suicide, mind you. I love it here, and I would be pleased to live here for a long time hence. Be that as it may, I still believe that we place far too much emphasis on these little measly bodies. We are far too judgmental about early death. As is true with so many things in life, the knowledge of when we will make the transition from this plane of existence to the next is not within our domain. That's simply not our business. I didn't choose when I came here, and I don't expect to choose when I leave. My business is to live every moment of this life fully, glorifying God in all things. God's business is to determine how long I need to be here. My business is to accept life as it is and manage in spite of it all, glorifying this Divine Intelligence right on. With this faith, there is no question but that healing will come. God's business is to determine how and when.

LEARNING TO TELL THE WHOLE TRUTH

It is time for those of us who are on the spiritual path to close the Embodiment Gap — that differential between what we say or think we are and what we really are. Fortunately, there is a way to do this for those who are willing. First we must resolve to do this, starting today. This moment. The best way that I have found to close the Gap is by becoming radically honest. It is no longer sufficient to just go along manufacturing truths to fit the circumstances of the moment. We must pause to search our souls for what the truth really is in every situation, large and small, significant and seemingly insignificant, even when such a process is not required by those with whom we may be interacting. If we are interested in acting like children of God, we must set standards of behavior much higher than any norm that we can expect to encounter in society. And the trick is, we must do this without becoming the least bit self righteous, and without withdrawing from society or feeling the need to make everyone else wrong who may not be adhering to *our* standards. Clearly, this is a standard that is far above religion.

The problem with religion is that it is usually judgmental, separatist and intolerant. I have searched far and wide and found few exceptions worth mentioning. This does not make religion bad. Religions comprise the best system that we have in society to serve the moral needs of the greater portion of people. They once served my needs and I'm glad we have them. Whereas there is no need to change religion, liberation is in realizing that it is possible for the sincere student of Truth to transcend religion.

If I had the power, I wouldn't change a thing on Earth. In all of its seeming imperfections, life on Earth is perfect just the way it is. **THERE IS NO SINGULAR ANSWER FOR THE MASSES, BUT THERE ARE ANSWERS FOR THE INDIVIDUAL.** As I have always stated, there are many paradoxes on the road to Truth.

Many lies are continuing to be dispensed in the name of Truth. Based on my rather rigorous observations, most of the ministers in metaphysics aren't doing any better than the students whom they are trying to teach. The truth of the matter is that there aren't any easy answers. This is what ought to be taught, whether the teaching is New Thought, metaphysical, mental, or orthodox Christianity. This doesn't change the fact that we are all divine beings. We really are, but we are never going to find the physical and material demonstrations that we too often flock to churches searching for. Don't think that you can visualize and make yourself well in any substantial, lasting way.

I once met a minister of a metaphysical religion who advertised herself as a healer, yet she had manifested cancer three times. Sure, she had used mental techniques (such as visualization) to cure herself, but an equally dramatic revelation is the fact that IT DIDN'T LAST! I mean, let's get real. God doesn't have to prove anything to us on our terms. Neither can God be coaxed into healing us because of the good deeds we are doing. That minister's case was no exception. I wish I had a buck for every minister that I know who has died from cancer or AIDS. In the last year alone, I can think of three or four just in New Thought alone. I won't even bother to count those in orthodoxy.

Now to many this may sound like judgment. I know, because it is so unthinkable in enlightened religious circles (New Age/New Thought/metaphysics) to publicly suggest that something is amiss among our leaders and troops. But I'm not announcing anything that ministers and students alike don't think and discuss privately and in confidence among friends. There is this degree of hypocrisy in the movement, but it is usually sloughed off as *normal* human behavior. My position is simple: Everything needs to be brought out in the open, and this kind of discussion has nothing whatsoever to do with judgment. Check out some of the language of Jesus if you want to witness harsh, but loving, criticism. When are we going to start being radically honest if not now? Also, look at where I'm coming from. I have already admitted that I have HS2. So, obviously, I'm not criticizing those ministers who manifested cancers and AIDS, and the ones who died, except to the degree that I'm also criticizing myself. Like them, I, too, am still trying to resolve certain inconsistencies between what I've been taught to believe and what is actually happening in my life. It only makes sense to compare the two and report the honest truth about what is found. There is no rancor in what I'm reporting. Whether it happens to hurt you or your religion or your favorite minister, or whether it happens to hurt *moi,* so what? We have to arrive at the point where it just doesn't matter. God is no respector of persons, and neither is Truth. I was not placed here to be nice. I was placed here to tell the truth. This is called getting the petty ego out of the way so that the light of Truth can be revealed in our lives. I'm not happy to have to report some of the situations that I have discovered.

The vast majority in the metaphysical or so-called New Age movement is putting on a big front. This movement is filled with some of the phoniest people you would ever chance to meet. Not only that, but just about every big name in metaphysics — present as well as historical — is suffering or has suffered from some intractable condition during his or her ascension in consciousness. If you read the history of the great names in the New Thought movement, you'll find that just about every one of them suffered from one disease or another: Ernest Holmes, Mary Baker Eddy, Phineas Quimby, Myrtle Fillmore, Charles Fillmore, Ralph Waldo Emerson, Malinda Cramer, George Washington Carver, Albert Schweitzer and others are examples. I have heard the stories of many contemporary metaphysicians, and the similarities are mystifying. This is not a knock, but it's a perspective that isn't highlighted to the same degree as all of the grandiose claims about physical healings and material demonstrations.

Now let it be known that I am neither a pessimist nor a doubter. Count me amongst the truest of believers in spiritual healing. There is no question but that spiritual healing is authenic. It is possible, it is real, and it happens. I strive not to be *against* anything, not even the misrepresentation and lying that is going on in the name of Truth. I am simply for Truth, and keeping Truth simple.

There are no accidents in God's Universe. There couldn't be liars unless there were people who needed to be lied to. For every liar, there is a gullible person who needs to be lied to, for life is always in perfect balance. Healings occur but they do not occur according to anybody's formula. Regardless of denomination or religious persuasion, each healing is custom made.

Percentagewise, I am sure that there are as many people being healed spiritually in conventional or orthodox religions as there are in New Thought or metaphysical religions. Spiritual healing is one of life's greatest enigmas. There is nothing that you can "do" to bring it about or to speed up the process. It's an issue of being good for goodness sake, of totally surrendering from ambition and desire and all concepts of healing. It requires that you move beyond the place where you may be working for a healing, praying for a healing, concerned about a healing, or waiting for a healing. It is purely paradoxical that you have to surrender even your *concept* of healing in order to be healed.

The thing that you have to do is honor God with each waking breath, not in a contrived — or even pious — manner, but because you have an overwhelming desire to do this. You have to learn how to honor God to such a high degree that you are seeing and experiencing divine goodness despite what may be happening to your cherished body. In doing so, you are busy doing what you know it is your mission on Earth to do, the same as you would be doing if you were so-called healed...or if you were happy...or if you were a billionaire. You must get to a point where you are doing the same thing that you would be doing if you were in heaven, and happily so. Then you would have indeed brought heaven to Earth, and you would discern no difference. At that point, there would be nothing to be healed *from.* I am always suspicious of people who would do wonderful things only *after* some condition is met. If God had a voice, He would ask: "Why aren't you doing it now?"

In stark contrast to what one might believe, "healers" — if there is such a breed — pay a great price to attain their special gift. And the only true healers are incredibly humble, compassionate people who have surrendered their wills to God's will. There is no way that such a one would ever use his or her power for commercial gain. Absolutely no way.

If you ever encounter one who is not humble, who is not compassionate, and who does not leave you feeling that you are totally and unconditionally loved, know that you are not dealing with a true channel for Truth and make haste. Sometimes it may be necessary for the Truth practitioner to be harsh with you, but the approach should never be personal or condemnatory. Instead, it should always be done with a spirit of love and total acceptance. Let me put it like this. As a spiritual practitioner, there are times when I must take a stand diametrically opposed to that of my client, even though the client in question may be a close, personal friend. The client and I may very well disagree, but if I'm going to be effective in my work, I had better not allow aspects of the personality to creep in and affect what I must say. My position on an issue cannot be bought or influenced by wealth or power or status. I don't care if I get paid or not — and many times I haven't been. All that matters is that the Truth be revealed.

I have met a number of contemporaries in the healing ministries who began by overcoming personal confrontations with life-threatening diseases. I think of people like Dr. Barbara King in Atlanta, Johnnie Coleman in Chicago, and of course, the late Norman Cousins (the latter, I never met). Whereas I'm not sure that Norman Cousins or some of the other contemporaries will be etched in the annals of history as healers, each has at least invoked the kind of mental clarity and spiritual faith that led to his or her own healing. Loosely speaking, one might say that they healed themselves, but we have to understand the limitations of such claims. Human beings don't heal; only God (also known as Universal Mind, the Absolute, the Creator, Infinite Mind, Divine Love or just Spirit) heals. Human beings can condition their minds and practice the kind of faith that is consistent with God's Truth, and in those rare moments when they are able to do this well enough, what we call physical healing *may* occur.

All of the truth teachers named have been the beneficiaries of a spiritual healing, because, when medical science had exhausted all hope, they allowed themselves to surrender totally in faith to the omnipotence of Spirit. In the case of Cousins, I'm sure his written, personal testimony has assisted in the healing of thousands.

Along these lines, let's examine a passage that I read in the textbook for a program in trans-personal development that is very popular in New Age, metaphysical and New Thought circles. I paraphrase: There are healers who have not healed themselves. But until these healers heal themselves, they have not yet learned the truth about God's healing power and about their own wholeness as children of God.

I have intentionally neglected to name the source, because I am not interested in embarrassing anyone or trying to deny any organization the right to teach in whatever manner it sees fit. The error that I am going to point out is quite prevalent in metaphysical teachings and can be found in many authoritative self-help source books.

The above-referenced passage comes across as being very soothing and "deep," as we say. It's certainly quite quotable. But let's examine it a little deeper. The writer of the above quote seems to be saying that many who are healers have not healed themselves for the simple reason that their faith is not yet whole. My response, as always, is so what?

Look closely at what is being stated. Better yet, look even closer at what is being *implied*: Until the healer heals himself, he (or she) has not learned the truth about God's healing power.... Though this may be technically true, where is the compassion? I still have a problem with teachings such as this. They can be utterly defeating to a person who is already depressed and suffering with conditions such as HS2 or AIDS. Such a message can also mislead devout spiritual students into fringe metaphysical practices, for it implies that Step 1 up the spiritual ladder is to heal yourself. It implies that your faith isn't whole yet, and that you do not yet have a sufficient understanding of God and the spiritual laws to take yourself seriously as a healer. But guess what: **NOBODY EVER HEALS ANYONE!** This is the first thing that we have to understand. I happen to know that the person who wrote the paraphrased passage suffered from much illness in this life, including mental illness. The truth is, we're all more or less in the same boat.

The effective spiritual teacher must not divide sincere truth seekers into camps of the "enlightened," or those who have made the principles work according to some external appearance, and the unenlightened. The latter group consists of those who are still grappling with afflictions and diseases (a large population). They, too, want to believe, but it's going to take effort and time. Now this is precisely the kind of negative message that far too many teachings are dispensing. It comes marquerading as enlightenment, but it's still negative. Where is the love? Where is the compassion? All who play at spiritual healing are not sincere, but the *sincere* ones who have not yet demonstrated outward signs just need more time and support — unconditionally. They are presently doing all that they know how to do.

As for me, I am not going to burden myself with any guilt about what somebody else thinks I may be doing wrong. Either this is a spiritual universe or it isn't. I believe in the Infinite and its absolute sovereignty over this universe, and I am consciously trying to live according to its Laws. If life is more complicated than this, then it's far too complicated for me and I will never be healed.

I stake my life on the claim that this thing has to be simple or it's not worth the parchment it's written on. It is not unconditionally loving to tell those who are *sincere* in their approach to Truth that they are doing something wrong.

Another implication in the referenced statement is that every student must experience some outward sign of healing. The faith spoken of in the *Bible*, particularly in the first verse of the eleventh chapter of Hebrews, is the kind where there is no evidence at all, and yet we are still told to believe.

When the experienced movie director begins work on a new project, the random fragments of film that she shoots and reviews during the first six to 12 months may not look much like a movie at all. If her vision can be likened to faith, it may seem that her faith has many holes in it. But eventually, if she sticks to her vision, the final, coherent product emerges and, lo and behold, the world proclaims the arrival of a new movie. In the director's mind, the movie existed two years prior, but the world had no way of knowing it for there was no outward evidence.

There are a number of issues here that can be instructive to explore. First of all, by what authority does the writer of the aforementioned statement speak? It is time for all of us to stop being intimidated by experts and authorities, whether it be the *Bible*, a metaphysical textbook written by some universally acknowledged authority, or the Holy Grail. Who needs these extra burdens? Please don't misunderstand what I'm suggesting. These people might very well be experts, but what does that have to do with your life or my life? In reality, very little.

The writer had to work out truth for himself just as the minister or rabbi has to work out truth for herself. And believe it or not, it was no different for Jesus. Even he, enlightened though he was, could not receive Truth by osmosis. So when the spiritual authorities speak, listen but realize that there is no need to be intimidated. Wherever you or I happen to be in our growth and evolution is exactly where we need to be − no apologies necessary. Not only that, but you and I have just as much right to teach from our own level of expertise as anybody else. Viewed from an ultimate perspective, none of us knows very much, so whom are we kidding? Compound all of the knowledge of all of the world's experts, Ph.D.'s, ministers, philosophers and nobel laureates and you still don't have very much. Together, they still couldn't make a seed grow or create life. Collectively, they still couldn't annihilate cancer or wipe out crime in the streets, so whom are we kidding when we lay these "heavy," absolute statements on people.

Most people are not all that confident and self-assured when dating. Most do not communicate all that freely, openly, or honestly during the early stage of a relationship. Of course, this was certainly the case during my dating experiences. Even those who are reason-ably enlightened and have the desire to be open will still discover that's it's a challenge to put their noble "shoulds" into practice. Given that this is the case when dealing with even the slightest personal problems between mates, the problem is magnified a thousand fold when you have HS2.

For instance, what might some of the problems be when planning something as simple as a weekend away together? If you have HS2, you may very well undergo all kinds of mental anguish trying to predict which weekend will be safe and how to control your anxiety and take care of your body so that you won't have an outbreak during the trip. Those who have HS2 will certainly be able to relate to what I'm talking about.

You might call up your date the night before and report that everything is all set for the two of you to have a perfect trip, but then as soon as you get on the road you begin to feel the all too familiar prodromal tingling, which signals the onset of an outbreak. Darn it! You certainly don't want to spoil this particular weekend. You are caught between wanting to have a good time and blowing the whistle on all the fun before the fun begins. You certainly want to do the right thing by your date, but your inner conflict is heightened by the fact that you aren't 100 percent sure that what you're feeling is the beginning of a genuine outbreak. You don't want to cancel the trip and later discover that the symptom is nothing more than a false alarm. You may be able to recall times when there was tingling and yet no outbreak occurred. What I have just described is a classic HS2 dating conflict.

The problem is confounded if, for whatever reasons, you haven't yet divulged this big secret that you have HS2 to your weekend date. Perhaps you're in a new relationship, or you just haven't found the ideal time to tell him or her yet. It's also possible that you have absolutely no interest in ever revealing this part of your life. Either way, you are now faced with the task of coming up with a decent alibi to explain your impromptu cancellation.

If you haven't yet told your mate, the conflict wreaks double havoc on your mind. The worst thing you could do would be to go forward with the trip where there is sexual expectation in the mind of your mate, and you, for some unexplained reason, fail to deliver. Of course, you can make up all kinds of stories to explain your failure to perform, but unless you are a better liar than I am, you are going to generate even more suspicion and distrust by your explanation. What is likely to ensue is a long, awkward, silent and unpleasant weekend.

You see, people are human, and no matter how well they understand, they do get disappointed. And no matter how strong or how honest you are, if you are normal you would rather do anything than be the bearer of bad news. This is one of the subtle ways that HS2 works on the psyche. Sometimes, fresh outbreaks can spring up so fast — even within minutes, or so it seems. In Chapter 7 under the discussion of HS2-related myths, we were exploring the question: Does stress cause HS2 activation? Wheras I'm not exactly sure about that, I am certain that HS2 outbreaks can cause stress.

So what is a person to do? This is when you are most vulnerable to making an horrendous decision. This is when, without even being aware of it, you are likely to begin rehearsing rationalizing arguments in your private mind, searching for an angle that would give you the green light. This is when you, an otherwise responsible, logical person, can be waltzed into making a one-time, irreversible mistake. Before you know it, you may find yourself in the position of subjecting your partner to risk and wondering how did you ever get into such a predicament. It's not only teen-agers who close their eyes before plunging into unsafe sex, thinking that they will be lucky. Adults at 20, 30, 40 and 50 do the very same thing — especially horny adults with HS2 who aren't willing to face the truth.

You started out sold on the idea of "safe" sex with the strong platform that, no matter what, you would never subject your mate to risk. If you had to lie to protect your mate, you'd lie. If you had to break the date without explanation, you'd do it. If your strange behavior and impulsive, inexplicable actions meant that you might lose your long-awaited chance to develop a relationship with this absolute, perfect partner — the mate of your dreams — then you'd just have to take that chance, because you just couldn't allow yourself to be in a position where there was the slightest chance of infecting your mate. These were your thoughts beforehand. But now, caught in the irresistible magnetic field of romantic closeness, looking into your mate's beautiful, alluring eyes and smelling the sweet perfume, touching skin so smooth and caressing silken hair, you find your objectivity rapidly yielding ground to primal desire. You are only moments away from making one of the worst decisions of your life.

Consider another case that could force you to compromise. Let's say that it's only been five days since the onset of an infection. Objectively, you know that you shouldn't even think about engaging in sexual activity until after seven days at the minimum, even though you don't "see" or feel any residual signs of infection. [For some people, infection cycles may last 10, 14, or even more days. Each must conduct himself according to his (or her) own experiences, body rhythms or doctor's advice.] Chances are you don't see any symptoms because your mind is in torment, and thus confused, and your body is burning because you want to have sex so badly. You may not believe that such a scenario is credible for an intelligent person, but I can vouch that it is. This thing about intelligence is one of the world's greatest myths. Believe me: Intelligence has nothing whatsoever to do with it, except perhaps, that the more intelligent you are the more guilt you are likely to feel. Intelligence can bring on some highly sophisticated guilt.

A MIND UNDER SIEGE BY THE LIBIDO WILL DISTORT ONE'S OBJECTIVITY EVERY TIME. IF YOU HAVE HS2, NEVER, NEVER, NEVER UNDERESTIMATE YOUR LIBIDO

Even if you don't have HS2, you would be wise to heed this advice.

Sex, even without the complication of HS2, has caused more than a few great men and women to weaken, and great empires to fall. Look at all that Samson risked just for one night of pleasure with Delilah. I could have just as well named any number of modern televangelists or politicians. When dealing with the libido, it doesn't seem that much is ever learned from history. Never underestimate the power of pleasure.

If you have HS2, you have to exercise good judgment long before you are in the throes of passion. By the time the fire is burning, it may be too late. During a period of infection, there must be NO foreplay — THAT'S CAPITAL N-O! — even if the infection is not located on a part of the body that you figure isn't likely to be touched by your mate during the activity. There are no areas on the body that you can say with certainty will not be touched during the wild, furious and spontaneous act of love-making. I'm not trying to be lascivious, but I have to tell it like it is.

From the moment you receive the faintest of signals that an outbreak is on the way, **THERE MUST BE ABSOLUTELY NO**

FOREPLAY! This point cannot be over-emphasized. The HS2 subject just can't afford to take that risk. Of course, we know that most medical athorities now consider it possible for the HS2 virus to be transmitted asymptomatically, but that is not the case that I'm discussing here. One source indicates that asymptomatic shedding only occurs one percent of the time, that individual episodes last about one day each on the average and that the amounts of virus present during those episodes are much less than during symptomatic recurrences. Thus it makes sense for me to focus most of my teachings on how to take responsibility for and avoid symptomatic transmission of HS2. There will always be circumstances which are beyond our control. All I'm asking is that we begin to take responsibility for the ones that we can control.

I understand how much store our sophisticated culture places on spontaneity in courtship and love-making, and I also understand how much we hate to give up even a single degree of our sacred freedom, but forget it! I don't care how spiritual the HS2 subject is, there is a harsh and impersonal side to life where certain higher laws have to be obeyed. The person who does not first learn to respect the nature of HS2 will never be able to overcome it. We are all eager to get to a higher place in consciousness where we won't have to respect these pesky little physical laws, but the road which leads there is *through* the disease, not around it. If the HS2 subject didn't need a disease for her soul to advance, she wouldn't have one.

Forget spontaneity; that is no longer an option. It took me a long time to accept that I couldn't be totally spontaneous with regard to sex any longer. It just didn't seem fair to me that at the tender age of 25 I was going to have to live my life restricted in the one area that I had not yet had the opportunity to fully explore.

Whether it is fair or not is of no consequence. This kind of discipline is a fact of life for HS2 subjects. This doesn't mean that life will be boring or unfulfilling. Nothing could be further from the truth. Our minds have all been corrupted by a society that places far too much emphasis on sex. Since the day that I formulated these new standards for myself and began to live by them, I couldn't be happier.

If anything, I feel liberated. No longer do I have to labor under the burden of feeling that I have to perform according to society's sexual expectations. There is no way to explain this to anyone's satisfaction who hasn't tried it, but believe me, it all works out.

To be happy, ultimately we must all learn to master life *in spite of* our conditions, and not whine, whimper, and rail about how unfair it seems. Society has a word to describe things which have already happened; It's called HISTORY! It includes that set of events which you can't go back in time and undo. It you have HS2, it's history now. Remember the serenity pledge. It is time now to turn your misfortune into an asset. Then, and only then, will you have no regrets later on, but you must be willing to exercise superior judgment and impeccable discipline at all times. I would have never been able to attract the wonderful wife that I have today if I hadn't made the decision to become totally honest and let the chips fall where they may.

Delilah was more deadly than a black widow spider and Samson knew it, but once he got a whiff of her passion he just couldn't say no. There's some Samson in all of us, be ye male or female. Realize one thing: Sometimes it's easier to say no on the telephone than in person. And if not on the telephone, try writing a note. I have used the latter approach many times to explain my situation to a woman rather than follow through with the date under the delusion that I would be able to control the situation, or that I would "tell her later." You know what is said about the best made plans of mice and men, and what the proverbial ill-fated road to hell is paved with. Well, all of this folksy lore applies here.

Now don't take this challenge too lightly — that is, the challenge confronting a person with HS2 of being totally disciplined in behavior and totally honest in confession. Take it from me. This is not to toot my own horn, but I am considered by friends to be the exemplar of a highly-disciplined person. That, I am. But let me tell you the truth. I have not always practiced the discipline that befitted my image, for I have taken some incredibly stupid risks. There, I've said it. If the truth be told, I've been more "lucky" than I've been smart. Hence, it's not so much what *I* have been able to do as it is Divine Providence that has protected me over the years. In other words, it is only by the grace of God that I have been protected from the worst fates when my personality self has been too weak to do the right thing.

How many stupid chances are we allowed during a lifetime? Are we granted nine lives like a cat, or just two or three? Just as it is true that a woman can't be a little pregnant, we must accept the fact that every lapse in correct discipline involves a degree of risk which could result in the worst possible outcome. There's no sense in railing against life when we get burned. Let's just confess the truth — that *we* were stupid.

GOD HASN'T DONE ME WRONG.
I DID MYSELF WRONG!

So far as our human ability is concerned, the best of us aren't much better than the worst of us. Let's face it: We need the invocation of an Absolute Power.

Speaking for a moment from a male perspective, sometimes when you try to exercise caution and good discipline, women may laugh at you. It's happened to me many times. They may not mean it the way you take it, but this is one of those tricky situations that you need to be aware of it. If you have HS2 there's a good chance that you're already overly-sensitive to every response made by your mate during your awkward attempt to communicate this unpleasant information. You've risked everything by hanging all of your fears and cautions out on the line; thus you're vulnerable in the worst way. An inappropriate laugh at this moment can totally deflate you. It may seem that she is trivializing something that is very emotional for you, but there is another possibility: She may not possess the skills to deal openly with such a serious issue.

It is a sad irony of modern life, but many women will strip off their clothes and lie down with you and yet be totally incapable and/or unwilling to discuss real, deep, sensitive issues with you. I know that most women are more adept at verbalizing deeper feelings and emotions than most men, but it would be a mistake to assume that this applies when it comes to exposing the darker, more unflattering sides of their personalities. Everyone has blind spots. At first, HS2 can be an unpleasant subject to broach for anyone, women included. Remember that no woman ever owned up to giving me HS2, and also that Elise, one of my most enlightened ex-girlfriends, gave me the slip rather than discuss her true feeling about HS2 with me.

This is only my opinion, but I have found that women are no more eager or honest than the average man when it comes to discussing past sexual histories. I'm not asserting that this is good or bad, only that men with HS2 should be aware of this. You have to choose your mates very, very carefully. Otherwise, you can be abused. If you aren't sure, don't make a move. Just sit back and wait. Of course, if you meditate and pray regularly, and rely on Spirit, It will reveal to you whatever you need to know.

Again, speaking from a male perspective, if you try to open up some space for honest communication and reap scorn or ridicule in return, one of your baser male impulses might be to try to show your mate how macho you can be, or even to make her pay. What you may be thinking is, "If she only knew what I was dealing with, she would understand why I have to take all of these precautions. I am attracted to her, but I don't want to put her at risk. I'm backing out for her own good and yet she's making fun of me. I ought to go ahead and show her how much of a man I really am. Hey! — she's asking for it. If she gets HS2 as a result of it, it serves her right for ridiculing me this way."

All I have to say to the man (or woman) who may be thinking this way is: "Don't do it!" You must do the right thing, yes, even if you are misunderstood and taunted. You have to spend some time working this stuff out in advance so that you will be clear on where you stand long before you are placed in such a position. You will meet a number of ignorant people along the way, and some who are just naïve. Some may "deserve what they get," but you need to be bigger than they. Protect them anyway, in spite of their ignorance, and then send them on their merry way. Just because people are ignorant doesn't mean that they don't deserve another chance. They do. Think of all the ignorant things you have done, the close brushes with death and how God has given you multiple chances.

I learned that it was important to make an absolute determination long before I got close enough to smell a woman's perfume. I learned to deal with truth as the first order of business for the evening. Often that would mean just going ahead and blurting it out before any other business of the evening was negotiated. Any hesitation on my part and there would be a good chance that I would never bring up the subject again. You know how life works: **THERE IS NEVER AN IDEAL TIME TO DELIVER BAD NEWS.** The longer you ponder it, the worse it gets, so you might as well go ahead and blurt it out right from the start.

When we're courting and the mood is good and everything is going smoothly, we hate to break the mood. Sometimes we think, "Ahh, I don't want to spoil things tonight. I'll bring it up tomorrow." As an HS2 subject, if you're going to be honest and act responsibly, you absolutely must be willing to be the bearer of bad news at times. There just isn't any other way. Today, I am very comfortable breaking moods if there is something on my mind that needs to be said. I fully understand the consequences of my actions. All things considered, breaking the mood and risking rejection by a mate or spouse is the least painful of all possible consequences.

This inability to be honest and possibly disappoint others is why so many people never admit that they have HS2. They mean well, but they just never quite get around to telling their mates. There are things in life for which there is never the perfect moment to disclose: telling someone that you have a criminal record, telling your date that you're married, or telling someone with whom you are falling in love and for whom you have tremendous sexual desire, "I hope you won't hold it against me, but I have HS2." Clearly, it would be even tougher to tell someone that you have the HIV virus, but that doesn't mean that it's easy to admit having HS2. Remember: Everything is relative, and no one's pain should be trivialized. A person who has a hangnail may be in more acute pain that I at the present time.

Some of the issues that I'm discussing, when looked at objectively, may seem trivial. But we aren't always objective. Suppose two people, one of whom has HS2, have been dating and have already been intimate for months before one of them musters up the courage to confess. Now here's how the mind works. If the party with HS2 only belatedly admits that he (or she) has HS2, one of his fears is that he will be called upon to go back and explain prior encounters when he may have subjected his partner to risk. I've been there, and I'm sure many sexually-active people with HS2 have been there. Even if the person is safe, it will not generally make a partner happy to hear that you haven't been honest with him or her during the preceding months of your relationship. His or her disappointment can vary from mild amusement to violent rage. Well, if it happens it's just something you'll have to live through, but immediate honesty is a price well worth paying if you want to have a clear conscience. Take it from me, total disclosure is the best policy and **NOW** is always the best time. Even if you did lie – or withhold truth – in the past, and regardless of how much time has lagged, do it today and let the chips fall where they may.

Given the current state of the dating game in our society and its implicit rules, it is so tempting for us to lie in our relationships. Even if you tell the truth, your mate may not reward you for it. In a situation where the other party is not yet ready to be dragged into an environment of honesty and accountability, he or she may even turn on you and make you the bad guy or gal rather than face the truth. That can really make you crazy, but it is the risk that you must take on your way to becoming a new person.

Whatever you do, don't make the mistake of over-analyzing your situation, trying to figure out every possible angle. "If I say A, she's going to say B, or maybe she'll react by doing C." You'll get your brain tied up in knots, plus you'll get a headache. Whenever you find yourself caught up in such an intellectual web, you can be sure that you're not coming from total honesty. The actions associated with truth and honesty are never intellectual or analytical. I would go even further to suggest that you strive not to be overly-apologetic. If you are being honest, there is no need to be apologetic.

PEOPLE WHO HAVE HS2 ARE NO MORE AT FAULT THAN PEOPLE WHO HAVE BEEN SLEEPING AROUND AND *HAVEN'T* ACQUIRED HS2.

No matter what is stated here, if an HS2 subject is lacking of a strong positive self concept, he (or she) is going to find himself whining and apologizing all over the place. Such an individual is going to be rejected on a regular basis, and possibly abused and treated badly, as well. No matter how smart or discriminating or smug people who are HS2-free may feel they've been, it's only by the grace of God that they haven't yet been infected. Remember, it is reportedly possible to acquire HS2 asymptomatically, and disregarding that possibility, it only takes one mistake to get caught. The irreducible truth is, there really is no such thing as safe sex. It is only by the grace of God that any of us are safe. Some may like to think that they've avoided HS2 or avoided HIV because of how smart they are and how well they've chosen their friends. Be that as it may, except in the case of the rare virgin, they have no grounds for gloating.

An important corollary of spiritual principle is this:

IT IS IMPOSSIBLE FOR ANYONE TO RESPECT YOU IF YOU DON'T RESPECT YOURSELF.

Admittedly, this is not an earth-shaking revelation. Neither is it original, but still, it needs to be reviewed and held fresh in consciousness. No matter how old and/or sophisticated we become, we will never be able to get away from grandma's wisdom. You're not a rat. You deserve to be treated with respect, and you should both expect and demand it. Instead of apologizing, let your love and honesty over the long run be your proof. You can feel proud of yourself because at least you're being honest. You can well believe that your mate has similar, painful, unpleasant and unresolved issues in his or her life. Those who pity, patronize, ridicule, judge or condemn you are simply immature individuals who have chosen to focus on *your* problems rather than work on their own. By casting themselves in a holier light than you, they are trying to buttress the walls around their insecurities at your expense. When I've been put in that situation, I have quickly come to the conclusion that I don't need such individuals in my life. Remember: You can't expect everyone to like you. Never try too hard to convince anyone to see things your way. After you've given it your best shot, if they still show no signs of leaning toward understanding or compassion (but not *sympathy*), simply and lovingly bid them adieu.

When people have complicated lives and complicated explanations for behaviors, it's usually because they have not yet learned to tell the simple truth. This may sound unbelievable, but test it for yourself. **THE MORE YOU MAKE IT A HABIT TO TELL THE TRUTH, THE SIMPLER YOUR LIFE WILL BECOME.** The belief that human beings are complicated, especially when they think of themselves as important figures, is pure myth.

You will find that this inability to be totally open and honest is one of the primary driving forces which causes many singles to switch partners frequently. Every time you pass up an opportunity to tell the truth, a little bit of mental residue is built up between you and the significant other in your life. After a while, the unresolved mental residue becomes too great to bear. The layers of complexity that have accumulated are suddenly too ponderous to explain, and you will feel compelled to flee. Fleeing is the road of least resistance. It represents the easiest solution for unloading the burden.

Now, obviously I'm talking about myself. During my irresponsible days there were times when I actually ended relationships with women rather than come clean. If you subject someone that you respect and care for to unnecessary risk, but haven't yet been able to muster up the guts or the discipline to tell that person, don't be surprised if you find yourself contriving reasons to end the relationship. Depending upon your soul's present level of development, it may be so much easier to run than to face up to unflattering aspects of your being.

Oh, I understand the reasons for being reticent. Once you come clean, you may have to face that dumbfounded look of pity that you get from people which translates to, "How could you do that to yourself? How could you be so stupid? I thought *you* were smarter than that!" It hits you like a dagger through the heart when someone you respect responds so ignorantly, but who is omnipotent enough to obliterate all ignorance? Many believe HS2 to be incurable. I'm not sure that I agree, but I do know that ignorance is eternal.

Another class of problem exists with those who are in non-exclusive relationships. If a person has HS2 and is sleeping around, things can get awfully complicated in a hurry. The same is true for any STD. After 14 to 21 days (a typical incubation period), an unethical individual can deny almost anything, and fabricate all kinds of scenarios for how something may or may not have occurred. It all begins when someone comes back and asks: "How in the hell did I get THIS?" Don't think that I am making this up. When I confronted my lady friend with the question of the hour, she denied everything. So don't feel like the Lone Ranger if you have been lied to.

Another subtle, and often subconscious, ploy used to avoid honesty is this: the old offensive smoke screen. You've heard the maxim that the best defense is a good offense. On one of those weekend trips when HS2 flares up, the disconsolate subject might blow up over some random trifle and start a fight. That way, he (or she) doesn't have to broach the subject of his infection, and he can use the disagreement and anger as a reason for not being interested in his partner sexually. I used this ploy about a million times before I was able to decipher what was really taking place in the subconscious layers of my mind. And believe me, it really is subconscious. Even after I finally learned how to be totally honest — well, about 99 percent of the time — I still had trouble identifying the onset of one of my anger/withdrawal cycles. This was one picture that just wasn't matching up with the image I held of myself. It's incredibly painful to face honestly. What's easier is to get weird or mysterious and demand that your partner "Give me my space!" under the guise of the old alibi about individual expression. This falls under the category of chicanery; it is not what I call being truthful.

If you have never had HS2, then think of one of those times when you may have been on the giving or receiving end of some other type of STD or infection, ranging from nonspecific urethritis or yeast infections to something more serious. Surely, every sexually active person has had one of these experiences. How did you handle that? Were you comfortable about informing the other party? You'll find some of the same psychological dynamics at play there as in the case of HS2.

Another twist to the problem of sexual ping-ponging occurs when someone you're seeing interrogates YOU because they suspect that you're the donor of THEIR disease or infection. It's very embarrassing to say the least. Wouldn't you agree? Yet it happens all the time in this modern world of musical beds. When you meet someone today with whom you haven't developed a trust or made a commitment, commonly-accepted sexual etiquette says that you can't just come out and ask him or her: "Are you sleeping with anyone else?" You may wonder, but you can't ask. As a man, I know that such an inquisitor will be considered to be possessive, insensitive, intrusive, nosey, jealous and very *uncool*. Not only that, but in 99 out of 100 cases, he can kiss his odds of consummating a relationship with that lady goodbye.

I realize that in this day of AIDS hysteria my point of view on this issue flies in the face of modern advice columns. Some are encouraging singles to interview potential mates about their sexual histories before becoming intimate. Naturally, I applaud the effort and agree with their goals. The only point I'm making is: lots of luck! We must face reality here. How many people really know themselves? There aren't that many people who are honest with *themselves*, no less being comfortable with their sexual histories, or being able to be honest about this area of their lives with a brand new partner. Chances are, the reason they have a new partner in the first place is that they weren't too honest with the last one!

Given the instantaneous, sitcom mentality of modern life, sexual histories can get awfully complicated in no time flat. That's why many guys put so much pressure on women during the initial weeks of a relationship. Subconsciously, they fear that if they don't hurry up and initiate intimacy there's probably some other guy waiting in the wings, perhaps an ex-husband or ex-boyfriend or a hot pursuer. Ask me how I know. Now I know that this doesn't sound either spiritual or enlightened, but I'm telling you, this is the way it is, perhaps less so as a man ages and matures. No man is ever going to admit to pressuring women, at least not while he's still trying to impress. This is just another part of our sexual legacy that needs to be told and understood. Also, this does not suggest that women aren't often the pursuers or aggressors during the early mating ritual. This story can play both ways, I'm sure. Nonetheless, if the truth be told, once you're past 15 there is often an ex-boyfriend, ex-girlfriend or ex-spouse in the picture during the initial stages of the dating game. When you're not on the scene, chances are — at least, you're likely to fear — one of these exes is. In the early stages of courtship, we are rarely, if ever, in control, and there are always more unknowns than knowns concerning our chosen mates' sexual pedigrees.

To give you a concrete example of how modern sophisticates deal with assaults on their fragile sexual images, a hilarious story from my past comes to mind. It's features a nasty little vermin, the presence of which causes great embarrassment: lice! There's no way that someone can lie about having been the source of lice. They are highly prolific little vermin that jump right into your crotch if you make contact with someone who is so infested. They seem to proliferate around college dorms. This happened to me once, and when I questioned the only source that I could have acquired these little suckers from, she still denied it! Sometimes it's hard for me to believe all of the predicaments that I've managed to get myself into over the years.

Now for the hilarious account. When I was living in Boston one summer after having graduated from college, there were these two little preppie female friends who were sharing an apartment in Cambridge. They were what you would call well-bred young ladies, having just recently graduated from Wellesley College — you know, high class, liberal arts and the whole shebang. Actually, they were friends of one of my favorite college roommates. I can't over-stress the point that my relationship with these women was totally platonic. They were interested in things like fine art, opera and culture, all things that were well above my head. But I give them credit for deigning to include me among their list of friends. But don't get me wrong. As a 23-year-old young man with perennially maxed-out hormones and no meaningful commitments, I would have jumped at the opportunity to become more than a friend, but I shouldn't dwell on fairy tales. They were just way out of my league. One of my assets is that I've always known my proper place in life.

Well, one day they called me on the phone in stark terror. Their entire apartment, including both of their mattresses, towels and all of their clothing were infested with LICE! They didn't even know what lice looked like. What had happened, they reckoned, was that a house guest had introduced these vermin into their apartment. An old college friend who had been sleeping her way around Europe throughout the summer had shown up at their door seeking a place to crash for a few nights, and of course, they had been accommodating. Now they were terrified by these little crabs that seemed to be pole vaulting all over the place. Lice were jumping from their mattresses into their hair with supernatural prowess. As I said, these were genteel ladies; they hadn't the slightest idea concerning how to handle things like this. In the meantime, they were afraid to touch their mattresses, go to sleep, shake hands with friends or do anything. They were basket cases.

After rolling on the floor with side-splitting laughter — after all, lice was not one of the world's most serious threats — I went over and assisted them in stripping down their mattresses and rounding up all of their clothes. Then we lugged everything they owned down to the local laundromat for a scalding wash. The next step was an embarrassing one for them, for they had to trek down to their friendly pharmacist for some crab treatment ointment. It's very difficult for a Wellesley grad to waltz into a drug store and ask for some ointment to kill crabs that are nesting in her pubic hair. The next few days involved a continuous cycle of spraying and washing and treating their prissy little bodies with...well, insecticide! Every spot on the body bearing hair had to be treated with this awfully repugnant stuff. Hair conditioner, it was not. It rendered the hair stiff and discolored. Still, their fear didn't subside for many moons. In the end, they could never feel comfortable sleeping on those mattresses again. They simply dumped the offending mattresses out on the street.

Ahh...life can be so unpredictable and comical.

Getting back to HS2 and how those of us who have it must learn to tell the truth, I should add that I do not believe that everyone is susceptible to HS2. As a matter of fact, I'm convinced that there are people who are not. Some people have no need for it on a soul level; therefore, they just aren't going to manifest it. They will, however, have equally frustrating or devastating challenges in other areas of their lives. From a universal, spiritual point of view, if there was nothing for them to learn by being on Earth, they wouldn't be here. It's just that simple.

In a theoretical sense I'm sure that almost everyone believes in telling the whole truth. Nevertheless, each of us needs to put teeth to the theoretical by examining it in the context of a real life situation. It is then that we sometimes fall short without even realizing that we have lied. Let me tell you about a very real situation that brought this issue to the fore for me.

There is one challenge that I am loathe to face and it is filling out medical questionnaires. I don't care if it's for a physician, dentist or insurance company, although of the three, I am slightly more cooperative when confronted with a physician's questionnaire. It's been my experience that some dentists and virtually all insurance companies ask far too many personal questions of an irrelevant nature. They tend to be of the "cover your rear end" variety. Whereas I have gone to great lengths to establish that I believe in being open, direct and straight-forward about HS2, I'm nobody's fool. And a fool is what anyone would be who fritters away his or her secrets to impersonal agencies and other bureaucracies of this sort. I know that these bureaucracies don't care anything about me as a person; accordingly, I have no interest whatsoever in cooperating with their ever-increasing demands for more and more information.

My present dental office has never asked me for irrelevant personal information, but a few years ago when I got the bright idea to become a standup comedian, I quit my engineering job and consequently became ineligible for continued dental insurance coverage. Naturally, within days after the grace period on my insurance lapsed, one of my teeth literally exploded in my mouth. There must be some kind of law — perhaps, one of Murphy's. Anyway, the timing could not have been worse.

I was forced to seek a more affordable dentist than the one I would have preferred if I had still been covered. All of a sudden I was operating on a strictly cash basis. I was shocked when the receptionist thrust this lengthy questionnaire into my face and directed me to fill it out in advance. Have you ever had any of the following diseases, it probed: heart disease, apoplexy, diabetes, herpes, cancer...wa-i-i-t a minute! Why in heaven's name does the dentist need to know if I have herpes? Of course the questionnaire didn't spell out whether it meant HS2 or HS1. Heck, virtually everybody has herpes simplex type 1.

The reason this bothered me so was that, one, I had no interest whatsoever in disseminating this information to these people, and two, I hate to lie to anyone for any reason, even to strangers. Clearly, I still have work to do in terms of my spiritual growth, because where that dental bureaucracy was concerned, I most certainly committed the sin of omission. I didn't volunteer the information that I had HS2, and although I felt justified in my action, I still felt guilty.

The dentist in question turned out to be a woman who belonged to the same church as I at the time. I probably would not have discontinued my patronage there had it not been for that one embarrassing issue that led me to compromise my integrity. At the time I considered other options rather than lying. I came awfully close to tossing the questionnaire back onto the receptionist's desk and walking out in protest. It's not beyond me to do that. There are many commonly-accepted mores and practices in this ever-degenerating "anything goes" society that I will never kowtow to. But there I was on that particular day visiting a new dentist's office under emergency circumstances with no job or insurance, and precious little money. You might say that they had me over a barrel. I needed my tooth repaired in the worse way, so I lied about my medical history.

What could the dentist have done if I had responded truthfully to that particular question? The thought occurred to me. Would she have refused to work on my tooth? Or, would she have donned a mask and extra thick rubber gloves and handled me like a leper?

Of course, now that the threat of HIV is widespread, many dentists routinely protect themselves in just that manner today, just in case. If they assume the worst, they don't have to ask their patients all of these potentially embarrassing questions. When I've gone to dentists who wear masks and rubber gloves in handling their patients, this hasn't bothered me. I don't want them putting a pair of dirty hands into my mouth anymore than they want to stick their hands into a contaminated mouth.

As I mentioned, I also had to weigh the fact that this dentist was an influential member of the church where, not only was I a member, but I was also quite active at the time. As a Sunday school teacher, fund-raiser, member of the faculty of the school of metaphysical instruction and licensed spiritual healing practitioner, I was highly visible and well-known in that environment. If I had revealed that I had HS2 to her staff, how far would that information have traveled?

I am not naïve enough to assume that the facade of professionalism is a sufficiently inviolate shield to protect me. I didn't just fall off a turnip wagon this morning. How well I know that dentists, doctors and other professionals are deflatingly human behind their antiseptic facades of objectivity. I have known too many of them personally to trust them across the board with sensitive information. An old college acquaintance who went on to graduate from the Harvard medical school and practice medicine is a pure drug addict. He spent most of his undergraduate years back at MIT stoned out of his mind. To put it bluntly, they are just as human and just as likely to gossip as anyone else.

On the other side of the ledger, I need to consider the plight of the poor dentist as well. Certainly, they are at risk when they stick their bare hands into the mouths of indiscriminate patients, or when they handle needles inside patient's mouths, or subject themselves to contagious, coughing, sneezing patients. Theirs is not an envious position. It would certainly gross me out to do what they do.

It makes sense that they would want to know if a patient has oral herpes (HS1 or HS2) before they work on him. If a patient has an active herpes ulcer on the lips or inside the mouth, I certainly wouldn't want to work on him at that time if I were a dentist. Still,

I am at peace with my decision to withhold questionnaire information because I am an ultimately responsible individual. First of all, I do not have oral HS2. That's one of the few things that I've never had. Thus the question is irrelevant to my situation. There is no way that I can pass on HS2 to a dentist. But — if I did have oral HS2, I would never plump myself down into a dentist's chair while having an active lesion, emergency notwithstanding. This falls under the same new resolve that HS2 subjects should make with respect to their mates, which is the commitment to truth, honesty and total disclosure. I know my body well and I don't believe in taking chances — not with my life, and not with other people's lives. No siree.

Here's where I draw the line. In the case of an emergency where even the slightest possibility of compromising the health of a dental or medical practitioner or professional could be exposed, it is imperative that you inform them in confidence *beforehand* and tell them in straight, unwavering and unequivocal language exactly what they're dealing with. If I were faced with that situation, I would inform my dentist or doctor even if there was no questionnaire. As tough as it would be to do, my conscience would never let me rest if I didn't do the right thing.

We have a responsibility in this life that none of us can afford to shirk. Even if it leads to the worst — i.e., suppose the dentist or doctor reacts ignorantly or fearfully, or allows the information to leak into the hands of the wrong person such that it causes us great embarrassment — then that is the risk we must take. It's a small risk, too, considering the consequences. There is plenty of time for me to recover from the blow, and besides, I can always find another dentist or doctor.

CHAPTER 9: VICTORY

Now that we have arrived at this point in our detailed exploration of the philosophical issues associated with having HS2, you are probably eager to explore the specific steps to victory. The fact that neither I nor anyone else can promise those with HS2 a physical cure or healing at this time cannot be over-emphasized. As I have established, the ultimate solution to the HS2 challenge is not physical. It is mental and spiritual. In addition to generalized exercises and processes shared in the previous chapters in narrative form, the specific exercises and processes detailed in this chapter can help every interested and sincere HS2 subject achieve more freedom, more happiness and an unlimited state of mental well-being.

TRANSFORMATIVE PROCESSES

To begin this process towards liberation, the essential questions of life must be pondered. What are these essential questions? If you haven't already completed this exercise, I suggest that you stop right now and prepare to write the below-listed questions on a 3 x 5 index card. Then tape that card to your bathroom wall or mirror, desk, or somewhere so that you will be reminded to ponder them daily. And ponder them you must, every day for the next month, year, decade, or however long it may take for answers to come.

1. Who am *I*?

2. What is the ultimate purpose of life?

3. From whence did I come?

4. Why do *I* exist?

5. Why am *I* here (on this Earth) and for what purpose?

6. What do *I* want from life and why? And is what I want from life consistent with what life wants from me?

Append any additional existential questions that may be important to you. If you are serious about healing, then it is essential that you approach each of the above questions seriously.

In Zen Buddhism, I am told that they have a device known as koans, which are paradoxical questions given to students on the spiritual path by certain master teachers to help them grow and expand beyond their present mental boundaries. The nature of these questions is that they appear to be simple and sometimes nonsensical, thus inviting quick and easy answers which, if given, totally subverts the process of growth and expansion.

Two of the most well-known koans are these: (1) What is the sound of one hand clapping? (2) If a tree falls in the forest and no one is there to hear it, does it make a sound?

The object is not to hurry up and answer the question as if you were taking a competitive college exam. This is real life that we're talking about here; you get no points for quick answers. And don't look to win any prizes or points for right answers, because there are none, at least not in any objective sense. Only you, the student, will know if the answer is right by the quality of your life *as* it unfolds. The teacher may not ever be able to tell you that. If your life is working out according to your liking, you are living out the correct answers to these ultimate questions...at least for now. Tomorrow — you may have to go back into contemplation and call for some new answers the same old questions. This is certainly not the kind of processes that they prepared you for in high school or college. This process is designed to put you in touch with the ever-expanding, ever-evolving nature of your spiritual life, which is forever expanding into newness.

Furthermore, no matter what answers you derive today, they may not suffice for tomorrow. This is the paradoxical nature of Truth. The sincere truth-seeker is a philosopher, and the philosopher's world is no place for lazy individuals. Every day that you awaken with breath in your nostrils, there is work to be done.

My primary thrust is not to have you go off and investigate koans just now. I simply wish to impress upon you how essential it is to devote some time on a regular basis toward the investigation of your life's ultimate questions. What do you really want in life and what are you after? After all, this is YOUR life. YOUR world has been tailored especially for YOU.

Spend a minimum of 15 to 30 minutes each day, twice a day, thinking about nothing but these issues. If you haven't already, begin to keep a journal and write essays on the answers — or questions — which come to you. These exercises are NOT optional for the student who truly wants to create a consciousness that is conducive to healing. Don't try to cover too much territory during each sitting. Remember: There is no time limit and you get no points for finishing quickly. It may prove most fruitful to work on one question per day — or per week. There are times when I lock onto a given question that's troubling my consciousness and carry it around for a month. I will contemplate it when I'm in the shower, while driving in my car, while walking, early in the morning before arising from my bed — whatever — until clarity finally comes. During that period of time, there is nothing more important in life than that single question. And this is how it must be for every sincere student of Truth. Victory does not come to those who approach these ultimate issues casually.

During the months or years that it takes to resolve these fundamental questions, forget about healing the body. Work only on opening the mind and expanding your consciousness. Work on finding out what you believe, and why you believe what you believe. Then set out to correct all errant and outmoded beliefs, i.e., beliefs that no longer serve you very well. All things in the outer world are the fruit of Universal Mind, and as such, follow the impressions made by thought. There is a medium that connects the individual to Universal Mind and it is thought. Learn to think clearly, consistently and truthfully, and you will be able to transform your consciousness. Transform your consciousness and your life will change automatically. By this method you will reap the golden reward: If you heal your consciousness, you don't have to worry about your body. By Law, it must follow suit.

Admittedly, this is not easy to do. As I've already pointed out, I haven't attained complete victory yet, but I'm well on my way. Evidence is accruing everyday. I have both witnessed and experienced enough of what the world calls miracles to be absolutely convinced of this principle, so much so that I could write a book on this subject alone and it would be wonderful. I have deliberately avoided focusing on physical healings in the present treatment to avoid the common New Age mistake of selling my message to potential aspirants based solely on hope. The metaphysical field is littered with people with mystical names, impressive titles and credentials, who sell hope backed up by false claims to desperate individuals. Look around you. The world is teeming with unhappy, diseased, suffering individuals who, still lodged in victim consciousness, are seeking the tiniest shreds of hope. It would be highly irresponsible on my part to attract people into this way of thinking under the delusion that they are going to be healed from HS2. Nothing could be further from the truth. At any given time, only a few will be ready to go in the direction that I am pointing.

Seekers of healings are so accustomed to doing things only for tangible gain, but in spiritual work there are no precise guarantees or promises. That you will be blessed, I have no doubt, but no one can say when or what form your blessing will take. How we wish, but nobody on this Earth can make absolute claims because no human is equipped to see the whole picture — a situation for which I am extremely grateful. Think about it: If you or I could see the whole picture, we would not be individuals. We would be God and it would be endgame.

For me to suggest that certain actions on your part will lead to a definite healing of the body would be the equivalent of plea bargaining with God. That would be no different than the outdated orthodox practice of sending up promises to some anthropomorphic deity that you will become a good person and conform to his will if only he will bless you in a certain prescribed way. There is no such deity or universe. That's why in this book I seldom refer to God as "He." God is not a person. IT is Spirit, and as such, cannot make decisions concerning your life. All It can do is bless you according to *your* thoughts and beliefs and your degree of conformance with the *Law*. That is, God's Law, or what is referred to in metaphysics as the Law of Spirit. This Law is impersonal. It is not punitive, although it may sometimes *appear* to be both personal and punitive.

One of our problems in understanding is that many times when we say *God* we actually mean the *Law* of God. There is a major difference. God, unlike humans, does not respond to human issues in a tit for tat manner. You know, "If you do this for me, I'll do that for you." Neither is healing a simple proposition of fulfilling certain requirements on somebody's checklist. Regardless, we often approach healing in this manner. We think because we've been good students or servants, read our scriptures, recited our affirmations, obeyed our parents, blessed those in need and forgiven our enemies, God should reward us with a healing. Admittedly, I, too, used to think this way. This is an orthodox concept, a limited concept and an incorrect concept. Those who think this way will continue to see a universe that is unjust, and they will continue to reap evidence which validates that belief. In other words, they will continue to be victims.

The truth is, I don't know what's going to happen *to* you or *for* you. For what may be the first time in life, you are being instructed to undertake a self improvement program that isn't promising you a single thing. We must all come to understand that God doesn't have to promise us any reward whatsoever for conforming to the natural order of the spiritual universe. It is our privilege to conform. Most people do not know it yet, but it is also our duty and our destiny. But beyond that, the best kept secret is: It is our choice! God created a perfect pattern to sustain life in this world and it is up to us to unravel the mystery of this pattern and then make the changes in our lives to conform to *it*. God does not have to bargain with us. The Infinite Knower can out-wait any and all of its creations. Long after you and I have departed from this plane of experience, God will still be God, gravity will still be gravity, the sun will still rise in the East, the Earth will turn, birds will sing and flowers will grow.

This revelation should be a cause for celebration, and not resignation or sadness. Why not approach life like any other challenging game. After all, that's all life is — one big, wonderful, educational game. When you play games such as Trivial Pursuit or Monopoly, your first move is to learn the rules so that you can increase your chance of winning. I see life the same way. I see nothing as good or bad, including HS2. Whatever cards I've been dealt, I figure there must be a way, utilizing the existing rules, to play the game of life and win. God is not sadistic. No matter your plight, you can be sure that Divine Intelligence has established a set of rules by which you can attain victory.

Learn to listen to yourself...not your namesake, but your true self. During contemplative moments, sometimes the questions that you raise will be more important than the answers. In seminars, lectures and panel discussions, I am always more fascinated by the questions raised by participants than the answers. Answers are too final, too direct and too limited, while a good question lingers in the air forever and expands the mind. Even the great mystic Jesus asked much better questions than he provided answers. Remember what he asked of the skeptic: "Who say ye I am?" And remember Saul of Tarsus' famous question: "Master, what wouldest thou have me to do?" How eloquent and how profound!

As you write in your journal, date each entry so that you can go back and review the progress, or at least the progression, in your thinking from week-to-week and month-to-month. If you follow these instructions, you will discover that the process is slow, tedious and extremely subtle, which, by the way, is wonderful. It may not seem as though you are making any measurable progress for months on end, but do not be deterred. Just remember to judge not by appearances. Fortunately (yes, fortunately!), there is no easy route. I would like to think that it's an indication of my spiritual maturity, but I am no longer interested in things that come easily. I have passed the test; I cannot be tempted. During the first two-thirds of my life, I wanted easy money, easy women and easy success — but no more. Today, I want to work for everything that I get. Conversely, if I haven't worked for a thing, I don't want it. That's why I never play the lottery or slot machines or respond to *Reader's Digest* sweepstakes. By practicing this over the years, I can now proclaim that I cannot be tempted. I am confident that I don't have to gamble to win. I'm not going to believe in games of chance, but I'm going to win anyway.

Regardless of appearances, you must continue to forge ahead. Your process may be interrupted by the discovery of books that you stumble upon at a bookstore or library or on a friend's bookshelf. Or a friend may suggest a book or meeting to you that you may feel moved to investigate. At the time, it may seem as if such a diversion has nothing to do with your main process, which is finding answers to your life's questions, but, in some cases, you will later discover that it does. However, you must also remain aware that, although friends may mean well, their suggested reading materials and advice may not be for you. One of the greatest challenges on the spiritual path is learning when to say no and how to say no to well-meaning cohorts. Remember, no one else really knows what is good for you. Only Spirit knows, and sometimes It will reveal it to you through others, be they friends or enemies. Yes, even your enemies. That's why it is so important to forgive and bless them, as well. So many of my blessings have come through people who thought that they were my enemies. They might have thought it, but I know that I don't have any enemies.

Enlightenment movements are filled with too many "nice" people — yes, nice and soft and unable to look at the mean, vile side of life, or to put meddling family and friends in their right places. That's right. As shocking as it may seem to say it, being "nice" has nothing whatsoever to do with growing spiritually. A steady diet of niceness, without a balance of toughness, will actually stifle your growth. Remember: God didn't place you here to be nice; Spirit created you here to be *true*. Every child of God has to learn to stand on his or her own feet, which is impossible if the student is hooked on always being "nice" or gaining the approbation of others. As you grow stronger and stronger in the Truth, you will need to rely less and less on other people's truths. Once we are strong enough, we must be free to tread our own paths and make our own mistakes.

You may wonder: But how will these stupid exercises help me? How do I know if they will work? Let me explain. I have no doubt but that, if you haven't been involved in transformational processes before, these exercises may seem silly and make you feel self conscious. You probably wouldn't want one of your parents or your boss to walk in on you while you're sitting there talking to yourself. In our sophisticated society, people get put away for that sort of thing. Nonetheless, if execution of these exercises makes you uncomfortable, that could be an indication that you are beginning to stir up an area of consciousness that has been blocking your growth. Lets face it; you've already tried everything that you knew to do and you've come up empty. The same was true for me. Growth is always painful and sometimes the therapeutic aspect of pain is camouflaged by embarrassment. To avoid discomfort we never enter into the pain, which means that the subconscious mental patterns remain unperturbed and unchanged. Consequently, we may not hurt any worse, but neither will we break through to new levels of happiness.

In life you must pay for what you get. Think of all the pain that you've amassed in your memory as a bank. If you wish to grow in consciousness, you must make a withdrawal from the bank of pain and pay for your own advancement.

By practicing these exercises, you are imposing new patterns upon your mind and literally cutting new grooves in your brain. Naturally, it will be painful at first and your entire being will protest. But when these new patterns become habituated and accepted by your mind without protest, transformation will follow. The process is subtle. Despite modern man's sophistication, our ability to tune into the finer mental vibrations is rather primitive and crude. The archetypal, successful professional in today's world — and this includes scientists, presidents, college professors, movie stars, politicians, CEO's and so forth — has to be addressed at the decibel level of a scream before anyone can get his or her attention. The only problem is, GOD NEVER SCREAMS. It whispers. Spirit communicates in a gentle and subtle, nearly inaudible voice. People have to be restrained to tune into its frequencies and levels. In metaphysics we call this the art of "lowly listening." These exercises will help you tune into the subtle registers of your being.

Let me backtrack for a moment. In stating that God never screams, someone may counter, "Yeah, but sometimes He sends the thunder and lightning." While it is true that thunder and lightning are not subtle, these are representations of natural law and not God as Conscious Being. There is a difference. It is true that some people do get struck by lightning, while others meet with great violence. Open the paper on any given day and examples of non-subtle manifestations of karma abound. I don't want to speak too harshly on this subject, because it is possible for any of us on the Path to manifest horrendous "accidents" that we think have no correspondent in our consciousness. I've certainly had my share. But this is nothing more than Law working itself out. Individuals who have gross consciousness such that they cannot hear the still small voice will oftentimes have to be awakened in the crudest fashion. We are here, not so much to succeed in business, purchase a nice home and buy a Cadillac, as to fulfill our divine destiny. If we don't do it consciously, the Universe will do whatever it takes to awaken us. Cancer, a horrible automobile accident or a bolt of lightning tends to arouse the consciousness of even the crudest individual.

There is an inverse relationship between what we regard as intelligence or I.Q. and the ability to master this process. The smarter you are and the greater your achievements in this world, the harder it will be to break your mind out of its old, high-threshold patterns. Don't be discouraged, however, for I ,too, come from the same mold. To arrive at where I am in consciousness, there has been so much that I have had to *un*learn.

When it comes to succeeding in these exercises, you don't have to know what the payoff will be in advance. You don't have to know what's going to happen to you or how everything is going to eventually turn out. If you do the highest thing that is within reach of your consciousness, I can assure you that there is an intangible "X-FACTOR" that will come to your aid. This is why it is virtually impossible for someone who isn't spiritually grounded to perfectly manage a condition such as HS2. Without this absolute moral foundation, your mind CAN and WILL rationalize almost any behavior that seems to satisfy the moment. I speak from painful experience. For years I tried to prove false this Truth by not obeying it. Plus I've observed the course the lives of so many of my "intelligent," "successful" and still unhappy friends have taken after they've spent years and years trying to make their inconsistent belief systems work.

By using the emotionally-loaded word *moral,* I am not referring to some other human being's judgment of what is right or wrong for you. No one can judge your behavior but you. Instead, I am referring to a **Universal Moral Pattern,** if you will allow, that is axiomatic with Truth itself. That such a universal pattern exists is one of the great undiscovered keys to successful soul development.

Working on your own terms, that intangible X-Factor will never come into play. This factor is the most amazing phenomenon *un-*known to humankind. When you are pressing forward to do the best that is within your power to do (which is the highest and best that you know how to do, based on your level of understanding), this Infinite Intelligence steps in. This is the mysterious X-Factor. All of a sudden your dentist will turn out to be amazingly understanding and compassionate, if it's a dentist that you need. Or if he or she rejects you and sends you out into the cold, you will immediately land in the hands of another dentist, and he or she will be perfect for you. Of course, the whole thing will seem totally fortuitous. You would have never been able to predict the chain of events that will have led up to it.

"Then," one might ask, "why does this system work?" That's a fair question. It is written that the natural man cannot receive or even know the ways of the Spirit, because they must be spiritually discerned. In other words there is an entirely different system of "government" which remains beyond our awareness until we turn to It in complete surrender. I know that this sounds spacey and unscientific in this modern technocratic world, but remember that I am a professional engineer who still harbors a great love for the field of science. Unlike increasing numbers of contemporary metaphysicians,

I am not going to attempt to prove the reality of spiritual power. It can't be proven according to the standards of science or the natural realm — never has been and never will be. And that's good. As for myself, I am at peace with this seeming paradox. The inhabitants of Earth comprise a spiritual melting pot. The souls that are incarnated here cover a wide band of consciousness and karma and spiritual growth potential. Everybody isn't meant to comprehend this principle at any given time on Earth. This is part of the perfection of God's Universe and mankind's role in it. Peace is ours to the degree that we understand this.

Because it can't be proven scientifically, it is impossible to package and sell spiritual power. You can't conduct clinical studies to statistically validate spiritual power. Terms like the *X-Factor, God, intangibility* and *faith* will get in the way and all further credibility will be lost so far as the average person is concerned. For that reason, I am not trying to sell this most perfect solution to everyone. Whosoever will, let them come. Let those who judge life based on the evidence of the five senses continue to suffer in their smug scientific ignorance. I am writing for that precious minority who, for whatever reason, are ready to advance. It may be one in a thousand, or only one in a hundred thousand. If so, so be it. Results, why's and how-for's are not my domain. It seems that few are chosen at any given time to recognize ultimate Truths, and if that's okay with God, it's certainly okay with me.

FIFTEEN STEPS TO LIVING SUCCESSFULLY WITH HS2

In this section I will summarize the steps involved in attaining victory over HS2. First, let me reiterate the major thesis of this book: You can live just as successfully with HS2 as you would have been able to live without HS2. At first this may seem like a ridiculous claim. But once you understand that life on Earth is nothing but a stomping ground for the soul as it continues on its greater journey, you will realize that no one can make it through life on this plane without some devastating challenges. Because none of us are objective, the other person's challenges never seem to be as excruciating as our own, but this is only a distorted perception. Everything is relative. Well...most things. As the venerable Shakespeare himself said: "Nothing is good or bad but thinking makes it so." The billionaire who is facing bankruptcy is just as devastated as the pauper on welfare or the woman suffering from a chronic disease. Likewise, this billionaire has just as much potential for spiritual transformation as anyone else as he sorts through his seemingly dismal options. He, on common footing with the despondent HS2 subject, stands in need of healing. Until we can understand this, we will never be able to see how we can live complete lives *in spite of* the conditions that confront us.

Following are the basic steps that I have followed and continue to practice assiduously to maintain a very high quality of life. I feel privileged to report that my life is characterized by joy, freedom, love, high self esteem and many levels of friendship.

(1) **RADICAL HONESTY:** Don't worry about what everybody else is doing and seems to be getting away with. You just be honest, moral, ethical and good. Why don't you resolve along with me to *always* tell the truth and *always* do the right thing, even if it means that you will lose whatever you may be trying to hold onto. Even if it means that you might have to suffer for your actions. Do those things that are going to help you in the long run – even beyond this life – as opposed to the short haul. Remember: This is not the *end* of your journey; it is only a stop along the way.

(2) **A SLOWER PACE:** It is time to stop trying to keep up with the world, whether it's a matter of keeping up with the Joneses or just trying to stay abreast with your friends. Consider the possibility that you may need to walk alone. If you have been living in the fast lane, perhaps it is time to shift gears, get a new set of friends and slow down. Obviously, whatever you have been doing isn't working to your satisfaction. You need some new thoughts, some new ideas, some new influences. You need to get a new perspective on the world, and the most effective way to get that perspective is to SLOW DOWN!

(3) DAILY SPIRITUAL READING: Most of us who have been on the path for any length of time have experienced moments of extreme clarity during which we have been able to sneak a glimpse into the very heart of reality, but those moments have been fleeting. One day our faith can be so strong that it's beyond words. The next day can find us so shaky it seems impossible that we could be the same person. During such times we may find ourselves struggling to remember how we felt during that elusive peak experience, not unlike a bowler trying to recall the exact motion of her hand and wrist during a previous hot streak, or a baseball player trying to recreate the swing that served him so faithfully during better days. While there is no surefire formula for remembering, we will discover that it is helpful to set aside some time for spiritual reading each day.

This is one of the most effective tools for taking me back to that place in consciousness where I like to be when negativity and doubt begins to rain down upon me. And it's not just random reading, but the rereading of the same chapters, verses, paragraphs, stories or passages in a few of my favorite books that accomplishes the task. Every time I review a familiar instruction, I find that I discover something new. It is a sad mistake to presume that we have digested the full meaning on any page of a good spiritual composition after having read it only once.

(4) QUIET TIME: The soul needs some quiet time each day. Plan to set aside some time each day for quiet contemplation, meditation and for simply being alone with your thoughts. Truth tiptoes in during the cool stillness of the evening. Psalm 46:10 instructs us: "Be still, and know that I am God." We can only know God or receive Truth when we take time to enter into the silence and still the mind.

It is so easy to get wrapped up in a lifestyle that is always swirling with noise and confusion, action items, shopping lists, people to call, places to go and television programs demanding to be watched. Even the most well-intentioned and spiritually-aware among us, if they let their guard down, will find themselves getting caught up in "busyness," where it seems that nary a moment can be sacrificed for being still. I have worked with many people in challenging life situations in which they had convinced themselves that it was impossible to find a single quiet moment during the day to devote to their healing. I understand this challenge as well as anyone, but regardless, if we want this pearl of great price we MUST make time for communing with the soul. If you can't steal away for 30 minutes — to play on the name of a well-known tune — *take five*. Never pass up five that are presently at hand while waiting for 30 that may never come. Take five here and five there, and fairly soon you will find yourself looking forward to those quiet moments for communing with Spirit just as you once looked forward to watching a good television program. It is imperative that we make time for God. Consider some old-fashioned wisdom: If you don't make time for God, God won't make time for you.

(5) DISCIPLINE: An ancient, but fundamental, metaphysical maxim states that order is heaven's first law. This is true. On the individual level, we might also add that it is impossible to grow spiritually without discipline, for discipline and order walk hand in hand. So let us begin to look at our lives from a new perspective each day and examine every action and response required of us as a new opportunity to grow by practicing good discipline. Do we really need to run with the same old gang tonight, or can we break rank this once to begin writing that article that we've been planning to write? Do I really need to watch that two-hour television movie tonight? Do I really need to stop by the happy hour with the same old gang on the way home from work tonight? What would it feel like to deny myself something that I had been planning to do all day? Is there any growth in this denial? Will I feel better about myself as a result? Will I be a better person? Is there a better way to utilize those two hours that will help me attain some of my professed goals faster?

I can only imagine that HS2 would be a disaster for someone who has no discipline. If you have HS2 and would like to live successfully in spite of it, it is absolutely essential that you cultivate the art of good discipline. Once you train your subconscious mind to better obey your will, you will understand that you don't have to cave in every time the libido calls, the same way that you don't have to eat cheesecake every time you get a craving. Mental power is not the whole enchilada, but it is a quantum leap towards true power. Because I have developed this kind of discipline, I know that I can trust myself to be in a relationship with a good woman. I now know that I will not be swayed by the heat of the moment to do something stupid which will jeopardize someone else's health. You can only know this when you make it a habit to practice being disciplined in small, as well as large, matters each day.

(6) **JOURNAL-KEEPING:** Another tool that should not be underestimated is that of keeping a spiritual diary or journal. It doesn't matter so much which of the many journal-keeping techniques you employ as long as you do it in a regular, disciplined manner. I prefer the common secretarial steno pad. However, when I am away on assignment or otherwise separated from my regular journal, I don't let that stop me. I will utilize whatever medium is available. Sometimes that will be in a loose-leaf binder; other times it will be on 3 x 5-inch note pads or even index cards. Okay, so I'm not always that organized, but the point is that you should never put off doing what you believe in. If you believe in the process of writing about your personal thoughts and experiences, you will never utter excuses for failing to do so. You will simply write. Doers do while talkers talk, and there's a world of difference between the two.

Now what are the advantages of keeping a spiritual journal? It is simply part of the process of becoming more aware. Plus it can serve as a sort of catharsis. There are many deep inner feelings about the experience of HS2 that you won't feel comfortable sharing with anyone else. You may not feel comfortable writing about them at first, but if you are committed to the process of becoming totally honest and releasing pent up feelings of shame, inadequacy, hurt, anger, and so forth, writing is a marvelous and effective way to set energies in motion that can lead to the desired breakthrough. As you commit your feelings to paper, you will discover that you will become clearer and more articulate about your feelings, as well as more enlightened in general. Believe me, the act of writing is truly a magical process.

One of the problems on the Spiritual Path is the difficulty of trying to assess our own growth. We are never objective in looking at our own lives. Sometimes it seems as if there is no payoff for all the diligence and hard work. There are times when for months on end it may even seem as though we are regressing. It is then that we can turn to our spiritual journals and review some of the thoughts, observations and processes that we were going through a year ago — or two years, or five years. When I do this, I will generally discover evidence that makes it clear that I have indeed made progress. Our written messages to ourselves, if uncensored, may be the closest we will ever come to being objective about ourselves. I am not afraid to commit some of my most private and/or troubling thoughts to paper. For the process to work most effectively, we must learn to be totally free with our words. It may take time and practice. Some may be afraid to do this for fear that someone else may intercept their journals and learn too much about their private thoughts. Granted, that is a valid concern for some people, but personally, I do not worry about it. This is my life and I must be about the Father's business. I refuse to let anything stand in the way of my transformation. If someone reads it, so what? I have chosen to trust in the Universe and the Laws that sustain me. Somehow I know that no one will be able to successfully perpetrate evil against me. Pity the soul of the person who tries.

(7) **COMMITMENT TO GOD:** As you work through these processes, you must strive constantly to remember your true priorities. Make the realization of God and Truth principles your primary goal, not the healing of HS2. Remember, we must approach Truth with a clean heart. We must not bear hidden or selfish motives. As harsh as it may sound to say it, remember that the Universe, by definition, is impersonal. Thus it is not important to the Universe that you be healed of HS2. Conversely, the Universe contains no desire that you be sick. It is not there to alter Its nature to cater to your or my whims. It serves us only to the degree that we adapt our ways to It. Whether we are what the world calls sick, or whether we are what the world calls well, we must somehow develop the conviction that our lives are part of a greater picture that did not begin with birth and will not end with death. If we commit ourselves

to God, then we can know that we will be in good hands regardless of what happens to this body in this particular life.

Each of us has a soul and that soul is the part of us that is rooted in the eternal. The experiences that we are enduring have been created to help us develop our soul to its maximum potential. We are living for the soul. Though we may suffer, the soul can yet grow and become stronger in God. The choice is ours. It all depends on how we interpret the experiences that we are having. Once we truly understand that we are forever walking with God, hand in hand, we will automatically see that there is indeed nothing to heal or pray to have changed. We are simply undergoing a process of life. We cannot fail and God is incapable of deserting us. So make a decision to cease giving power to any other thing, including HS2. The immortal state to which everything will return is perfect love and perfect health, not disease. Therefore, do not react to any condition as if it were real in any eternal sense. Rely only upon God.

(8) DISEMPOWERING THE HUSH WORD: Be careful not to buy into society's conspiracy in making the word *herpes* verboten. Why allow such a simple, six-letter word to have so much power over your life? While it is true that words do have power, you and I have a lot more control over what they mean in our lives than we may have ever thought possible. In essence, words convey ideas that plug into concepts that have already been programmed into our subconscious about what they mean. To prove this to yourself, take a few moments to do this simple exercise. Close your eyes for a few seconds. Then imagine that you have a lemon in one hand and a knife in the other. Take the knife and slice the lemon into two halves. Now lay the knife down. Take one piece of the lemon and bring it to your lips. Now imagine yourself squeezing the lemon and sucking the juice. How does it taste? How does it make you feel? Open your eyes. Notice that there is no lemon actually present.

Your see, it did not matter that there was no lemon present. I'm sure you were able to feel the sensation of the astringency sucking your jaws together. This proves that there is great power inherent in your imagination, as interpreted through your subconscious mind. I have gotten seasickness from being tossed about in the ocean on fishing boats. Because the experience left such a profound impression on my subconscious mind, today I can induce seasickness on demand by simply imagining that I'm on the ocean and "seeing" those waves rolling up and down...up and down...up and...well, you get the point. Oh, it's not a pleasant feeling. The subconscious mind is just that powerful. In fact, it is the most powerful tool available to the individual for transformation — or enslavement.

We can use this powerful ally to help us overcome automatic subconscious reactions to HS2 by changing the mental program that we have about the word *herpes*. After all, herpes is nothing but a word. It contains six innocent letters: e, e, h, p, r and s, when placed in alphabetical order. By selecting different combinations of these letters, I can immediately spot 21 singular forms of different words contained within the word herpes. Can you see them? They are eh, he, her, she, see, pee, ere, esp, re, rep, hep, here, pe, per, peer, seer, seep, spree, sheep, sheer and sphere. Chances are, you never thought about herpes this way, huh? Isn't it quite a versatile word? It's quite egalitarian when it comes to the sexes, as it contains "he," "her" and "she," which is a "sheer" reminder that everyone is your "peer." So if you stop acting like "sheep," and call upon your God-given "esp," through this experience you will learn how to "see." By keeping your feet planted "here," you can become a full-fledged "seer," "ere" your consciousness expands and encompasses the whole "sphere."

Look at all of the beautiful words that can spin off from the word herpes. None of these words are negative, are they? Why is that? More than likely you don't have any kind of reaction to words like *sheep, peer, sphere* or *seer*. Thus in the future one way to look at herpes is that there are 21 times more positive words wrapped up in these six letters than anything that you may construe as negative. It's all a question of how you look at it. It's up to you.

There's even more that you can do to desensitize yourself to the word. Why not devote some time either daily or weekly, depending on your particular need, doing the following exercises.

* Recite the word *herpes* out loud anywhere from 25 to 100 times, preferably with your eyes closed, allowing yourself to look through the word and beyond the word until the word begins to appear meaningless and devoid of power or sting. Any word that you look at long enough begins to lose its original meaning. At that point you can assign to it your own, truer meaning, one that is more appropriate.

* Now, let us take the sting out of the word. Recite the following sentences at least 25 times: *Herpes, like the word "cold" or "pneumonia," is just a word. I am not ashamed to say the word "herpes." Herpes is just a word.*

* Based on your strong faith in God, you now have a basis for reciting the following statement 25 times: *Herpes is not incurable, because all things are curable. I therefore accept that herpes is curable. God is the cure for all conditions. Since God lives within me, everything I need for perfect healing already exists within me. I accept God. Therefore, on some level, I accept my healing. All things are curable in the Mind of God.*

(9) COMING OUT OF THE CLOSET: One of the areas of greatest confusion in all of spiritual practice surrounds the issue of whether it is better for the student of Truth to pray in secrecy and remain in the closet or to tear away with tires smoking and take on the world. Of course, when one is the recipient of a miracle or some other wonderful blessing, it is his or her tendency to want to shout it from the mountaintop. Conversely, let the same person be visited with some form of social blight and he or she will gravitate towards the other extreme. When things aren't going well, we tend to want to hole up in the closet and hibernate. When we don't have good news to trumpet, the kind that will shine a flattering light upon ourselves, we shrink from facing the dragon. The dragon is anything that we privately fear, for private fears, like the dragons of our worst nightmares, tend to loom larger than life. I have found that the best way to destroy any dragon is to turn around and face the beast, eyeball to eyeball. **WE NEED TO**

EMERGE FROM THE CLOSET!

For those who have HS2, the best way to destroy the dragon is to pick a good friend, someone whom you trust and know that you can confide in, and tell him or her all about it. I'll never forget the first time that I did this. Somehow I knew that I was suddenly free and that I would never be the same again. And I was right; I have never been the same again. Up to that point, I had gone to great extremes to make certain that no one would ever find out that I had HS2. However, after breaking the ice, I refused to ever worry about the issue of disclosure again. I was liberated. Believe me when I say that a great weight was lifted from my shoulders.

This type of fear is so preposterous when you think about it. How can anyone harm you by knowing that you have HS2? What can they do with the information? What is the worst thing that could happen as a result? Even if it happened, assuming there are no legal ramifications, I guarantee you it wouldn't be as bad as you may expect. After you get over the shock (which is just your reaction to a previous rigidly-held attitude), you might discover that it was a blessing. My belief in myself, the truth of my being and the light that I represent is so much greater than anyone's disbelief in me could ever be. I defy anyone to try to undermine me by misusing the information that I have shared with them in faith. It would be impossible for them to win. Those who stand on Truth are protected by the Law of Spirit, and no evil shall prevail against them. Darkness can never overcome the light. When you stand on divine principle, there is no reason to fear anything or anyone. No one can prevail who is foolish enough to attack that which is aligned with Spirit.

(10) MASTERING RELATIONSHIPS: The mastery of Step 10 begins with Step 1. Again, honesty is not only the best policy, it's the *only* policy. Granted, the management of relationships represents one of the most frightening challenges for singles with HS2, because it is awfully difficult to totally confide in anyone with whom there has not been enough history to develop a complete trust. You may not be committed to your significant other, and that significant other may not yet be committed to you. What kind of training has the average person had concerning how to broach the truth in such a situation? The risk may or may not be as great in the case of married persons, depending on whether HS2 preceded the marriage or was introduced into the union as a result of infidelity. In either case, as with single people, honesty is the only policy. Even if the price is steep, it is better to tell the truth and get on with the process of cleaning up your life for the future, at least that is this writer's opinion.

No one has to tell you that there is tremendous risk in practicing a policy of honesty. Your fear that a disgusted or aggrieved mate might reject you and go on to spread gossip about you is not groundless. It could very well happen. It has happened to me. However, as I stated in Step 9, no one has the power to harm a student of Truth by spreading malicious gossip. Through your faith, just know that. Since I didn't waver from Truth when the going got shaky, the tarnish did not stick. It all worked out for my highest good in due time. Remember, there is only one prerequisite: You must stand firmly on the platform of Truth. Learn the Laws of Spirit and invoke them in all of your actions. In few cases is this ever done. Once I stopped worrying about the possibility of rejection and the relationships that I stood to lose, and once I stopped worrying about what others thought and unpleasant fates that could befall me, circumstances began to change immediately. Fairly soon thereafter, I became a happily married man (not that marriage is necessary for happiness).

They say that the Marine Corps is looking for a few good men. Likewise, God is forever looking for a few firm believers. Circumstances and conditions will always look threatening. This is the way the world is ordered, but it is all an illusion. It is not *the* Truth. Openness and honesty really do work but they must first be employed, even in the face of all odds. Most of the people who are afraid that these principles won't work haven't tried them.

Whether one is single with HS2 or married with HS2, the same principle applies. Let's say that a person is married and acquires HS2 as a result of having an affair. That doesn't make his or her case unique. Now I understand how he (or she) might worry himself to death trying to figure out ways to explain away his predicament. He is right to suspect that his relationship may not survive such a shock, but whether it will or won't should not be his primary issue. His primary issue should be to clear his slate by telling the whole truth — that is, if he is interested in surrendering to Spirit. Otherwise, he's on his own. If he has the kind of faith that I have been addressing, he will understand that, once he has confessed the truth, the rest is up to Divine Law. Even if he loses a particular mate, it will be the best thing that could have possibly happened to him, and in the long run he will gain someone or something even better, and he will be happy.

(11) **HYGIENE AND RESPONSIBILITY:** Enough can't be said about the importance of practicing good personal hygiene when one has HS2. I haven't addressed this issue in terms of specifics in this book because there are sufficient articles and health care books already written on this subject. Regardless, a responsible person in this context is a hygienic person. As I mentioned, when a person acquires HS2 or any other persistent condition, he or she automatically gives up a number of degrees of freedom. Such an individual can no longer afford to live haphazardly, or practice slovenly, unkempt habits. From that moment forward, these individuals must become aware of where they place their hands, which towels are used for which parts of the body, how these towels are dispositioned after their use, etc. For example, I know from many years of observation that many people, both men and women, have not developed the habit of washing their hands in a way that is hygienic after using the toilet. This has to change if the HS2 subject hopes to avoid unintentional spreading of the condition.

It's amazing how much suffering can be avoided if we are conscious, concerned and disciplined. On my job as an engineer, I have observed otherwise intelligent people who emerge from the bathroom without washing their hands. There are those who only sprinkle a little light water over one or both of their hands, depending on how much of a rush they're in. Then there are those who wash their hands well, but seem to be allergic to soap. I've watched grown men entering and leaving the bathroom at various establishments over the past 20 years, and you won't believe what I have found. Some have been middle level and upper level managers. Sometimes when they are in a hurry, they will bolt through the bathroom without touching a drop of water! The implications are simply frightening.

Individuals who want to practice being responsible must decide from this day forward to ALWAYS wash their hands copiously with soap and warm water. When traveling long distance in the car, they shouldn't be ashamed to carry a mini bar of soap and some towels with them at all times. Surely you know how skimpy supplies can be and how filthy facilities often are at freeway rest stops and service station rest rooms. It is better to be ridiculed as a methodical, uptight old fuddy-duddy than to be sorry for the rest of your life. Or worse, to have a loved one pay for your neglect. I've been laughed at and ridiculed on a regular basis for being such a meticulous old fuddy-duddy, but so be it. Those who have laughed have no idea why I am so meticulous. Safe-guarding the health of those whom I love is not their responsibility. It's mine.

The student of Truth shouldn't make the mistake of thinking that just because she (or he) is spiritual, natural laws don't apply to her. I have met more than a few sad cases in metaphysics who thought that they were immune to germs and viruses, and even seatbelts.

HS2 subjects must also learn to reprogram their subconscious minds to replace risky, but unconscious, habits such as rubbing their hands in their eyes, scratching their groins or butts, etc. They must even learn to train their minds not to do these things in their sleep. At first this may seem like too much to deal with, but I'm proof that it can be done. If it seems as if a lot of spontaneity is taken out of the lives of HS2 subjects, you're absolutely right. They have forfeited certain degrees of freedom. There are changes that individuals need to accept when they have HS2. Refusal to do so means that they aren't taking the experience of this condition seriously, and in many cases they will end up sorry.

When others are present in the household, it is even more important to practice good hygiene. Don't be ashamed to firmly dictate to loved ones what the new rules of the game are: the towels that they cannot use, periods of time during an outbreak when you don't wish to be "explored," or even prefer to be left alone.

Even as I write, someone is surely asking this question: If I am supposed to be so spiritual, and if God protects those who practice living only according to principles of Truth, doesn't it smack of a lack of faith to be overly concerned with contagiousness? The answer is a resounding NO! This is one of the gravest and most common mistakes made by students of Truth. When something such as HS2 occurs in your life, it is of paramount importance to take it seriously. These conditions are situations that are taking place in time and space, which is where we reside. We may suspect that the physical realm is not real, but it the one that we must both deal with and master if we wish to advance. In the realm of time and space, seldom is there an instantaneous healing. What students need to do is deal with their condition as a hard and fast fact, while working toward the healing that is yet to come. This way, they won't be jeopardizing their health and that of their loved ones while the healing is manifesting. If some minister or self-appointed spiritual guru levies an attack on you for not relying more on sheer faith, just realize that that's their trip, not yours. Then turn around, pick up your feet and keep on truckin'. Don't deal with airy-fairy healers and pie-in-the-sky absolutists, and for God's sake, don't try to be one. Those types will land you in a world of trouble.

A story that has never been written is about the mountain of trouble that religious and spiritual devotees get themselves into. Unnecessary trouble, too. And it happens for one reason: They tend to think that just because they have faith, they don't have to exercise common sense. I've seen metaphysical students purchase cars without having money to make the monthly payments, or even without having steady employment. I've seen them borrow money under the same circumstances; start businesses without proper preparation or a plan. They think that to be spiritual is to be totally spontaneous, and that spontaneity and common sense are conflicting values. This is why they often end up in so much trouble. In most cases I have seen nothing but disappointment and heartache derive from this kind of living. It's time for spiritual aspirants to stop kidding themselves.

Remember: There is a reason why we acquired HS2 in the first place. It was not an accident. There are lessons that have to be learned, one of which is to learn how to manage this great challenge by developing greater discipline and training our subconscious minds to break old habits and form new ones. Having any disease is a masterful way to learn a lot of new principles about Truth, or else embody the ones that we already know. I believe that when the lessons are effectively learned, there will no longer be a need for the actual condition to remain with us.

(12) **RESPECTING THE CONDITION:** Though you may be highly advanced on the Spiritual Path, and though you may be the proud bearer of a monumental faith, it would be an error to deny the impact of HS2 on your life. It would be an error to fail to regard this condition with a healthy respect. This does not mean that you should fear this condition, or just lie down and yield to it. You should not and you must not. There is a world of difference between healthy respect and surrendering. To be an intelligent person who has bought into the delusion that you have always had control over your life, and then to awaken one morning and discover that your God-given free will has been usurped by HS2 can send you into a state of permanent shock. I have observed the way close friends have reacted to this discovery, speaking of the few who have admitted it. In some cases they never actually admitted it, but only hinted.

One tough, streetwise friend of mine who has HS2 used to trivialize the condition and summarily dismiss it with a patented laugh of derision. He tried to give me the impression that HS2 was not a significant problem, and that, of course, just about everybody had it anyway. The unspoken message was that any guy who fretted about HS2 was nothing more than a wimp or a chicken at heart. By declaring HS2 to be trivial, he never had to sit down and enter into a serious discussion about it. To protect himself from pain and insulate himself from the need to be responsible, he cleverly shifted the responsibility back on everyone else. If a woman contracted HS2 as a result of sleeping with him, you know, it just wasn't any big deal. And, were she to blame him, he would consider her to be childish, immature and naïve concerning the harsh realities of the world. In my eyes this macho ex-friend of mine was plainly ignorant. He was a guy who had no respect for the deleterious potential of HS2. Unfortunately, there are irresponsible people like him running loose in the streets and operating without a conscience. In most cases they are nice enough people, but they have been assaulted by life and forced to bear a certain level of hidden pain that they don't know how to talk about. So they do the next best thing. They trivialize the pain and try to make others feel silly or inadequate for wanting to discuss it.

Then there is this female acquaintance who is well-advanced on the spiritual ladder. She, too, has HS2. She confided as much in me a few years ago during a rare, vulnerable moment, but I've never been able to get her to reopen the discussion since. She has weaved herself a lifestyle and cultivated an aura about her which says, "I'm pure; I'm enlightened; I'm clean-living; I'm other-worldly; I am much too dedicated to the spiritual pursuit to be concerned with everyday human concerns and mundane earthly matters. Of course, I'm healed. Anyone who walks as close to God as I do has got to be healed." In the meantime, she won't put herself in a position where she would ever have to deal with sexual desire again. She keeps all potential suitors at arm's length. I'm sure she's not anywhere even close to being "healed." In fact, she is in full-fledged denial. There's too much denial and repression, and more than a healthy proportion of anger. It is apparent to me that there's a great gulf between her carefully manufactured image and her true feeling, an Embodiment Gap which has given rise to a mountain of fear and guilt concerning the possibility that she might be found out.

Each of these people has failed to pay simple respect to HS2 by just acknowledging its existence and its nature. Those who will not first acknowledge that water is wet and rivers are deep stand a good chance of drowning. Speaking for myself, granting the proper respect to HS2 was an essential step toward my liberation. By doing so, I was able to buy myself some needed time. I don't have to pretend to be healed when I'm not. All the pressure has been taken off me now, leaving me room to work naturally and develop incrementally in consciousness until perfect healing can ensue according to God's own natural way. In the meantime, I have no stress, guilt or shame to weigh me down and force me to distort reality.

I remember an old gospel song that the late Rev. James Cleveland used to sing, in which he ad-libbed: "I'm not what I wanna be, but thank God I'm not what I used to be." And this is the attitude that we must foster. We must be honest about what we are right now. I've read about people who are enlightened, but I'm not there yet. (I'm not what I wanna be.) And it's still all right. I am what I am. Right now I'm a person who is experiencing HS2. That's my plight in life and that's what I have to deal with. But I don't have to be what I used to be, thank God. I can be a more wonderful person with HS2 than I ever was in the past, even before I acquired HS2. So why don't I get on with the business of becoming that person, without trying to hoodwink anybody, or deny anything, or hide anything, or trivialize anything, or ignore anything, or heal anything or transcend anything. Let me learn how to manage HS2 and protect myself and those whom I love. Maybe this is all that I need to learn right now.

(13) GIVING THANKS AND APPRECIATION: We must not allow our minds to become so dominated by HS2 that we lose appreciation of life and all of its splendor and beauty. Take time out each day to look around and behold life's myriad wonders and treasures. When we think about it, most of us would agree that our problems pale in comparison to life's splendor. This is true even when our problem is HS2. It is so much easier to reiterate our problems than to count our blessings. This is as true for me as it is for you. But if we are going to change our lives and become pure, clear channels for God's love, we must begin to bless everything. We must begin the practice of searching for reasons each day to utter spontaneous prayers of thanksgiving for every good thing that comes into our experience. There is so much to be thankful for. We have the sun and the rain, the moon, seasons that change, flowers, air to breathe, and an endless variety of foods to eat. Most of us have jobs for which we could be thankful every day, and we have use of a portion of God's Intelligence, without which we would not be able to enjoy all of life's pleasures.

When we arrive at the point where our cup of gratitude runs so full as to overflow, we will find ourselves daily bursting into spontaneous streams of praise and thanksgiving for that which we have already received, and generally take for granted. When was the last time that you burst into spontaneous praise and thanksgiving? Such a suggestion may seem preposterous to some who are grappling with the practical problems associated with HS2. One who sees himself as a victim will find it difficult to give thanks. "What for?" he or she may wonder.

This reminds me of an experience I had recently with the proprietor of a business that I often patronize. He must have been having one of those days because he immediately began to unleash a volley of opinions on me concerning what a lousy job he thought the President of our country was doing. Though he railed on and on, I did not initially challenge his opinions. But each topic kept branching into two new ones. One of the businessman's strongest beliefs was that American society was steadily headed downhill and that everything that is happening to our society was predicted long ago by one Nostradamus. Of course, I challenged this belief on the basis that the universe could not possibly be predestined. In defense of his point of view, he proceeded to drag me through discussions of Armageddon and Revelations, as well. In the end this whole circuitous argument boiled down to a discussion about the validity of miracles. On one hand he was hoping that one would amble along and save us from ourselves, yet when I explained to him what miracles actually were, he didn't believe in them at all.

When I suggested that the United States would not become a third rate power and the world would not be destroyed because there exists this inherent righting power for good in the universe, he conceded that there is only one thing that could thwart the seeming inevitable: a miracle. He went on to explain that something truly momentous, supernatural and unexpected would have to come along and change the course of things. When I suggested that his very awakening that morning was a miracle, he totally disagreed. He even became angry, for he thought that I was putting him on or that I was attempting to trivialize the conversation. He protested, "No, no, man, I'm not talking about everyday events like waking up. That's not a miracle. Everybody does that! That's just *natural*. I'm talking about *real* miracles."

To my way of thinking, when I contemplate what is required to fall asleep each night, the complete loss of consciousness and escape to that nether world beyond my control — a state where, for all I know, I could just as well be dead — and then to be brought back intact, conscious, refreshed and in possession of a continuous stream of memory such that I am able to pick up my thoughts where I left them the night before, I have to see this process as a miracle. The businessman's reply was, "That's just a common occurrence which happens to everybody." Oh-me-oh-my, if this man only understood.

Well, it's a good thing that God isn't human. If He were, He would be awfully insulted. Just let one little thing go awry with this finely-tuned body/machine that we are inclined to take so much for granted. Then we will instantly realize what a miracle it is to keep this body functioning "normally."

Like David's praises to God in the 100th Psalm, let us condition our minds to see the miracles in everything and give thanks for something every single day, no matter how lousy the world or the government or our plights in life seem to be. If you have a job, why not occasionally shout out to the rooftops: "Infinite Knower, I thank you for my job." Even if you are not making enough money and feel that you have been mistreated or passed over for a promotion, give thanks anyway. When you go to the throne of grace each day to give praise and appreciation, don't adulterate it by mentioning the negative (not enough money, no promotion, no healing), and don't ask God for anything. Just make this a time for pure praise and appreciation. If you find this difficult to do, then you can be certain that some intensive processing needs to be done in this area of your life. Work at it until it becomes natural for you.

If you have a car, you can give thanks for that, yes, even if it's a mechanical wreck. You can give thanks for your home, clothes, family members, friendships, co-workers, boss, mate, savings in the bank. A favorite of mine is to give thanks that the Creator has chosen to live its life through me and that I get to live at this special moment and appreciate all of this grandeur and splendor. I'm thankful for having the ability to appreciate things. Every time I eat, I cannot take a bite without giving thanks to God. He did not have to provide apples, oranges, tomatoes, beans and wheat, or fish in the sea. And until the day arrives that scientists in the laboratory are able to create apples, wheat and fish (which would be the first of never), I will continue to give thanks to God.

Instead of concentrating on being healed or getting rid of something, we would fare much better if we would shift our energy toward appreciating the near endless list of marvelous things that God is already doing for us. The more we bless a thing, the more fruit it will return unto us. And the more we appreciate life, the more life will bless us in return. Our purpose for being is to discover, accept and align ourselves with this **Ubiquitous Pattern of Goodness** that is already here. When we can do that so completely that we find ourselves forgetting that HS2 even exists, HS2 *will* cease to exist.

(14) FORGIVE THYSELF: So much has been said and written about the need to release hostility and forgive others for what they have done to us or against us, and the need to ask God's forgiveness for what we have done to or against others. If you are still seething with anger and directing hostility towards someone for giving you HS2, it is time to forgive and let go. It is imperative that you get on with your life, and the only way to do that without carrying excess baggage is to forgive. I don't care if that person has badly mistreated you, lied to you or even refused to acknowledge what he or she allegedly did to you. Granted, this can leave a person in a troubled, seething state. I know how it feels. It has happened to me, too. Regardless, all you need to know at this juncture is that there is a Power that you can turn to that can right all wrongs and work everything out for you. And it's even better than that. This Power will also work things out for those who have mistreated you. Our attitude must be for everyone to be liberated and blessed — the ones who have hurt us, as well as we ourselves.

There is no need to worry, for none shall escape having to face up to the fruits of their own sowing. It may not happen in *your* lifetime or under the scrutiny of *your* observation. You and I must simply learn to trust in the Law of God. This is the key to our own freedom. The moment we release those whom we view as having harmed us, and wish them well, we shall feel a great weight lifted from our shoulders. I often tell people that I'm not in the punishment business. I can't afford it.

The universe is perfectly just; this I know. Therefore, I accept before God that, on the highest possible level, no mistake has been made and no wrongful deed, committed. I deserved every experience that has come my way, which includes HS2 on the down side, as well as a prosperous, successful life filled with many happy moments on the up side. They all play their parts in the symphony of life, and I shall no longer judge one as being better or worse than the other. If I had not acquired HS2 from a woman by the name of Katey, it would have come by way of Jamille. So what's the difference? Why blame one person or another? They were no more than channels or messengers, and why kill the messenger? Indeed, everyone who comes into my life is part of a bigger picture that is far beyond his or her control. If I'm rightfully aligned with God, no one can harm me regardless of intent. And if I'm not, then anybody can. So why don't I just get right with God? It is useless and spiritually retrogressive to shoot our messengers and channels.

Once we understand higher Truth, the whole idea of forgiving someone will seem ludicrous. I can't remember the last time that I've had to forgive someone. It's been so long. In Truth there is no one to forgive. When I used to have a problem with unforgiveness — which meant that I was holding an active grudge against someone — I did not understand these universal spiritual principles. Once I began to understand principle, I immediately realized that there was no one to forgive. All belong to God, and we are all growing through ignorance, and out of our ignorance, into a consciousness of greater understanding as fast as we possibly can. It's a matter of understanding more than forgiveness. If they knew better, they would do better. And if we had known better, we would have done better.

Despite all that I said about Sophia and Marsha — ex-girlfriends from my negative, worldly past — if either one came to me today with an open mind and a sincere desire for friendship, I would be right there for her. I hold no grudges, for we have all erred in the past.

The flip side of the forgiveness question is when we ask God to forgive *us*. This one is easy. Again, it's all a question of understanding. Once the individual understands how the universe is constructed and the true nature of the absolute, all-loving Infinite Spirit, it becomes axiomatic that God cannot forgive us. The belief that we need to be forgiven is the only thing that has to be forgiven. Why else would it be that many who believe in forgiveness never seem to accomplish the goal of being forgiven? They carry their burdens around for decades, if not their entire lifetimes. Although the *Law* of God will return punishment to us for our misdeeds, God or Spirit Itself is pure love, and thus, cannot hold anything against us. Once we rise to a height where we can see the truth and erase every notion from our minds of engaging in evil, in that selfsame moment we are forgiven. Since God cannot withhold forgiveness, we are automatically forgiven in the selfsame moment when we accept forgiveness. So simply accept forgiveness and get on with your life.

(15) SURRENDER! After we have read so many books about Infinite Spirit and our relationship to It, and after we rise to a level of understanding the spiritual connection that binds us back to the Source, there comes a time when we must put all intellectual processes aside and simply surrender. Accept. Let go. While no single sage may know all of Truth, there is planted within everyone certain truths that continue to surface through human consciousness with unrelenting regularity. Though it is not often put in direct phraseology, one thing that is known to all deep down within is that each of us comes from God and is somehow on his or her way back to God. The same door that we came through when we entered this Earth is the same door that we must pass through when we depart. There is not a man or woman alive who does not intrinsically know that one day he or she will have to give up the struggle to satisfy human desires and begin living according to the Divine Plan. We all both know — and some fear — this. But still, we put off that day as long as possible. We put it off for the simple reason that in a world filled with so many pleasures, things to do, places to go, temptations to be explored and sensations to be sampled, surrendering to God is viewed

as the least pleasurable activity of all.

Life is as life must be. Though we lament the way things are, nothing is ultimately out of order. So we keep on living, ignoring our destiny and living our lives, each according to his or her own estimation of what makes sense. Or better still, according to what we can comfortably get away with. As we proceed through the years of young adulthood, the 20's and 30's, and perhaps, even longer, we ask few questions of the Universal or the Eternal Order for fear that (1) the answers might come too swiftly, and (2) that they might make sense. We are not so much afraid that there aren't answers to the eternal questions as we are that they might descend upon us with such inexorable force as to prematurely divert us from fulfilling plans of our own desires.

We would each like to know that there is a God, but there is that human part of us that does not want It to tell us what to do. We are nonplussed by the notion that Its Will requires us to surrender a great portion of our will before we can achieve perfect alignment with It. If It were a person, we would quickly protest that the prevailing Universal Rule is unfair. Being civilized and of sane mind, which, for the western majority, means that we are acculturated into the western Judeo-Christian ideal, we are unwilling to mount such an irreverent protest to the Infinite. And like the once-warned, headstrong children that we are, we take the more socially-acceptable recourse towards the same end. We ignore It. We continue on the trail of our own volition, ignoring universal traffic signs along the way.

Finally, we arrive at a dead end. Or a detour. Or we hit some unexpected bumps in the road and find that we cannot proceed as planned. These snags will materialize under different names. They may come as divorce; drug addiction; the death of a loved one; a long-term, abusive dependency; cancer; HS2; or some other intractable condition that does not lend itself to a three-day cure. It will come as the kind of challenge that forces us to cease living as we desire and venture deep within our souls, deeper than we ever planned to go at this juncture along the way of our eternal journey. It is then that our soul will shout out: What is it all about? Why are we here? What is God's Will? What do I have to do to bring my will into alignment with the Universal Plan?

The answer will be found to be the same as all mystical wayfarers have discovered: We must surrender. It is my carefully reasoned conclusion that this is where life leads each one of us. There is no formula for how it is to be done, nor is there a definite timetable. And there is no sense in my trying to prescribe one. After all, no one ever has or ever will surrender individual will before his or her time is due. This is not something that one can do intellectually.

Now, by no means am I suggesting that to surrender is to come under the domination or control of a particular church, denomination, order or organization. Different avenues serve different people. It's a personal thing between each individual and the one Universal Spirit, Creator and Presence. If we are honest and sincere, and if we ask the right questions of the Infinite, we will be guided from within to take the right road and do the right thing. The process is not nearly as mysterious as we may think. I am speaking from the premise that there is something within each one of us — yes, even the worst of us — that already knows *the* Truth. Our personality or ego selves may not know, but there is that something within each of us, made in the image and likeness of God, which knows. All we have to do is come to the point of absolute resolve where we are ready to give up the pursuits of self interest that have brought us to the precipice, and behold, enlightenment will surely come.

It may not be today; it may not be tomorrow; it may not be this year, but I say to everyone who has known the anguish of HS2, the time will surely come when you will be confronted with the choice of continuing in your anguish or surrendering to God. If you choose correctly and choose for the right reason, you will come to know success and freedom and joy and peace. Indeed the greatest secret of all is that you will transcend the lessons of HS2, and — I am convinced — come to know perfect health.

Good luck and may God bless you. Have a wonderful, meaningful, fulfilling life. You deserve it!

INDEX

ABOUT THE AUTHOR

Bernard Jackson was born and raised in Augusta, Georgia. Following graduation from high school, he attended the Massachusetts Institute of Technology, where he earned bachelor and master's degrees in chemical engineering. In 1976 he journeyed to Los Angeles to practice standup comedy and study script writing, technical writing and publishing. There, he also worked as an engineer in the aerospace industry. Even more important, in Los Angeles he began his spiritual quest. He enrolled in numerous metaphysical courses under some of the great teachers in the modern New Thought movement, culminating with his graduation as a licensed practitioner of spiritual healing under the United Church of Religious Science. As a practitioner, he served on the faculty of the Guidance Metaphysical Bible College, received clients, and conducted workshops and seminars in spiritual awareness, growth and development.

In 1986 he surrendered his practitioner's license, became independent and founded a New Thought, spiritual publication, THE UPSTAIRS JOURNAL. Since then he has written many articles on the practical, everyday application of spiritual and metaphysical principles. In addition to honoring regular speaking engagements at local New Thought organizations, he recently founded **The Institute for Practical Spiritual Living,** a non-hierarchical teaching and practicing spiritual order that provides a worshipful alternative to formal church services.

BOOK ORDER FORM

If you would like to order additional copies of *WHAT DOCTORS CAN'T HEAL*, please use the convenient order form below. Bulk purchase inquiries invited.

Make check or money order payable to: **STRICTLY HONEST.**

Mail to: 815 N. La Brea Avenue, Suite 187
          Inglewood, CA 90302

          310-419-2284 (Los Angeles area)
          1-800-578-2284 (anywhere in the U.S.)

Please print:

Your Name _____

Address _____

City/State/Zip _____

Phone _____

___ Copies x $16.95 each $ _____

$1.40 Sales Tax ea. (Calif. residents only) $ _____

$2.10 Postage and Handling, each $ _____

Total (U.S. funds only) $ _____

Please allow 4 weeks for delivery.
Foreign orders: Please write for price quotation.